The Medicine of Less

The Sim-Bo Diet™ for Restoring Rhythm Through Food, Simplicity, and Daily Practice

By Dr. Choi

Doctor of Acupuncture and Oriental Medicine

Certified Emperor's Cupping Therapist®

Functional Nutritionist

Precision Acupuncture, Inc.

Long Beach, California, USA

Published by Precision Acupuncture, Inc.
Long Beach, California, USA

The Sim-Bo Diet™ is unrelated to the clinical SIBO diet used in clinical discussions of small intestinal bacterial overgrowth. "Sim-Bo" refers exclusively to "Simple and Boring," Dr. Choi's dietary and lifestyle framework for biological simplicity, metabolic order, and inflammatory-load reduction.

Disclaimer:

This book is written for educational and informational purposes only. It is not intended as medical advice, diagnosis, treatment, or a substitute for care from a qualified healthcare professional. This book does not diagnose, treat, cure, or prevent any disease.

Readers should consult a qualified healthcare professional before making changes to diet, exercise, supplements, lifestyle practices, or prescribed medication. Readers should not discontinue, reduce, or alter prescribed medication without appropriate medical supervision.

The author and publisher are not responsible for adverse outcomes arising from the use, misuse, or misinterpretation of the information presented in this book.

The clinical case studies presented in this book are based on the author's clinical experiences. They are presented for educational purposes. Identifying details have been altered or combined to protect confidentiality. Names, occupations, and timelines may also have been changed, combined, or obscured to protect patient privacy. Medication changes, when appropriate, should always be coordinated with the prescribing clinician; Sim-Bo was not used as a unilateral substitute for prescribed care. Supplement changes, herbal prescriptions, acupuncture, cupping, medication decisions, and treatment plans were individualized and monitored clinically.

First Edition — 2025
Printed in the United States of America

For my patients—
who trusted simplicity, practiced rhythm, and reminded me that healing often begins when the body finally feels heard.

For my family—
who have stood beside me, strengthened me, and never withheld their prayers and love. They have made me realize the truth that we barely have enough time in this life just to love.

Table of Contents

Preface....6
Introduction: Returning to Physiological Intelligence....9

Part I - The Modern Health Crisis....13
Chapter 1. From Infection to Inflammation: How Disease Evolved...14
Chapter 2. The Hidden Epidemic: How Inflammation Drives Modern Illness....29
Chapter 3. The Cost of Convenience....40

Part II - Food as Medicine....52
Chapter 4. Understanding Nutrients: Food as Biological Language...53
Chapter 5. Protein: Friend or Foe?....65
Chapter 6. The Truth About Animal Protein....79
Chapter 7. Fat, Sugar, and the Inflammatory Cycle....92

Part III - The Sim-Bo Diet™: Simplicity as Healing....108
Chapter 8. The Philosophy of Simplicity....109
Chapter 9. The 3:2:1 Formula for Healing....124
Chapter 10. Brown Rice: The Healing Grain....140
Chapter 11. Fruits: Nature's Targeted Medicine....157
Chapter 12. Vegetables: The Cleansing Current....171

Part IV - The Science of Natural Healing....185
Chapter 13. The Gut: Where Immunity, Metabolism, and Mood Converge....186
Chapter 14. The Antioxidant Defense System....202
Chapter 15. Targeted Supplements: Strategic Support, Not Substitution....219

Part V - Living Without Medication....235
Chapter 16. Mind and Emotion: The Missing Medicine....236
Chapter 17. Movement as Medicine....249
Chapter 18. Sleep, Sunlight, and Circadian Healing....264
Chapter 19. The Six-Month Sim-Bo Transformation Plan....279

Part VI - Beyond the Body....293
Chapter 20. Beyond the Diet: Simplicity as a Life Architecture....294

Appendices....305
Appendix A. Nutrient Reference Architecture....306
Appendix B. The Sim-Bo Materia Medica....313
Appendix C. The Sim-Bo Clinical Formularies: Recipes and Procurement....320
Appendix D. Scientific and Philosophical Foundation....324
Appendix E. The Biological Lexicon....328

About the Author and Cover Designer....341

Preface

Modern health is facing a quiet crisis of rhythm.

We live longer than previous generations, yet many people spend those additional years fatigued, inflamed, metabolically unstable, and increasingly dependent on medication. Modern medicine has achieved extraordinary victories against acute infection, trauma, surgery, and emergency care. Those victories are real. They should not be diminished. But the dominant illnesses of our age are often not sudden invaders from the outside. They are slow disturbances from within: chronic inflammatory load, metabolic confusion, digestive depletion, disrupted sleep, emotional strain, and the gradual loss of natural timing.

Years ago, on a quiet afternoon in my clinic, a woman in her mid-forties sat across from my desk and began to weep. She unzipped a heavy purse and emptied its contents onto the table between us: a dozen prescription bottles, each carefully prescribed by respected specialists.

Wiping her eyes, she looked at me with exhaustion and said, "I take every single pill as I'm told. So why do I feel like my vitality is fading a little more every day?"

That moment stayed with me.

Her medications were not careless. They were not irrational. They were part of a system designed to control measurable risk, manage symptoms, and prevent crisis. But stabilization is not the same thing as vitality. Her distress signals had been quieted enough for her to function, yet the deeper question remained unanswered: why had her physiology lost its capacity to feel well?

The fire was being contained, but the house was not being rebuilt.

This book grew from decades of clinical observation: many modern illnesses are not caused by a lack of medication alone, but by the progressive loss of natural order. When we eat in excess, move too little, sleep irregularly, breathe shallowly, live under constant pressure, and disconnect from the timing systems that govern repair, the inner conversation between organs, hormones, nerves, immune cells, microbes, and metabolism becomes distorted. The body does not suddenly fail. It compensates, adapts, warns, and eventually exhausts itself.

True healing begins when that conversation is restored.

The restoration is not sentimental. It is physiological. A predictable meal changes insulin response. Morning light changes circadian chemistry. Slow breath changes vagal tone. Walking changes glucose uptake, lymphatic movement, and vascular shear. Sleep changes immune memory. Emotional honesty changes the endocrine atmosphere in which every organ works. Sim-Bo gathers these ordinary acts into one disciplined pattern so they stop competing and begin cooperating.

Originally, I planned to call my nutritional method the "Simple Diet." My intention was straightforward: strip away the noise of modern eating and return metabolism to a clean, predictable baseline. I began giving patients food plans anchored in brown rice, vegetables, fruit, hydration, steady meals, and the deliberate removal of dietary chaos.

Then a pattern emerged.

Patient after patient would look at the plan, sigh, and say some version of the same sentence: "Dr. Choi, I'm sure this works, but this diet is just so boring."

At first, I smiled. Then I realized they had named the principle better than I had.

One afternoon, after hearing the same complaint from a highly stressed executive, I leaned forward and said, "You are right. It is boring. But your nervous system has been riding a chemical rollercoaster for years—hyper-palatable foods, stimulants, stress, constant novelty, and irregular days. Boredom is not the problem. Biological boredom is what your body has been asking for."

That day, "Simple and Boring" became Sim-Bo.

What began as a patient complaint became the central philosophy of my work: when food becomes simple enough, digestion no longer has to defend itself against every meal. When daily cadence becomes predictable enough, the nervous system stops scanning for threat. When life becomes less chemically stimulating, vitality has room to return.

The Sim-Bo Diet™ is not a rejection of medicine. It is a return to physiology. It honors the lifesaving power of acute care while asking a different question: what daily conditions allow inflammatory load to fall, metabolic regulation to improve, and repair systems to operate again?

The answer is not exotic. It is not hidden behind expensive technology.

It also does not require the patient to become a full-time manager of health data. The sick modern person is often already exhausted by management: appointments, prescriptions, supplements, test results, wearable metrics, dietary theories, alarms, reminders, and conflicting advice. Sim-Bo cuts through that noise. It gives the patient a repeatable center. When the center holds, clinical observation becomes clearer, professional care becomes more coherent, and the patient stops confusing stimulation with progress.

It begins with recognizable food, meaningful movement, trustworthy sleep, calming breath, and a daily structure simple enough to repeat.

This book connects molecular science with ancestral cadence, clinical observation with practical discipline, and the science of inflammation with the lived practice of simplicity. Each chapter builds a single architecture: remove unnecessary noise, restore readable patterns, and give repair systems the space to reorganize.

The goal is not to abandon conventional care. The goal is to live in such a way that physiology requires less rescue.

Introduction

Returning to Physiological Intelligence

The Shift from Rescue to Regulation

For much of human history, the greatest threats to life came from the outside: infection, injury, famine, exposure, contaminated water, and poor sanitation. Modern medicine changed that story. Antibiotics, vaccines, surgical technique, emergency care, public health, and pharmaceutical innovation saved countless lives and transformed the human future.

That achievement deserves respect.

Yet a new pattern has emerged. Many of today's most common illnesses do not begin as sudden external attacks. They develop through repeated internal strain: excess intake, poor food quality, chronic psychological pressure, disrupted sleep, toxic exposures, sedentary habits, digestive imbalance, and loss of daily order.

This is the defining health paradox of our time: lifespan has expanded, while healthspan often contracts. Survival improves; vitality weakens.

Inflammation as an Unresolved Alarm

The immune system was designed to respond to injury and invasion. Inflammation is one of its essential tools. When tissue is damaged or infection appears, inflammation protects, cleans, and prepares the terrain for repair.

The problem begins when the alarm does not resolve.

Low-grade, persistent inflammatory activity can disturb vascular function, insulin sensitivity, mitochondrial energy, joint integrity, neurological stability, digestion, and mood. It may first appear as fatigue, stiffness, brain fog, poor sleep, digestive sensitivity, weight gain, anxiety, or a slow decline in resilience.

Inflammation is not an enemy to be crushed. It is a message to be understood. The deeper question is not only how to suppress the symptom, but why the alarm is still sounding.

Food as Biological Instruction

Food is more than fuel. Every meal carries instruction. It influences glucose response, insulin demand, bile flow, microbial fermentation, mineral balance, neurotransmitter tone, oxidative stress, immune behavior, and gene-regulatory pathways.

The modern problem is rarely a simple shortage of calories. It is confusion of instruction. We consume more stimulation than nourishment, more novelty than cadence, more density than clarity. Ultra-processed food can deliver intense taste and abundant energy while stripping away the fiber, water, minerals, texture, bitterness, color, and pacing that help metabolism interpret the meal.

The Sim-Bo Diet™ begins by removing noise. Brown rice, vegetables, fruits, hydration, and predictable meal timing return food to a form physiology can read. Digestion becomes less defensive. Appetite becomes clearer. The nervous system receives fewer danger cues. The immune system has fewer reasons to remain provoked.

This is not deprivation. It is simplification with purpose.

The Progress Paradox

Modern convenience has reduced physical hardship, but it has also reduced internal coherence. Electric light extended the day while weakening our relationship with darkness. Refrigeration and global food distribution made food constantly available while disconnecting eating from season and hunger. Automobiles shortened travel while removing daily motion. Digital technology expanded information while fragmenting attention and rest.

We gained speed. We lost cadence.

Human physiology still depends on older laws: morning light, evening darkness, movement by day, rest after effort, hunger before eating, satiety after nourishment, breath during stress, and sleep for repair. When those laws are ignored long enough, the system adapts at a cost. Glucose becomes unstable. Hormones lose timing. The gut becomes irritated. The nervous system remains guarded. The immune response becomes overactive in some places and under-responsive in others.

That pattern is biological disconnection.

Healing Through Subtraction

Modern health culture is built around addition: more supplements, more tests, more protocols, more devices, more hacks, more complexity.

Many overloaded systems do not need more input. They need less interference.

The liver needs a lower chemical load. The gut needs microbial balance and digestive rest. The nervous system needs safety, breath, timing, and stillness. The immune system needs fewer reasons to stay inflamed. Sim-Bo begins with this governing law: simplicity reduces friction, cadence restores communication, and discipline gives repair systems time to work.

The Sim-Bo Standard

Sim-Bo is not minimalism for its own sake. It is a clinical standard of readability. The meal must be simple enough for digestion to understand. The day must be steady enough for the nervous system to trust. The environment must be quiet enough for appetite, fatigue, pain, sleep, and mood to become legible again.

A complicated protocol can impress the intellect while exhausting the patient. A simple pattern can look ordinary while giving physiology what it has been missing for years: repetition, proportion, warmth, fiber, hydration, light, movement, breath, and rest. The method does not ask the patient to become perfect. It asks the patient to become consistent enough for repair to gather momentum.

In this sense, boredom becomes an intervention. It reduces novelty. It lowers decision pressure. It removes the constant biochemical negotiation created by food engineered for stimulation. Once the daily pattern becomes stable, the patient can finally detect cause and effect: which meal calms, which food congests, which schedule protects sleep, which relationship tightens breath, which movement restores circulation.

Medicine and Maintenance

Pharmaceutical medication is one of the great achievements of modern civilization. In acute crisis, infection, trauma, surgical care, and appropriate risk management, it can be lifesaving.

Medication alone cannot restore the daily patterns of eating, sleeping, breathing, digestion, movement, repair, and felt safety. When medication becomes the only strategy for a chronic lifestyle-driven condition, symptoms may improve while the terrain that generated distress remains unchanged.

This book does not shame medication use. It clarifies what medication cannot replace.

Food still matters. Sleep still matters. Movement still matters. Stress chemistry still matters. The gut still matters. Daily order still matters.

This distinction protects the dignity of both systems. Medicine is strongest when danger must be stabilized. Daily practice is strongest when the terrain must be rebuilt. The mistake is asking one to perform the work of the other. A prescription can lower pressure, suppress pain, or reduce risk; it cannot chew slowly, sleep early, walk after meals, breathe through anger, prepare vegetables, or create a quiet evening. Those acts remain the patient's medicine because they are the patient's participation.

The Return to Partnership

The purpose of this book is not fear. It is literacy.

Pain, fatigue, cravings, anxiety, insomnia, reflux, stiffness, weight gain, and brain fog are often forms of communication from a system trying to adapt under pressure. The first act of healing is listening. The second is removing what keeps the alarm active. The third is building a life simple enough, steady enough, and disciplined enough for the nervous system to trust.

That is the purpose of the Sim-Bo Diet™.

Not to dismiss emergency care. Not to glorify suffering. Not to chase perfection.

But to restore the daily conditions under which physiology becomes less inflamed, more orderly, more resilient, and more alive.

Healing begins where unnecessary complexity ends.

This is the quiet discipline of the entire work: to make life simple enough that physiology can speak, and steady enough that the patient can answer. The result is not a rejection of modern medicine, but a return to partnership with the living system that medicine is trying to protect.

Part I

The Modern Health Crisis

The defining health challenge of our era is no longer only the sudden invasion of an acute pathogen. It is the slow disruption of internal regulation: chronic inflammation, metabolic dysfunction, stress physiology, sleep disturbance, and the loss of biological cadence.

Modern life changed the conditions under which the human organism now lives. Convenience reduced many external hardships, but it also introduced new forms of biological friction. From infection to inflammation, from scarcity to excess, and from natural order to chronic dysregulation, the modern medical landscape was quietly remade.

Chapter 1

From Infection to Inflammation: How Disease Evolved

The Changing Face of Disease

When historians describe the progress of civilization, they often measure it in inventions: fire, wheels, electricity, microchips. Yet there is another, quieter timeline that tells an even deeper story: the history of disease.

Every era has had its signature affliction. In the Stone Age, people died from trauma, exposure, and malnutrition. In the nineteenth century, infectious diseases ruled: tuberculosis, cholera, typhoid, smallpox. By the twenty-first century, the dominant threats had changed again. Now they carry modern names: diabetes, cardiovascular disease, depression, arthritis, neurodegeneration, cancer. The battlefield moved from outside the body to within it.

Two hundred years ago, infection was an unavoidable companion of life. People fought invisible enemies without understanding bacteria or viruses. When antibiotics became widely available in the twentieth century, humanity celebrated the conquest of infection as a victory of reason and science. That victory was real. But as epidemics of acute infection declined in many industrialized societies, another pattern rose quietly: metabolic dysfunction, chronic inflammation, and lifestyle-driven disease.

Today, many people are not struck down by sudden illness. They are gradually worn down by systemic imbalance. In many chronic conditions, the organism is not invaded by pathogens; it is strained by excess, stress, poor food quality, disrupted sleep, and disconnection from natural cadence. This is the paradox of progress: longer survival, but often weaker vitality.

The Birth of Modern Medicine

Modern medicine was built on crisis. The emergency room, the antibiotic, the vaccine, the surgical theater: each is designed to rescue life when acute danger exceeds ordinary resilience. For traumatic injury, infection, surgical emergencies, and acute organ threat, this system is one of humanity's great achievements. It can restart a stopped heart, sterilize a lethal infection, rebuild a shattered bone, and intervene when minutes matter.

Yet chronic illness usually does not scream. It whispers. It develops across years as small disturbances accumulate: rising blood pressure, irregular glucose signaling, gut irritation, fatigue after meals, sleep fragmentation, subtle pain, emotional exhaustion. By the time the diagnosis appears, the underlying terrain may have been distorted for decades.

The culture of modern medicine grew alongside the culture of industry: identify the problem, apply a targeted fix, repeat. This model is powerful in emergencies. It is less complete when the condition is produced by the daily architecture of life. Human biology is not a mechanical assembly of isolated, replaceable parts. It is an interdependent system of organs, hormones, nerves, immune cells, microbes, electrical signals, and metabolic pathways. When one pathway is artificially suppressed, another may compensate. When one symptom improves without changing the environment that produced it, another symptom may emerge elsewhere.

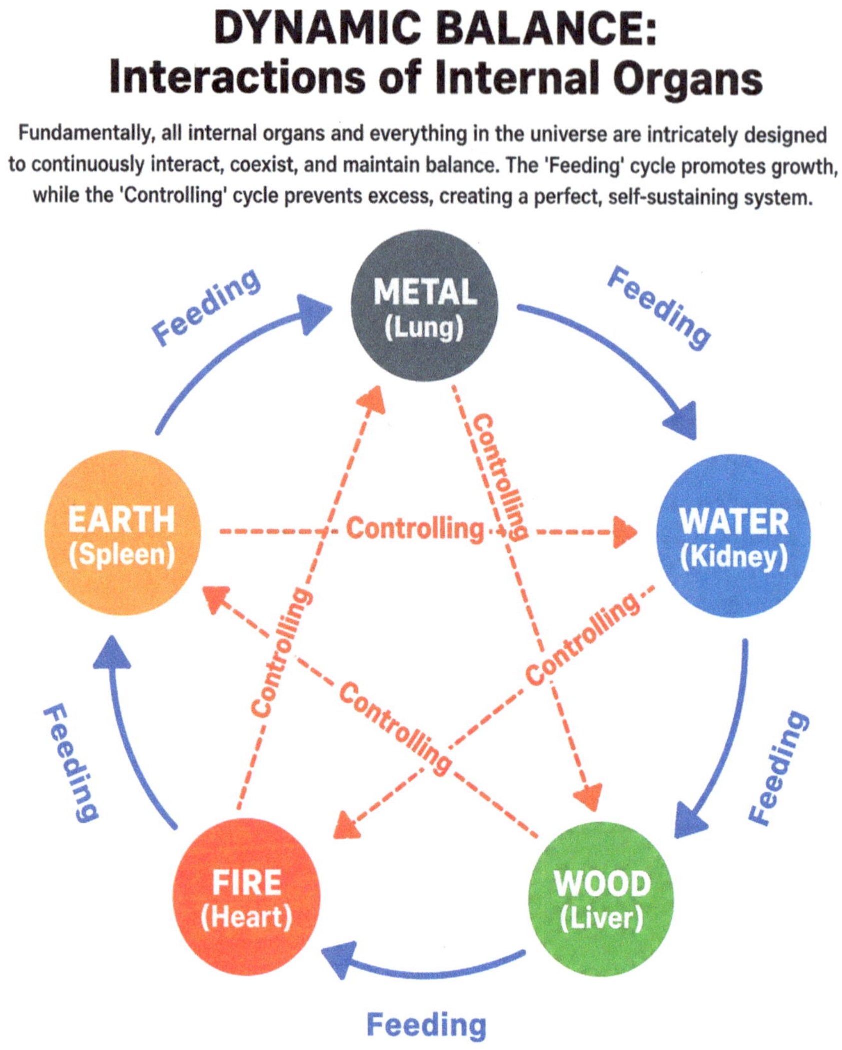

Figure 1. Dynamic balance: interactions of internal organs.

Medication can reduce risk, relieve suffering, and stabilize dangerous numbers. It should never be dismissed when it is clinically necessary. The problem begins when medication becomes the only long-term strategy for a chronic, lifestyle-driven condition while diet, stress, sleep, movement, digestion, and inflammatory load remain unchanged.

The question, then, is not merely how to extend life. The deeper question is how to live with enough physiological coherence that life does not require constant rescue. Human physiology was designed for dynamic regulation, adaptation, and repair. Medication can support risk control, but it cannot replace the daily conditions that make regulation possible.

Industrialization and the Dietary Revolution

If infection was the defining disease threat of the pre-industrial age, metabolic dysfunction is one of the defining patterns of the modern one. The turning point did not occur only in hospitals. It occurred in factories, mills, kitchens, offices, transportation systems, and food laboratories.

When grain milling became mechanized in the nineteenth century, the humble wheat berry was stripped of much of its bran and germ, the nutrient-rich layers that once accompanied the starch. White flour became a symbol of refinement, and with that refinement came the first quiet separations between calories and nourishment. Later, refrigeration, canning, chemical preservatives, global shipping, and industrial processing made food more available than ever, but often less biologically complete.

By the twentieth century, a person could eat three full, calorie-dense meals a day and still be poorly nourished at the tissue level. Modern eating solved the problem of scarcity for many people, but created a new problem: abundance without cadence, density without clarity, stimulation without satiety.

Protein soon became another cultural obsession. Postwar prosperity, athletic culture, and bodybuilding imagery elevated meat, milk, and eggs as symbols of strength. Protein is essential, but human physiology is efficient. The goal is not maximal intake; it is sufficient intake, clean source, proper timing, and metabolic appropriateness. Excess does not automatically become strength. It can become another demand on digestion, filtration, and inflammatory regulation.

Source and context matter. Highly processed meats and feedlot animal products, especially when embedded in a diet high in refined starch, sugar, oxidized fats, and low fiber, may increase inflammatory load. High-quality animal protein can have a targeted clinical role in some circumstances, including tissue repair, frailty, or digestive rebuilding. For long-term metabolic maintenance, the Sim-Bo philosophy favors a plant-dominant framework built on grains, vegetables, fruits, fiber, and steady cadence rather than chronic excess.

Industrialization also changed the quality, quantity, and context of fat consumption. Traditional diets used fats in forms the cellular machinery generally recognized: whole foods, seasonal animal fats, nuts, seeds, olives, coconuts, and other minimally processed sources. Modern processing introduced large volumes of refined seed oils into packaged foods, fried foods, and restaurant cooking.

The issue is not merely the presence of linoleic acid or any single fat molecule. The issue is the industrial setting: extraction, refining, storage, repeated heating, oxidation, and consumption within ultra-processed food patterns. Under those conditions, unstable lipids can contribute to oxidative stress and lipid peroxidation, damaging membranes and increasing metabolic strain.

Industrialization changed not only what we eat, but how we live. Machines replaced labor once performed by muscle. Urbanization compressed daily activity into sitting, driving, and screen work. A physiology built for varied daily movement became sedentary while continuing to receive abundant fuel. The imbalance between intake and expenditure created fertile ground for insulin resistance, mitochondrial stress, vascular strain, and metabolic fatigue.

From Infection to Inflammation

Inflammation is one of the body's oldest and most intelligent defense mechanisms. When you cut your skin, the area turns red, warm, and swollen. Blood vessels widen. Immune cells arrive. Chemical messengers coordinate repair. When the wound heals, the signal should resolve. In that setting, inflammation is not the enemy. It is the repair crew.

The problem begins when the alarm does not turn off. Chronic inflammation is not the dramatic flare of a visible wound. It is a low, persistent signal that keeps tissues on alert long after the original need has passed.

For most of human history, inflammation was usually tied to short-term threats: trauma, infection, exposure, injury. Today, the same immune language can be provoked by repeated internal irritants: excess calories, unstable blood sugar, oxidized lipids, stress hormones, environmental toxins, sleep disruption, sedentary living, and unresolved emotional strain. When inflammatory signaling remains active too long, it can begin to damage the tissues it was meant to protect.

At the molecular level, this chronic state is marked by inflammatory mediators, oxidative stress, mitochondrial strain, and the slow aging pattern often called inflammaging. The essential point is simple: acute inflammation is protective; chronic unresolved inflammation becomes corrosive.

Unlike an infection, chronic inflammation cannot be solved by killing a single invading organism. The trigger is often not one germ to eliminate, but a pattern of provocation to reduce. The solution begins with order: consistent meals, reliable sleep, daily movement, emotional regulation, and a cadence the immune system can recognize as safety.

The Silent Saboteurs

Several forces keep the inner alarm active.

Dietary excess is the first. The modern palate is trained toward overstimulation: salt, sugar, unstable fats, artificial flavors, and engineered textures that excite reward pathways more intensely than whole foods. This can distort appetite signaling, amplify cravings, and encourage eating beyond genuine need. Highly processed foods often deliver dense energy with reduced fiber, minerals, water, and phytonutrients, increasing metabolic workload while providing less biological clarity.

Stress is the second. The hormones that once helped human beings escape immediate danger now circulate in response to traffic, financial pressure, screens, deadlines, family tension, and unresolved fear. Cortisol and adrenaline are useful in short bursts. When chronically elevated, they can disrupt digestion, alter vascular tone, disturb sleep, increase blood sugar, and impair immune regulation. Over time, the nervous system may become guarded even when no immediate danger is present.

Sedentary living compounds the problem. The lymphatic system has no central pump comparable to the heart. It depends heavily on muscular contraction, diaphragmatic breathing, walking, posture, and daily movement to circulate fluid, immune cells, and metabolic waste. When movement declines, stagnation increases. Even gentle daily walking can support circulation, glucose regulation, mood, and inflammatory balance.

The absence of digestive rest is another often-ignored saboteur. In a world of constant access, many people eat from early morning until late night. Digestion is metabolically expensive. When food intake is continuous, the system receives little time for repair, cleanup, and metabolic recalibration. Periods of digestive rest, including clinically appropriate time-restricted eating, may support metabolic flexibility and cellular cleanup pathways. More intensive fasting practices require individualized assessment and professional supervision.

Sleep deprivation is the final accelerant. Deep sleep is a nightly repair program. Without it, inflammatory signaling rises, glucose regulation worsens, appetite hormones shift, and cellular repair becomes less efficient. Artificial light, late screens, irregular schedules, alcohol, stress, and nighttime eating can all distort circadian timing, leaving physiology in a state of internal jet lag even when the person never boards an airplane.

Together, these forces create a feedback loop: poor food quality increases inflammatory load; inflammation disrupts hormonal signaling; disrupted hormones increase cravings and fatigue; fatigue reduces movement and worsens dietary choices; poor sleep magnifies the entire cycle. Medication may control one part of the loop, but only a broader change in daily pattern can alter the architecture of the loop itself.

The Hidden Cost of Progress

Progress is rarely free. Every modern convenience carries an invisible exchange.

Refrigeration freed humanity from constant food scarcity, but weakened our relationship with seasonality. Electricity extended the productive day, but reduced the restorative authority of darkness. Automobiles shortened geographic distance, but removed much of the need for functional daily movement. Digital technology opened infinite access to information, but fractured attention and disrupted sleep hygiene.

We have gained comfort at the expense of biological coherence.

Our environment now changes faster than physiology can adapt. The human genome carries ancient expectations: natural light by day, darkness at night, periods of exertion, periods of rest, hunger before eating, satiety after nourishment, stress that resolves, and community that regulates emotion. Modern life often provides the opposite: constant stimulation, constant food access, constant sitting, constant light, and stress without physical discharge.

This mismatch defines the modern condition. Our physiology still carries ancient expectations; our attention now lives inside a digital machine. We are overfed and undernourished, stimulated and under-rested, digitally connected and often emotionally isolated. In that conflict, inflammation becomes a physiological language of imbalance.

The Emotional Roots of Physical Disease

Emotions were once treated as separate from the hard science of medicine. That separation is increasingly difficult to defend. The fields of stress physiology, psychoneuroimmunology, neuroendocrinology, and microbiome research all point toward a consistent pattern: thoughts and feelings influence immune behavior, hormonal rhythm, digestion, vascular tone, breathing, sleep, and pain perception.

Anxiety, grief, anger, shame, loneliness, and unresolved fear are not merely private mental events. They have biochemical consequences. Chronic emotional states can influence blood pressure, breathing depth, vagal tone, digestive secretion, immune signaling, and microbial balance. These are not poetic metaphors; they are measurable pathways through which the nervous, endocrine, immune, and digestive systems communicate.

When emotional strain persists, the gut can become more reactive, sleep becomes lighter, pain thresholds shift, and inflammatory signaling may remain elevated. Depression, anxiety, digestive distress, and inflammation can merge into a self-reinforcing loop. Breaking that loop requires more than positive thinking. It requires nourishing both the physical terrain and the psychological environment in which that terrain lives.

A Lesson from Simplicity

Across cultures and centuries, many of the healthiest populations have shared a pattern of moderation. In places such as Okinawa, Sardinia, and traditional rural communities across the world, long-lived elders often remain active not because they follow complicated protocols, but because ordinary life contains medicine: plant-rich meals, slow eating, sunlight, daily movement, manual work, community, rest, and purpose.

Simplicity is not deprivation. It is precision. When life becomes too complex, the nervous system spends energy managing noise. Simplifying food, schedule, movement, and emotional environment returns that energy to regulation and repair. Human physiology strongly prefers cadence. Repair becomes more efficient when daily inputs are predictable.

The Sim-Bo principle, short for Simple and Boring, emerged from this clinical observation. Patients overwhelmed by complex, multilayered health regimens often fail not because they lack intelligence, but because the regimen itself becomes another stressor. When they adopt a plain, consistent pattern centered on brown rice, vegetables, fruits, hydration, and predictable timing, the system often stops reacting defensively.

In many patients, digestion becomes steadier, inflammatory symptoms begin to soften, and energy becomes more predictable. What appears boring to the palate may be deeply calming to the cellular machinery.

Metabolic Peace

At the cellular level, true health resembles peace. Each organ communicates continuously with the others through hormones, nerves, immune signals, microbial metabolites, and electrical patterns. Chronic inflammation creates static in that conversation. The Sim-Bo approach is designed to reduce that static.

Whole foods support a steadier glucose curve. Natural fiber slows absorption and feeds beneficial microbes. Phytonutrients and antioxidants help buffer oxidative stress. Predictable meals reduce digestive confusion. Regular sleep and movement coordinate metabolic timing. None of this depends on a single miracle nutrient. It depends on lowering friction and allowing regulation to re-emerge.

In clinical practice, patients often report early changes in joint comfort, digestion, skin clarity, sleep quality, and energy stability. Over longer periods, some also show measurable improvement in metabolic markers, including lipid patterns, insulin sensitivity, blood pressure trends, and liver enzyme patterns. These changes are not magic. They are the visible consequences of a less overloaded system.

The liver and kidneys, no longer overwhelmed by constant excess, have more opportunity to perform their filtration and regulatory roles efficiently. The immune system, less occupied with daily dietary and stress provocation, can redirect resources toward repair. Clarity returns because chemical chaos declines.

The Cycle of Interference

Why do so many people resist simplicity? Because complexity creates the illusion of control. It feels sophisticated to chase the newest supplements, specialized diets, wearable metrics, and biohacking algorithms. Yet every new layer of management can become another form of interference if the foundation remains unstable.

Human physiology does not need to be micromanaged. It needs conditions under which it can self-organize.

Think of a forest after a storm. No gardener instructs the surviving trees how to heal. They receive sunlight, water, soil, and time. The same principle applies to tissue repair. Remove irritants. Provide clean fuel. Restore cadence. Allow rest. Under those conditions, order can return without constant force.

Pharmaceutical medication can be necessary when risk, infection, trauma, pain, or organ stress exceeds the system's immediate capacity to recover safely. The problem arises when medication becomes the only long-term strategy for a chronic lifestyle-driven condition and the underlying terrain remains unchanged.

Anti-inflammatory medications can reduce pain, but they may also mask feedback that would otherwise prompt changes in posture, movement, workload, or diet. Acid-suppressing medication can be appropriate and necessary, but long-term use should be periodically reviewed because stomach acid has important digestive and protective roles. Lipid-lowering medication can reduce cardiovascular risk in appropriate patients, but a lower number on a lab report does not eliminate the need for metabolic repair.

None of these interventions are inherently wrong. They are incomplete when used without addressing the biological conditions that made them necessary. True healing is not mere chemical suppression. It is biological adaptation supported by the right environment.

Restoring the Dialogue and Purpose-Driven Vitality

The first step toward living with less dependence on medication is listening. Pain, chronic fatigue, anxiety, reflux, stiffness, cravings, and insomnia are not enemies to be silenced automatically. They are signals. They are forms of communication from a system under pressure.

When those signals are ignored repeatedly, the system escalates from whisper to shout. Medication may quiet the alarm when necessary, but the deeper work is to ask why the alarm is sounding.

Listening means noticing which foods provide clean energy and which leave you exhausted. It means recognizing how stress shortens breathing, how certain relationships tighten the chest, how late meals disrupt sleep, and how inactivity changes mood. It means respecting the cycles of light and dark, hunger and satiety, movement and stillness, effort and recovery.

Healing is not merely the absence of disease. It is the restoration of capacity. We do not pursue metabolic flexibility only to extend life in passive comfort. We pursue it to have the stamina required for meaningful work: raising a family, serving patients, leading a community, studying deeply, creating art, practicing faith, mentoring the next generation, or meeting the demands of a difficult calling. Physical simplicity provides the biological foundation for demanding service. You cannot pour from an empty, inflamed vessel.

The Evolution of Responsibility

If infection defined the medical challenge of the nineteenth century, and inflammation defines much of the chronic-disease pattern of the twenty-first, then the next evolution of medicine must include responsibility: the active, informed partnership between the individual and their own physiology.

Responsibility is not blame. Blame paralyzes. Responsibility restores agency. Each meal, each hour of sleep, each movement pattern, each repeated thought, and each stress response participates in internal chemistry. Once a person understands this, dependency begins to shift. Healing stops being passive reception and becomes daily participation.

Health will always require skilled clinicians, emergency care, surgery, medication, diagnostics, and professional judgment. But it also requires a patient who understands that the most powerful signals are often repeated quietly every day: breakfast, breath, light, movement, sleep, and emotional regulation.

The Return to Balance

History is coming full circle. Long before modern hospitals existed, the wisest healing traditions understood the unity of diet, environment, movement, sleep, and mental state. They recognized that recovery depends on the whole pattern of living, not merely the suppression of one symptom.

Modern science now describes these relationships in different language: microbiome sequencing, circadian biology, mitochondrial function, insulin signaling, inflammatory mediators, vagal tone, epigenetics. The vocabulary has changed, but the principle is familiar: the organism heals best when its environment supports regulation.

The great challenge of our era is not the discovery of new information. It is the disciplined application of what is already known. Most people know they should eat whole foods, move daily, sleep more, and manage stress. The real question is why we do not. The answer lies in inertia: advertising, convenience, habit, exhaustion, social pressure, and the constant seduction of novelty.

Changing that momentum begins with one uncompromising choice repeated until it becomes ordinary. When a person chooses a simple bowl of brown rice, vegetables, and fruit over a highly engineered snack, the act is not merely dietary. It is a vote for biological order. It is a small refusal of the inflammatory age.

Conclusion: From Fire to Flow

Inflammation is not your enemy. It is an ancient attempt to restore order. The goal is not to extinguish it artificially at all times, but to help it resolve appropriately: to turn destructive fire back into restorative flow.

When underlying triggers are reduced, energy circulates more cleanly, waste clears more efficiently, tissues have more opportunity to repair, and the nervous system receives fewer danger signals. That is the definition of true health: dynamic, responsive balance rather than static, medicated perfection.

We are among the few generations in history with the potential to live well beyond previous limits, yet many people do so under the weight of constant medication, fatigue, and chronic inflammatory load. It does not have to be that way. By understanding how we moved from an era dominated by infection to an era shaped by inflammation, we gain the knowledge required for the next step: a conscious return to biological harmony.

Healing begins where unnecessary complexity ends.

Clinical Case Study 1

Reducing the Modern Inflammatory Load

Patient: Robert M., 48-year-old male

Chief complaint: severe chronic fatigue, persistent hypertension, post-prandial gastrointestinal distress, caffeine dependence, and reduced stress tolerance.

Clinical Presentation

Robert illustrates the modern shift from acute external threat to chronic internal load. He was not fighting an obvious infection. He was living inside a pattern of metabolic stress: hyper-processed food, irregular meals, heavy caffeine intake, sedentary work, poor sleep, and sustained psychological pressure.

His medications were not failures. They were controlling measurable risk and suppressing distress signals. But they did not address the daily pattern that kept generating the signals. The clinical goal was not to reject medication. It was to reduce the physiological load that made constant intervention necessary.

Vitals and Traditional Asian Medicine Assessment

In traditional Asian medicine, terms such as Spleen Qi Deficiency, Damp-Phlegm, Liver Qi Stagnation, and Internal Fire describe functional patterns rather than isolated biomedical diagnoses. They are used here to explain the clinical reasoning behind the treatment strategy.

Vitals: resting blood pressure measured at 152/94 mm Hg at intake.

Tongue: swollen and scalloped, with a greasy yellow coating suggestive of Damp-Phlegm and heat accumulation.

Pulse: wiry quality in the Liver position with weakness in the Spleen position, consistent with stress constraint overlying digestive depletion.

Functional assessment: chronic dietary excess, stress physiology, impaired digestive resilience, inflammatory load, and autonomic nervous system strain.

Traditional pattern assessment: Spleen Qi Deficiency with Damp-Phlegm, complicated by Liver Qi Stagnation transforming into Internal Heat.

Plan and Intervention

The treatment plan was structured to reduce inflammatory load, calm sympathetic overactivity, improve digestive cadence, and rebuild daily consistency. The approach combined dietary simplification, acupuncture, cupping, herbal support, caffeine reduction, walking, breath regulation, and sleep timing.

The Sim-Bo Dietary Prescription: *3:2:1 ratio*

3 parts grains: warm, slow-cooked millet and brown rice to provide stable complex carbohydrate and reduce dietary volatility.
2 parts vegetables: dark leafy and bitter greens to increase fiber, minerals, phytonutrients, and digestive regularity.
1 part fruit: yellow and orange fruits, eaten apart from heavy meals when needed, to support gentle sweetness without destabilizing the meal structure.

Targeted acupuncture: LR3 and LI4 were used to regulate constraint and sympathetic tension; ST36 and SP9 were used to support digestion, fluid metabolism, and resilience.

Emperor's Cupping Therapy®: myofascial decompression was applied along the posterior Bladder meridian to soften guarding, support local circulation, and assist lymphatic movement.

Herbal medicine: a modified Jiawei Xiaoyao San formula was used within scope to support Liver Qi movement, reduce heat signs, and assist digestive regulation. Herbal use was reviewed for clinical appropriateness and potential contraindications.

Lifestyle cadence: caffeine was reduced gradually, meals were placed on a predictable schedule, evening screen exposure was reduced, and daily walking with diaphragmatic breathing was prescribed as a non-negotiable consistency practice.

Twelve-Week Clinical Response

Resting blood pressure improved from 152/94 mm Hg to 118/76 mm Hg during the twelve-week follow-up period.

Medication changes were coordinated with the appropriate prescribing clinician.

The greasy yellow tongue coating was substantially reduced, and the tissue color appeared healthier and less congested.
Post-prandial bloating resolved during the twelve-week follow-up period.
Energy became more stable, and the patient no longer relied on

synthetic caffeine to function through the day.
Sleep quality, stress tolerance, and digestive predictability improved subjectively by patient report.

Clinical Reflection

Robert's case does not prove a universal formula. It illustrates how strongly physiology may respond when dietary load, stress pressure, digestive dysfunction, and inflammatory triggers are addressed together. Chronic illness is not always inevitable decline. In many cases, it is a sustained protest from a system living outside its regulatory design.

The clinical lesson is not that medication has no value. The lesson is that medication alone may not rebuild regulatory baseline. When food, stress, digestion, movement, sleep, and nervous system tone are brought into alignment, the conditions for repair become more favorable.

Transition: From History to Biology

The history of disease has changed. For centuries, medicine focused primarily on threats that entered from the outside: infection, contaminated water, injury, famine, and exposure. Modern science transformed that battlefield.

But as acute infection receded in many parts of the world, another pattern emerged. Chronic inflammation became one of the defining biological languages of modern illness: not a sudden invasion, but a sustained internal alarm.

History now yields to chemistry. Inflammation is not a moral failure and not a mysterious enemy; it is a protective process trapped in overuse. To understand modern disease, we must understand how that alarm is triggered, why it refuses to resolve, and how daily life teaches it either danger or safety.

Chapter 2

The Hidden Epidemic: How Inflammation Drives Modern Illness

The Fire That Never Sleeps

In the architecture of biological life, inflammation begins as protection. When the skin breaks, when a pathogen enters, or when tissue is injured, the immune system initiates an exact repair sequence. Blood vessels dilate. Permeability increases. White blood cells move toward the site. Chemical messengers call for containment, cleanup, and rebuilding. Heat, redness, swelling, and pain are not random symptoms; they are the visible signs of a living system defending its host.

The acute response is not the enemy. It is the repair crew. It isolates danger, removes damaged tissue, neutralizes threat, and prepares the terrain for renewal. In health, the alarm rises, the work is performed, and the message resolves. Specialized pro-resolving mediators cool the response so tissue can return to homeostasis.

The crisis begins when resolution fails. Modern life rarely provokes the immune system with one clean, visible wound. It provokes it with repetition: hyper-processed food, unstable blood sugar, environmental toxins, emotional strain, sleep deprivation, alcohol, sedentary hours, and a nervous system that rarely receives the cue of safety.

A brilliant process designed for short-term repair becomes a source of slow injury when it remains active for years. Chronic inflammation is unresolved protection: a persistent internal alarm that keeps tissues locked in defense long after the original threat should have passed.

When Defense Becomes Damage

The human immune system was built for precision defense, not perpetual occupation.

Its rapid-response forces—macrophages, neutrophils, cytokines, complement proteins, and other immune mediators—were designed to act with timing and restraint. In the ancestral environment, many threats were intense but temporary: a physical trauma, a sudden infection, a short famine, a brief escape from danger. The inflammatory response rose, completed its work, and receded.

Modern triggers behave differently. They are subtle, repetitive, and unresolved. A person may not feel acutely ill, yet the internal terrain may still be receiving danger cues from poor food quality, chronic psychological pressure, disrupted circadian timing, alcohol, pollutants, and constant digital stimulation.

Stress hormones mobilize stored energy. Adrenaline shifts blood flow away from digestion and toward readiness. Interleukins and tumor necrosis factor coordinate immune communication. Cortisol attempts to regulate the response. When this chemistry never fully resets, the same mediators meant to protect the organism begin irritating the vascular lining, joint surfaces, intestinal barriers, neural circuits, and mitochondrial engines.

The conscious complaint may be fatigue, stiffness, brain fog, digestive irregularity, or anxiety. The deeper pattern is unresolved immune activation, oxidative strain, and the loss of regulatory cadence. Chronic inflammation rarely announces itself with a fever. It reshapes health quietly, year by year.

The Web of Modern Disease

Persistent immune activation is a shared pathway, a master amplifier, and an unseen force inside many major modern illnesses. The diagnostic names differ, but the grammar repeats: chronic irritation, oxidative stress, impaired repair, and a failure of resolution.

When the immune alarm persists, it changes vascular integrity, glucose handling, lipid metabolism, microbial ecology, sleep quality, pain perception, mood, and tissue repair. What appears on a chart as separate disease often arises from one disturbed internal conversation.

Cardiovascular Disease

In cardiovascular disease, inflammation explains how vascular injury, endothelial dysfunction, LDL retention, oxidative modification, immune-cell recruitment, and plaque formation interact over time. The danger is not cholesterol traveling through a calm vascular system; the danger is cholesterol moving through an inflamed, oxidatively stressed, metabolically unstable arterial environment.

When the arterial lining is stressed by high blood pressure, elevated glucose, smoking, oxidative load, poor sleep, or chronic stress chemistry, repair signals intensify. Over time, unresolved repair can contribute to plaque instability, vascular stiffness, and the final sudden event that seemed to appear from nowhere.

Diabetes and Metabolic Syndrome

In diabetes and metabolic syndrome, excess energy intake, repeated glucose surges, ectopic fat, adipose dysfunction, mitochondrial strain, and immune activation gradually erode insulin sensitivity. Insulin is a messenger of storage, repair, and survival. Metabolic chaos forces that message to speak too often, too loudly, and without recovery.

The loop becomes self-reinforcing. Unstable glucose increases oxidative stress. Oxidative stress injures mitochondria. Mitochondrial inefficiency reduces metabolic flexibility. Fatigue and cravings rise. More dietary excess follows. The result is not a failure of willpower; it is a regulatory system trapped in overuse.

Arthritis and Joint Disease

Arthritis is not one disease with one doorway. Osteoarthritis, rheumatoid arthritis, psoriatic arthritis, gout, and other joint disorders differ in origin and mechanism. Yet inflammatory tone often determines how much pain, swelling, stiffness, and limitation the patient ultimately experiences.

In autoimmune patterns, immune cross-reactivity can turn protection toward tissue attack. In metabolic patterns, uric acid, insulin resistance, excess weight, oxidative stress, and low-grade immune activation degrade the joint environment. Joint pain is not merely local wear. It is an ongoing conversation between mechanics, immunity, metabolism, and repair capacity.

Neurodegenerative Disease

The brain has its own immune surveillance system, strongly shaped by microglial cells. These cells clear debris, respond to injury, and maintain neural order. When chronically primed by systemic inflammation, poor sleep, vascular strain, toxins, or metabolic instability, they can shift from guardianship into overactivation.

In that state, the brain becomes more vulnerable to neuronal stress, synaptic disruption, impaired debris clearance, and cognitive decline. Genetics, vascular health, protein aggregation, sleep quality, toxin exposure, and age all matter. Chronic inflammatory chemistry acts as a powerful amplifier of vulnerability.

Mood, Motivation, and Depression

Mood is not sealed inside the skull. In many patients, depression travels through immune chemistry, microbial metabolites, sleep fragmentation, endocrine disruption, glucose instability, and mitochondrial fatigue before it becomes a thought.

Inflammatory cytokines influence the kynurenine pathway, tryptophan metabolism, neuroendocrine tone, pain perception, motivation, and cognitive energy. A person may experience sadness, apathy, anxiety, or loss of drive not because the mind is weak, but because the internal terrain has become chemically hostile to resilience.

Depression has many doorways. The nervous system lives inside the immune, endocrine, digestive, and metabolic field. To heal mood deeply, the whole terrain must be considered.

The Gut: Ground Zero

Nowhere is chronic immune activation more intimate than in the gastrointestinal tract. The gut hosts trillions of microbes that digest complex fibers, educate immune cells, generate short-chain fatty acids, maintain the intestinal barrier, and communicate continuously with the nervous system.

When microbial balance is disrupted by repeated antibiotic exposure, industrial emulsifiers, refined sugar, alcohol, low fiber intake, chronic stress, or poor sleep, the intestinal lining becomes more reactive. Tight junctions lose precision. Barrier permeability increases. Bacterial fragments such as lipopolysaccharides, along with incompletely digested food particles, can enter circulation and intensify systemic immune alert.

This process is often called leaky gut; the more precise language is increased intestinal permeability and metabolic endotoxemia. The immune system reads these fragments as danger. The bloodstream becomes a messenger of alarm. Brain fog, joint pain, mood instability, skin irritation, fatigue, and digestive unrest often travel with this pattern.

The gut is one of the oldest borders between the outer world and the inner immune system. Every meal, every medication exposure, every stress response, and every disrupted night speaks to this border. When the diet is simplified and digestive friction decreases, cognition often clears, energy steadies, and physical resilience returns with surprising consistency.

The Future of Psychoneuroimmunology

The future of psychoneuroimmunology will not divide the mind from the gut, the immune system from mood, or inflammation from thought. It will treat cognition, emotion, microbial ecology, mucosal integrity, sleep architecture, and endocrine cadence as one living network.

Clinical models will increasingly expand beyond neurotransmitter manipulation alone. Psychobiotics, mucosal-barrier therapies, microbiome modulation, metabolic repair, anti-inflammatory nutrition, circadian stabilization, and nervous-system regulation will become central tools for patients whose symptoms arise from gut inflammation, immune dysregulation, and metabolic endotoxemia.

The most sophisticated care will ask a better question: What internal environment is the mind being asked to live inside?

Inflammation and Energy Production

A chronic immune alarm is a thief of cellular energy.

Inside each cell, mitochondria convert nutrients into ATP, the fundamental currency of biological work. ATP powers thought, movement, detoxification, immune repair, digestion, cardiac contraction, hormone synthesis, and tissue renewal. When oxidative stress rises, mitochondrial efficiency falls.

Inflammatory cytokines and reactive oxygen species can impair mitochondrial communication, reduce energy efficiency, and increase oxidative load. Under inflammatory stress, cells rely more heavily on less efficient metabolic pathways. The system works harder for less usable output.

Patients describe this state with striking accuracy: "I am running on empty." Energy production is not absent. It is inefficient, strained, and poorly regulated. The liver loses reserve for filtration and metabolic processing. The brain struggles to sustain executive function. Muscles fatigue early. Even immunity becomes dysregulated because perpetual defense consumes immense energy.

A physiology under chronic alarm has little energy left for growth, learning, repair, creativity, or joy.

Why We Miss the Signs

Low-grade immune activation is easy to miss because it rarely looks dramatic in the beginning. Morning stiffness, bloating after meals, afternoon crashes, stubborn weight gain, poor sleep, anxiety, and mild pain are normalized as aging, ambition, busyness, or ordinary stress.

Modern healthcare is strongest when disease is diagnosable, measurable, and urgent. It is less equipped for the whispering stage of dysregulation, when routine labs appear acceptable, symptoms remain vague, and lifestyle patterns are still the dominant drivers.

This is where observation becomes medicine. How do you feel after a specific meal? How quickly do you recover from stress? What happens to sleep after late eating, alcohol, conflict, or screens? How stable is your energy without caffeine? These signals do not replace medical testing; they add a crucial layer of intelligence. The whispering stage is where change carries the greatest leverage.

The System Under Alarm

Imagine a city under perpetual emergency. Sirens sound day and night. Roads are blocked. Resources are hoarded. Repair crews never leave. Eventually, the machinery designed to protect the city begins damaging the infrastructure it was meant to save.

Chronic immune activation works the same way. Vascular tone changes. Hormonal coordination weakens. Pain thresholds drop. Sleep becomes lighter. The nervous system begins reading ordinary internal sensations as threat. The digestive tract becomes reactive. Joints become louder. Mood becomes brittle.

This is not merely a collection of isolated symptoms. It is a breakdown of internal communication. The immune system is not evil. It is exhausted from being asked to defend a world that never stops provoking it.

The Triggers We Can Influence

Not every immune trigger is fully within personal control. Genetics, infections, trauma, autoimmune predisposition, work schedules, environmental exposure, medication history, and socioeconomic strain all matter. Still, many inflammatory inputs respond to the repeated architecture of daily life.

Food is one of the most immediate levers. Every meal sends instruction to immune tone. Hyper-processed carbohydrates, repeatedly heated oils, low-fiber meals, excess alcohol, and constant snacking increase metabolic strain. Whole grains, fibrous vegetables, fruits, legumes, adequate hydration, and slow eating support bowel regularity, microbial balance, antioxidant defense, and calmer glucose handling.

Stress is the second major lever. The nervous system can respond to psychological threat with many of the same pathways used for physical danger. Breathwork, prayer, meditation, emotional honesty, and deliberate pauses do not erase life's burdens. They reduce sympathetic drive and allow inflammatory chemistry to settle.

Movement functions as mechanical communication. Skeletal muscle contraction supports glucose uptake, vascular flow, lymphatic movement, mood regulation, and the release of myokines that influence immune behavior. Movement does not need to be violent to be effective. Walking, mobility work, resistance training, and diaphragmatic breathing all tell the organism that it is alive, capable, and safe.

Sleep is non-negotiable. During deep sleep, glymphatic exchange increases as interstitial space expands, allowing cerebrospinal fluid and interstitial fluid to exchange more efficiently and support clearance of metabolic waste. Growth hormone rises. Tissue repair accelerates. Appetite signals recalibrate. Skipping sleep is not a badge of productivity; it is a withdrawal from the repair account.

The Chemistry of Calm and the Reallocation of Energy

When inflammatory inputs are reduced with consistency, measurable markers begin to move. In some patients, hs-CRP decreases, blood pressure trends stabilize, glucose regulation improves, digestion becomes more predictable, and joint discomfort softens. These shifts are not instant and not universal. They are the visible consequences of a system no longer forced to defend itself at every meal, every night, and every stressful hour.

The gut microbiome can shift toward species associated with mucosal resilience, including Akkermansia muciniphila, while fiber-feeding microbes generate short-chain fatty acids such as butyrate that support barrier integrity and immune regulation. The key is not chasing one magic microbe. The key is building a dietary and circadian environment in which native ecology can recover.

Calm is not passivity. Calm is efficient allocation of energy. When the immune system no longer monopolizes ATP for constant defense, energy becomes available for thought, repair, movement, libido, learning, leadership, creativity, and service.

The immune system rewards trajectory, not perfection. One extra hour of sleep, one fiber-rich meal, ten minutes of walking, one deliberate breathing pause—each is a vote for order. Repetition turns that vote into a new metabolic reality.

Restoring Signal and Cadence

How do we live inside an inflamed world without becoming inflamed ourselves? Not through neurotic avoidance. Through deliberate order.

Human physiology is built around cycles: eating and fasting, movement and rest, light and darkness, engagement and silence, stress and recovery. When those cycles are protected, the nervous system interprets predictability as safety. At the cellular level, safety is the opposite of unnecessary inflammation.

Begin with the basics. Replace chaotic, hyper-processed meals with single-ingredient foods. Pause for diaphragmatic breathing before reacting to stress. Move every day. Protect darkness at night. Keep meal timing stable enough for digestion to anticipate its work.

These acts are ordinary, but their chemistry is not. They tell the living system: the emergency is over. Protection may resolve. Repair may begin.

The Hidden Epidemic Revealed

Chronic immune load is woven into ordinary routines: caffeine used in place of sleep, meals engineered for entertainment rather than nourishment, sitting accepted as the default posture of life, and digital stimulation mistaken for connection.

The foundational step toward living with less dependence on medication is learning to interpret inflammation as feedback rather than fate. Medication can reduce risk, stabilize symptoms, and save lives. For chronic patterns, it works best when paired with a life that no longer keeps provoking the same alarm.

The goal is not to reject medical science. The goal is to build an internal environment so coherent that physiology requires less rescue. Inflammation is the message: something in the terrain must change.

Conclusion: A New Kind of Immunity

True immunity is more than resistance to a passing winter cold. It is resilience: the capacity to encounter stress, injury, infection, grief, exertion, and uncertainty without losing physiological coherence.

Food calms the chemistry. Sleep restores the cadence. Movement clears the channels. Breath settles the nervous system. Simplicity reduces the noise.

The immune system is not trying to destroy you. It is trying to communicate. The work of healing is to reduce unnecessary provocation so protection can resolve into repair.

Clinical Case Study 2

Reducing Complexity to Restore Rhythm

Patient: David K., 35-year-old male, technology executive.

Chief Concerns: Severe decision fatigue, chronic sleep-maintenance insomnia, generalized anxiety, erratic digestive distress, and a persistent "wired but tired" state.

Clinical Presentation

David represents a pattern increasingly common in high-functioning patients: the pursuit of health optimization becoming another source of physiological strain. In an effort to improve performance, he had built a frantic routine around macro-tracking, extreme fasting windows, constant wearable-metric checking, and twenty-two isolated supplements.

Each intervention appeared logical in isolation. Together, they created psychological load, digestive confusion, and constant decision pressure. He was not lacking discipline. He was lacking cadence. His nervous system had no stable pattern to trust.

The clinical priority was to reduce complexity, restore predictable meals, calm autonomic vigilance, support digestive resilience, and rebuild sleep architecture.

Initial Findings and Assessment

Blood Pressure: 112/70 mm Hg, within normal range. His broader presentation suggested depletion and nervous-system overactivation within the Traditional Asian Medicine framework.

Tongue: Pale and quivering, with a thin peeled coating, consistent with Blood and Qi deficiency complicated by agitation.

Pulse: Thin, rapid, and choppy across multiple positions, with weakness in the Heart and Spleen positions.

Functional pattern: chronic mental exertion, irregular nourishment, disrupted sleep, digestive instability, and guarded autonomic tone.

Treatment principle: reduce friction, support Spleen Qi, nourish Heart Blood, calm the Shen, restore digestive timing, and rebuild sleep continuity.

Plan and Intervention

We reviewed his supplement list and discontinued non-essential products in a structured, supervised manner. The objective was not to villainize supplementation, but to remove unnecessary inputs until the true clinical baseline emerged.

The Sim-Bo Dietary Prescription used the 3:2:1 ratio: three parts warm brown rice and millet for steady complex carbohydrate; two parts grounding root vegetables and steamed leafy greens for fiber, minerals, and digestive regularity; and one part fruit, including jujube and tart cherries in the evening, to support a calmer circadian pattern.

For fourteen days, meals were intentionally identical and placed at the same times. This was not punishment. It was therapeutic predictability. The intervention removed decision fatigue and gave the nervous system a stable daily architecture.

Targeted acupuncture included HT7 and PC6 to support emotional steadiness and reduce sympathetic overdrive, with SP6 and ST36 to support digestive motility and physiological reserve.

Emperor's Cupping Therapy® was applied along the upper and middle back to reduce myofascial restriction, support local circulation, and assist relaxation of the paraspinal tissues associated with stress physiology.

Gui Pi Tang was used within the Traditional Asian Medicine framework to support Spleen Qi and Heart Blood, with the clinical goal of improving sleep continuity, emotional steadiness, and digestive resilience.

Follow-Up Observations

Sleep improved from three to four fragmented hours to seven and a half to eight hours of more continuous rest.

Digestive symptoms became more predictable, with daily bowel movements and reduced urgency.

The "wired but tired" pattern softened into a quieter mental state, with improved executive focus and less emotional reactivity by patient report.

Tongue presentation became more stable, with improved color and a healthier coating.

Non-essential supplements remained discontinued, while core nutrition was maintained through whole foods.

Clinical Lesson

David's case illustrates a central clinical lesson: more intervention is not always better. In driven patients, improvement often begins when unnecessary complexity is removed and the nervous system receives predictable daily instructions.

The obsessive pursuit of optimization can become another form of stress when it multiplies variables faster than physiology can interpret them. Sim-Bo reverses that error. It removes noise, restores cadence, and allows the system to hear its own regulatory intelligence again.

Transition: From Fire to Friction

The internal alarm does not arise in isolation. It is fed by the world we have built around ourselves: effortless food, endless screens, motionless work, speed without pause, and stimulation without recovery.

The fire has chemistry, but it also has architecture. To cool it, we must examine the culture that keeps feeding it.

From the hidden epidemic of inflammation, we now turn to the cost of convenience.

Chapter 3

The Cost of Convenience: How Frictionless Living Disrupts Cadence, Metabolism, and Attention

The Convenience Paradox

Every generation has believed that technological progress would make human life easier, and in many practical ways, it has. We no longer gather firewood to survive the winter or wash every garment by hand. We can eat, work, purchase, communicate, and broadcast our voices across continents with almost no physical exertion.

Yet as physical resistance disappeared from ordinary life, baseline health became harder to preserve. Convenience has saved us time, but it has quietly stolen our vitality.

The systems designed to liberate us from labor—combustion engines, ultra-processed food, instant communication, digital outsourcing, and automated commerce—have altered the conditions under which metabolism, attention, digestion, sleep, and social connection operate. We live inside a strange dissonance: calories are plentiful, but nourishment is thin; information is infinite, but attention is fractured; physical comfort is abundant, but resilience is harder to maintain.

Ease carries an invisible price. It is rarely paid immediately. It accumulates as chronic stress load, weaker attention, metabolic strain, emotional exhaustion, and disrupted daily order. Many external shortcuts reduce exertion while shifting the cost inward, toward glucose regulation, nervous system tone, digestion, and immune balance.

The Birth of Effortless Living

The Industrial Revolution changed far more than economics and manufacturing. It changed the daily relationship between work and survival.

Before widespread electricity, the human day was governed by sunlight, darkness, weather, and the turning of seasons. People rose with the dawn, worked with their hands, and rested when darkness made labor difficult. Securing food required continuous movement:

harvesting, grinding, carrying, hunting, preparing, cooking, and cleaning. That work was not merely inconvenience. It was one of the mechanisms that synchronized internal clocks with external reality.

When machines took over, necessary exertion began to disappear. Work migrated from fields and workshops into chairs, cars, and screens. Elevators reduced climbing. Automobiles erased walking. Delivery systems removed the small daily rituals of acquiring and preparing meals. Digital tools compressed tasks that once required movement, memory, conversation, and waiting.

At the same time, caloric density rose sharply. Refined flour, sugar, industrial fats, and packaged snacks made energy instantly available. The ancient survival equation—energy expenditure required to obtain energy intake—was fractured. For the first time in human history, large populations could consume abundant, energy-dense food while remaining nearly motionless.

Modern culture traded cadence for speed. Physiology still operates on older codes: light and darkness, hunger and satiety, exertion and rest, work and recovery. When culture accelerates beyond those codes, regulation becomes difficult.

The Addictive Design of Processed Living

Modern ease is not merely an accidental byproduct of progress. Much of it is engineered.

Industrial food manufacturers and digital designers both exploit reward prediction. Hyper-palatable combinations of refined salt, concentrated sugar, unstable fats, and artificial flavors stimulate reward pathways more intensely than ordinary whole foods. Over time, the nervous system begins to anticipate the reward before the food is eaten. A colorful package, a delivery app, or a familiar smell becomes a cue for craving.

Digital systems use the same vulnerability. News feeds, short videos, social alerts, and algorithmic suggestions deliver small, rapid, unpredictable rewards. These rewards are not earned through completion or meaningful exertion; they arrive instantly, repeatedly, and with almost no resistance.

Repeated exposure to this loop disorders attention, satiety, and motivation. Ordinary analog experiences begin to feel dull by comparison. Reading a long book feels difficult. A simple meal feels insufficient. Silence feels uncomfortable. The brain is trained to expect novelty every few seconds. The arrangement saves minutes, but it costs mindfulness.

Technology is a contract. In conscious hands, it educates, connects, heals, and expands human capacity. In unconscious hands, it replaces natural pauses with engineered compulsion. The contract must be renegotiated.

The Metabolic Price of Comfort

Each labor-saving comfort appears harmless in isolation. Over a lifetime, passive design reshapes metabolic behavior.

When a person sits for hours without interruption, skeletal muscle activity falls. Glucose uptake becomes less efficient. Lipid handling slows. Muscular inactivity weakens triglyceride clearance and gradually contributes to poorer metabolic flexibility, insulin resistance, and vascular risk.

Labor-saving design has sharply reduced ordinary sources of Non-Exercise Activity Thermogenesis, or NEAT: walking, standing, carrying groceries, climbing stairs, pacing, cleaning, gardening, and manual chores. These low-level activities once contributed substantially to daily energy expenditure, lymphatic movement, and glucose regulation. Formal exercise is valuable, but a brief workout cannot erase a day otherwise spent motionless.

Ultra-processed meals add another internal load. Designed for speed, shelf life, and maximum palatability, they remove the physical and sensory work of food: washing, cutting, cooking, chewing slowly, and stopping when satisfied. They deliver rapid energy with reduced structure.

Sleep timing is also affected. Artificial light and late-night screens extend the day beyond its natural boundary, disturbing circadian cues. Sleep restriction and circadian disruption alter hunger and satiety patterns, including ghrelin and leptin dynamics. Over time, cravings, weight gain, blood pressure changes, fragmented sleep, and baseline anxiety become more likely.

Society often mistakes these symptoms for normal aging. In many cases, they are the metabolic receipt for a life stripped of useful difficulty.

Stress in Disguise and Allostatic Load

Most people associate stress with obvious crises. But some of the most persistent stress in modern life is quiet: unfinished tasks, constant digital alerts, fragmented attention, schedule pressure, emotional overload, and the expectation of constant availability.

Stress physiology describes the cumulative wear and tear from repeated adaptation as allostatic load. The modern nervous system leaps from demand to demand without completing the natural cycle of activation and recovery. A notification arrives. A message waits. A meal is eaten while staring at a spreadsheet. The day becomes a chain of interruptions rather than a cadence of exertion and completion.

Cortisol is an essential survival hormone. It mobilizes energy, sharpens alertness, and coordinates adaptation. Injury begins when survival chemistry becomes the atmosphere of daily life. Blood sugar becomes more volatile. Digestion loses efficiency. Sleep architecture weakens. Immune regulation becomes less stable. A person may appear productive to the outside world while the autonomic nervous system remains in chronic readiness.

Convenience was marketed as a stress reducer. In practice, it often removed the natural pauses that once forced recovery: waiting for a meal to cook, walking between places, working with the hands, or ending the day when darkness arrived.

The Silent Architecture of Isolation

Convenience has also redesigned human connection.

Where communities once prepared meals and shared labor, many people now eat alone while staring at screens. Where cooperative survival once required face-to-face contact, automated services increasingly replace human interaction with digital transactions.

Loneliness is not merely emotional. It is associated with measurable changes in stress physiology, immune communication, sleep quality, and inflammatory load. Human beings are cooperative mammals. A familiar voice, physical presence, shared meals, ritual, and trusted community help regulate the vagus nerve and create signals of safety.

Digital connection has value, but it cannot fully replace embodied presence. The nervous system reads safety through proximity, tone of voice, repeated trust, eye contact, shared work, and the physical experience of belonging.

The Hidden Hunger for Effort: Hormesis

Human biology requires resistance. Not punishment. Not exhaustion. Recoverable effort.

Hormesis describes the principle that brief, manageable stressors trigger adaptation. Strength training, walking uphill, heat, cold, fasting windows, and physical labor become useful when matched to age, constitution, medication status, metabolic reserve, and clinical risk. The key is dosage: enough resistance to awaken adaptation, not enough to exhaust the system.

Modern culture often worships efficiency, but efficiency without physical challenge creates fragility. When every task is automated and every discomfort removed, metabolism receives fewer instructions to remain agile. Muscles soften. Bone density declines. Attention fragments. Emotional tolerance narrows.

We are engineered to lift, stretch, pull, carry, chew, walk, breathe, and recover after exertion. When daily life asks almost nothing of the muscles while flooding the mind with abstract digital pressure, a mismatch emerges. Many patients end the day mentally exhausted but physically unused. They are tired, yet sleep does not restore them, because the exhaustion is neurological rather than the clean fatigue of honest labor.

The prescription is the deliberate return of embodied action: walking instead of driving, cooking instead of ordering, lifting, carrying, cleaning, stretching, and breathing with full diaphragmatic participation. These acts restore the severed dialogue between motion and reward.

The Convenience Economy and Cellular Confusion

In a single generation, slow cooking was displaced by an industrial food system built for shelf life, portability, and hyper-palatability. The same logic now appears inside the wellness economy, where synthetic vitamin stacks, powdered greens, meal replacements, and protein bars are marketed as equivalents to whole food.

They are not equivalent.

Real food arrives inside an architecture: water, fiber, minerals, polyphenols, intact cell walls, natural texture, and digestive pacing. That architecture governs absorption speed, satiety, microbial fermentation, and glycemic response. A processed powder may contain isolated nutrients, but it lacks the structure that teaches metabolism how to receive them.

This creates Cellular Confusion: the mismatch that occurs when concentrated fragments arrive without the fiber, water, texture, and timing that normally guide digestion. Mechanical hunger may be briefly satisfied while the deeper need for structure remains unmet. The person eats enough, yet the system still searches for coherence.

Real nourishment requires presence: washing, cutting, smelling, chewing, tasting, pausing, and stopping. These steps are not romantic decorations. They are the first phases of digestion. Restoring the physical act of preparing and eating food is not primitive; it is sophisticated physiology.

Breaking the Convenience Cycle: The Luxury of Intentional Effort

Passive living has enormous cultural momentum because it feels instantly gratifying and the economy rewards speed. Breaking the cycle does not require fleeing to the wilderness. It requires inserting small, strategic doses of useful resistance into the day.

Walk to complete errands when distance allows.
Carry your own groceries.
Take the stairs.
Stand while taking phone calls.
Wash a few dishes by hand.
Cook one simple meal each day from raw, single-ingredient food.
Step outside into natural light before checking your phone in the morning.
Leave quiet gaps between tasks instead of filling every pause with a screen.

None of these acts are heroic. Together, they retrain metabolism toward participation.

The Future of Luxury

As artificial intelligence and digital outsourcing expand, hyper-convenience will eventually lose its glamour. The next true form of luxury will be the freedom to remain embodied.

The rarest people will be those with enough time to cook, walk, lift, garden, pray, read deeply, sleep in darkness, gather around a table without a screen, and protect their attention from constant extraction. As machines absorb more ordinary tasks, the ability to choose meaningful effort will become privilege—and medicine.

The Sim-Bo principle is direct: when appropriate physical work replaces unnecessary automation, physiology responds. Heart rate rises naturally. Peripheral circulation improves. Contracting muscles release anti-inflammatory myokines. The nervous system receives the primal instruction that life is not merely being consumed from a chair; it is being lived through action.

Technology is a tool, but it is also a contract. The terms must serve the organism. A good tool extends capacity; a poor bargain replaces capacity. Modern health depends on renegotiating that bargain with discipline.

The Psychology of Enough

At the root of our addiction to speed is the manufactured fear of scarcity. We chase efficiency because we fear there is not enough time, success, approval, energy, or safety. That phantom shortage drives overproduction, overconsumption, and over-stimulation. It depletes the human spirit while pretending to optimize it.

Simplicity begins with the radical realization that enough is already available. When the mind stops chasing endless optimization, the nervous system drops its defensive posture. Appetite becomes more honest. Breath deepens. Decisions clear.

The Sim-Bo philosophy refuses to define health as a sterile metric to be hacked. Health is the restoration of regulatory order. Unexamined ease is interference. Once that boundary is redrawn, energy returns to the tasks that actually sustain life: nourishment, movement, sleep, relationship, repair, and purposeful work.

Reclaiming the Cadence of Effort

Reclaiming physiological order begins with redesigning daily life around exertion and rest.

Begin with the morning. Instead of waking and immediately surrendering attention to a phone, start with natural sunlight, hydration, gentle stretching, and a few minutes of quiet orientation. Let physiology set the tone before the algorithm does.

During work hours, respect the natural cycle of focus and fatigue. Step away every ninety minutes. Stand, breathe diaphragmatically, and mobilize the spine. Allow attention to ebb and return rather than forcing the nervous system into exhausted output.

After meals, walk gently for ten minutes. This simple practice supports gastric emptying, steadier glucose handling, circulation, and mental reset. Before bed, dim bright lights, end work, remove screens, and give circadian biology permission to initiate sleep.

These are not punishments. They are guardrails. Consistency is built by repeating cues the nervous system can trust.

The Return to Meaningful Labor

Human beings are builders, caregivers, and active participants in the physical world. We are stabilized by the visible evidence of our own work: a cleaned room, a home-cooked meal, a watered garden, a swept floor, a completed walk.

In a culture of frictionless design, the physical evidence of living can disappear. Work happens invisibly inside screens. Food arrives in a bag. Social contact becomes text. Memory, navigation, and entertainment are delegated to machines.

Meaningful labor restores dignity to health. It transforms exercise from a punishing aesthetic chore into participation in life. There is a difference between running on a motorized treadmill while watching a screen and walking through a trail under natural light. Both may burn calories; one also restores spatial orientation, sensory richness, vagal tone, and connection with place.

Work that serves life, rather than merely speed, builds resilience. When the mind understands why physical work matters, movement stops being a calculation of calorie expenditure. It becomes regulation.

The True Cost

The ultimate cost of hyper-convenience is not measured in dollars. It is measured in the loss of bodily awareness.

Every intrinsic human action outsourced to a machine—moving, cooking, remembering, navigating, connecting—gradually weakens a capacity earlier generations practiced daily. Over time, these small surrenders create dependence: technology to think, stimulants to wake, screens to self-soothe, sedatives to sleep, and medication to function through pain.

Convenience must serve health rather than replace the behaviors that create it. Every micro-decision—cook or order delivery, walk or drive, breathe or scroll, stand or sit—tilts physiology toward either dysregulation or resilience.

Earned comfort feels different from passive comfort. Food tastes better when prepared with attention. Rest deepens when preceded by honest work. Sleep arrives more easily when the day contains natural light, movement, and satisfying completion. A system starved of meaningful work often celebrates its return.

Conclusion: Choosing Effort as Freedom

Frictionless ease was marketed as the ultimate path to freedom. In many logistical ways, it succeeded. But when ease replaces movement, cadence, cooking, real human connection, and meaningful labor, baseline health becomes harder to maintain.

The antidote is deliberate, joyful re-engagement with the physical work of being alive. Each conscious act of effort is a small rebellion against biological passivity.

Physical effort is not the enemy of freedom. It is one of the conditions that makes true freedom possible. To live with less dependence on medication in a hyper-convenient world is to restore a practical partnership with physiology.

Vitality is rarely found in a shortcut. It is built through resistance, awareness, timing, and repeated intention.

Clinical Case Study 3

Restoring Circadian Rhythm in Reflux and Metabolic Strain

Patient: Marcus T., 42-year-old male, senior software architect.

Chief Concerns: Persistent reflux symptoms, chronic morning nausea, central adiposity, elevated fasting glucose, late-night eating, and significant morning lethargy. He described waking with a "poisoned" sensation: nausea, heaviness, and no appetite until late afternoon.

Clinical Presentation

Marcus illustrates the metabolic cost of a life organized around screens, caffeine, late meals, and disappearing boundaries. His workday depended on black coffee and adrenaline. Food arrived in fragments: processed snacks at the desk, minimal daylight, long hours of sitting, and one large meal around 10:30 PM while staring at a screen.

The issue was not only food quality. It was timing, volume, sympathetic overdrive, and the absence of digestive cadence. Large late meals worsened gastric distension, delayed emptying, nocturnal reflux, and morning nausea. His digestive system was asked to perform heavy labor at the exact hour circadian biology was preparing for repair.

The clinical objective was not to reject acid-suppressing medication when clinically appropriate. It was to correct the daily pattern that kept provoking reflux: late-night caloric loading, screen exposure, erratic meal timing, sympathetic activation, and loss of an evening shutdown ritual.

Vitals and Traditional Asian Medicine Assessment

Vitals: Blood pressure elevated at 138/88 mm Hg, consistent with autonomic stress load.

Fasting Blood Glucose: 114 mg/dL, in the prediabetic range and consistent with metabolic strain.

Tongue Presentation: Red tongue body with a thick, sticky yellow coating concentrated at the center and root.

Pulse: Slippery and rapid at the right middle position.

Primary Pattern: Food Stagnation generating Stomach Heat. The late, heavy intake overwhelmed digestive timing, producing fullness,

reflux tendency, heat signs, and morning nausea.
Secondary Pattern: Spleen Qi Deficiency with Damp Accumulation. Sedentary digital work and erratic nourishment weakened transformation and transportation, contributing to central adiposity and sluggish digestion.

Plan and Intervention

Marcus committed to a structured twelve-week Sim-Bo circadian overhaul.

Sim-Bo Dietary Prescription, Circadian Shift: His largest 3:2:1 volume meal was moved to midday, aligning food volume with stronger digestive capacity. Evening meals were simplified to light vegetable broths and steamed greens. Caloric intake ended by 7:00 PM.
Morning Support: Warm millet and pumpkin puree were used at breakfast to provide gentle nourishment, stabilize appetite, and support digestive cadence.
Therapeutic Meal Timing: Coffee was tapered. Breakfast and lunch became predictable. Nighttime eating was replaced with a shutdown ritual of dim lighting, diaphragmatic breathwork, and screen reduction.
Targeted Acupuncture: ST44 and LI11 were used to clear Stomach Heat patterns; CV12 and ST36 were used to support digestive regulation, stomach function, and peristaltic rhythm.
Emperor's Cupping Therapy®: thoracic Bladder-meridian cupping was used to decrease protective tension, support local circulation, and relax the paraspinal region associated with digestive strain.
Herbal Medicine: Bao He Wan was used within the Traditional Asian Medicine framework to support food-stagnation patterns and digestive movement. The clinical goal was to reduce fullness, reflux tendency, and morning nausea while restoring meal timing.

Clinical Changes Over Twelve Weeks

Reflux Symptoms: Severe nightly reflux and daily antacid use were reported at baseline. By twelve weeks, reflux symptoms were markedly reduced during follow-up; medication status was reviewed with the appropriate prescribing clinician.
Morning Nausea: Daily nausea, heaviness, and lack of appetite resolved during the follow-up period, and natural morning hunger returned.
Body Weight and Adiposity: Weight decreased from 212 lbs. by 18 lbs., with visible reduction in central adiposity.
Fasting Blood Glucose: Fasting glucose improved from 114 mg/dL to

88 mg/dL.
Tongue Presentation: The red tongue body with thick, sticky yellow coating improved to a healthier color with a thinner coating.

Case Reflection

Marcus's case demonstrates that timing shapes metabolic outcomes. He was not simply suffering from random excess acid. He was living in a pattern that repeatedly forced digestion to work against circadian order.

When late-night eating was replaced with predictable daytime meals, lighter evenings, warm simple foods, walking, breathing, and targeted Eastern therapies, his symptoms and markers improved during the follow-up period. The clinical lesson is central to the Sim-Bo philosophy: timing determines response. Even high-quality food can become burdensome when eaten in the wrong volume, at the wrong hour, under an agitated nervous system state.

Convenience did not make Marcus freer. It made him dependent on rescue strategies. Restoring the physical work of daily life—cooking, timing, stopping, walking, breathing, and deliberately ending the day—helped restore the conditions under which digestion could regulate.

Transition: From Habit to Biology

Convenience begins outside us: in the chair, the screen, the car, the delivery app, the microwave, the disappearing walk. No shortcut remains outside for long. Repeated long enough, every external pattern becomes internal chemistry.

The question is no longer only how modern life reshaped our habits. The question is what those habits are made of. Food is not inert material. It is molecular instruction. It becomes blood, membrane, hormone, enzyme, neurotransmitter, and thought.

Amino acids construct tissue. Fats build membranes and carry hormonal instructions. Carbohydrates influence energy and metabolic timing. Vitamins, minerals, fiber, water, and oxygen act as essential cofactors in the living architecture.

When the language of food is coherent, physiology receives clearer instructions for repair. When that language is distorted by extreme processing, additives, chaotic timing, or excess, the message becomes inflammatory noise.

From the cost of convenience, we enter the language of nourishment.

PART II

Food as Medicine

Human physiology does not live by calories alone. It reads structure, timing, sequence, texture, mineral density, microbial consequence, and energetic demand.

A calorie can arrive wrapped in fiber, water, minerals, bitter compounds, aroma, temperature, and chewing. It can also arrive as refined starch, liquid sugar, industrial oil, synthetic flavor, and artificial urgency. The arithmetic may look similar on a label. The biological instruction is entirely different.

Food is not a passive substance dropped into a furnace. It is directive. It becomes blood, membrane, enzyme, hormone, neurotransmitter, bile, mucus, collagen, immune protein, mitochondrial current, and microbial fuel. Every meal participates in the architecture of the person who eats it.

The Sim-Bo method enters nutrition at this level. It removes excess novelty, excess processing, excess supplementation, and excess decision-making so physiology can read the meal without static. A plain meal is not primitive. It is legible.

Chapter 4

Understanding Nutrients: Food as Biological Language

Food as Instruction, Not Just Calories

Modern nutrition often begins with arithmetic: calories, grams, percentages, serving sizes, and macro targets. Arithmetic can guide research, clinical planning, and therapeutic accountability. But arithmetic is not the full language of nourishment.

A meal delivers biochemical instruction through glucose response, bile flow, gut peptides, mineral charge, redox balance, microbial fermentation, receptor activity, immune tone, and gene-regulatory pathways. Its meaning is shaped by source, preparation, sequence, temperature, chewing, stress state, sleep debt, digestive capacity, and the hour of the day.

This is why a bowl of brown rice with vegetables, eaten slowly in calm attention, does not behave like a sweetened beverage consumed in a car under stress. The calorie count may appear comparable. The directive is not.

Reductionist nutrition sees a label and believes it has seen the food. It has not. A label cannot measure chewing time, satiety, microbial response, digestive warmth, nervous-system readiness, or the way a meal lands inside a depleted patient. Those hidden variables determine whether food becomes nourishment, storage, irritation, or repair.

The Sim-Bo approach begins with food simple enough to observe. When meals become predictable, patterns become visible. The patient learns what steadies energy, what congests digestion, what clouds thought, what calms appetite, and what disturbs sleep.

Food is, above all else, communication.

The Native Tongue of Physiology

Long before human beings isolated vitamins, mapped molecular structures, or sequenced the microbiome, they knew that food changed resilience. Fresh greens restored strength after depletion. Warm broths steadied recovery. Fermented foods altered digestion. Starvation changed mood, temperature, fertility, and thought. These were not primitive superstitions. They were early readings of nutritional language.

Modern science now names part of this process nutrigenomics and epigenetics: the study of how nutrients and dietary patterns influence metabolic pathways, gene expression, and cellular behavior. The human organism is not a combustion engine. It is a living interpreter, continuously turning physical matter into tissue, immunity, memory, movement, and repair.

Food becomes architecture: muscle, bone, skin, enzymes, hormones, immune proteins, connective tissue, neurotransmitters, cell membranes, and the matrix that holds organs together. It also becomes instruction: build, conserve, mobilize, cleanse, store, defend, calm, or inflame.

One meal is rarely destiny. Repetition is destiny. Repeated meals create the terrain in which insulin acts, mitochondria generate energy, inflammatory mediators rise or settle, microbes flourish or fade, and tissues decide whether to repair or defend.

When food remains close to its natural matrix, digestion reads it with less confusion. When it is refined, denatured, stripped of fiber, repeatedly heated, or engineered for hyper-palatability, the syntax breaks. The system receives energy without pacing, stimulation without satiety, and density without order.

This is why timing matters as much as ingredients. A clean meal eaten chaotically once in a while cannot create the same regulatory cadence as a steady pattern repeated daily. The genome listens to the environment that daily nourishment creates.

Macronutrients: The Grammar of Energy

Proteins, fats, and carbohydrates form the major grammar of nutrition. Each carries a distinct function. Each can restore order or create strain depending on source, dose, timing, preparation, digestive capacity, activity, and clinical stage.

Protein: Structure and Signal

Protein builds the visible and invisible structure of life. It supplies amino acids for enzymes, antibodies, connective tissue, muscle, transport proteins, peptide hormones, and repair machinery. Without adequate protein, resilience weakens.

Protein also carries a growth directive. Amino acids, insulin, energy status, exercise, and growth factors converge on mTOR, one of the great nutrient-sensing pathways of human physiology. When tissue must rebuild, this signal is valuable. When abundance is constant and recovery pathways are never given space, growth can crowd out repair.

The clinical art is adequacy, not excess. Too little protein weakens structure. Too much poorly timed, poorly sourced, or poorly digested protein increases digestive demand and shifts the terrain toward growth when cleanup is needed. The essential question is never simply, How much protein? It is: for whom, from what source, at what stage of healing, with what digestive strength, and with what daily workload?

Fats: Master Messengers

Fats are master communicators. They form cell membranes, support bile flow, carry fat-soluble vitamins, protect nerves, contribute to steroid hormone synthesis, and shape inflammatory tone. The brain is lipid-rich; every membrane depends on the quality of the fats that repeatedly enter the diet.

Omega-3 fats help generate pro-resolving lipid mediators. Whole-food fats arrive with texture, minerals, antioxidants, fiber, and natural satiety. Refined oils used repeatedly in packaged and fried foods bring a different instruction: speed, oxidation, easy excess, and weaker structural intelligence.

The modern problem is not the existence of fat. It is the industrial handling of fat: extraction, refinement, storage, heating, dose, and the processed-food matrix in which these oils are consumed. In their traditional settings, fats nourish membranes and hormones. In distorted settings, they become friction.

Fat also slows the meal. It changes gastric emptying, bile demand, satiety, and the pace at which carbohydrate enters circulation. In whole-food meals, this can stabilize energy. In engineered foods that combine fat with refined starch, sugar, salt, and flavor chemistry, it can mask satiety and invite excess.

Carbohydrates: Timing, Fiber, and Metabolic Cadence

Carbohydrates are context-sensitive molecules. In intact form—brown rice, millet, oats, legumes, sweet potatoes, whole fruits, and fibrous vegetables—they bring glucose with fiber, water, minerals, resistant starch, polyphenols, and digestive pacing. This structure slows entry into circulation, feeds microbes, and creates steadier energy.

Refined carbohydrates and liquid sugars arrive as speed. They ask the pancreas to answer quickly and repeatedly. Over years, that tempo can distort glucose regulation and weaken metabolic flexibility.

This is why whole grains and starchy vegetables can be clinically useful even in a program designed to reduce inflammation. The question is not whether carbohydrate exists. The question is whether it arrives with fiber, minerals, structure, warmth, and timing. Brown rice is not merely carbohydrate. In the Sim-Bo system, it is a stable anchor.

Micronutrients: Master Regulators

If macronutrients form the grammar of energy, micronutrients are the master regulators. They appear in smaller quantities, yet they determine whether enzymes ignite, nerves fire, muscles relax, thyroid hormone converts, collagen forms, glutathione protects, and mitochondria produce steady current.

Magnesium teaches the nervous system how to release tension. Zinc governs taste, epithelial repair, immunity, and the boundary surfaces of the body. Vitamin D behaves less like a simple vitamin than a hormonal conductor, influencing immune and skeletal patterns through receptor-driven gene regulation. B vitamins help convert food into usable metabolic current. Iodine, selenium, copper, manganese, chromium, potassium, sodium, calcium, and iron each hold a small key to a large gate.

Deficiency rarely announces itself with one clean symptom. It whispers through fatigue, poor stress tolerance, altered taste, brittle immunity, muscle tension, sluggish cognition, poor wound repair, skin changes, and unstable mood. These signs require clinical interpretation, but the principle is simple: calories without micronutrient order create abundance without command.

The deeper solution is not an endless cabinet of isolated pills. It is a diet whose architecture naturally delivers minerals, vitamins, fiber, water, and phytochemicals in forms the digestive system can recognize. Targeted supplementation has its place when need is clear. It must support the foundation, not impersonate it.

Digestion: The Translation Process

When food enters the mouth, translation begins. Chewing breaks structure. Saliva begins starch digestion. Stomach acid unfolds proteins. Pancreatic enzymes dismantle carbohydrate, fat, and protein. Bile emulsifies lipids. Intestinal villi absorb. Microbes ferment what human enzymes cannot. Every organ adds a necessary phrase to the sentence.

When translation falters, the message distorts. Insufficient acid, stress-impaired secretion, rapid eating, low bile flow, enzyme weakness, dysbiosis, poor motility, and low chewing can leave food incompletely processed. The result appears as bloating, reflux tendency, stool irregularity, food reactivity, heaviness, and microbial imbalance.

Efficient digestion depends on autonomic cadence. The gut works best when the nervous system receives cues of safety: regular mealtimes, warm recognizable food, adequate chewing, upright posture, calm attention, and a pause after eating. Rush and anxiety pull blood flow and attention away from digestion. The meal is swallowed, but not fully received.

Sim-Bo uses simplicity before complexity. A predictable meal lowers interpretive demand. The stomach receives familiar food. The pancreas anticipates the workload. The microbiome receives fiber with rhythm. The nervous system is spared novelty, urgency, and overstimulation at every plate.

Warmth matters. Many depleted or stressed patients tolerate warm cooked foods more easily than cold, raw, or highly complex meals. A bowl of warm rice and vegetables may seem ordinary. Clinically, it can lower digestive effort and restore the first language of nourishment: safety.

Metabolic Flexibility: Reading the Directive

Once nutrients cross the intestinal barrier, the next interpretation begins. Glucose is coordinated through insulin and uptake pathways. Amino acids move toward repair, enzymes, immune proteins, or fuel according to need. Fatty acids become membranes, hormones, stored energy, or usable fuel.

Metabolic flexibility is the capacity to shift between these sources without distress. After a meal, a resilient system uses circulating glucose cleanly. Between meals, it draws from stored energy. During activity, it mobilizes fuel. During rest, it repairs.

Inflammation, sleep loss, chronic stress, low muscle mass, excess snacking, late eating, and stimulant-driven appetite suppression disrupt this capacity. What a patient experiences as weight gain, fatigue, cravings, poor exercise tolerance, or brain fog may be the outward expression of confused metabolic instruction.

Simplicity restores legibility. Repeated meals at stable times allow metabolic pathways to anticipate demand. Movement gives glucose somewhere to go. Sleep lowers stress chemistry. Fiber gives microbes a steady substrate. The system becomes less reactive because the daily pattern becomes easier to read.

Physiology's Survival Priorities

Human physiology follows hierarchy. In depletion, illness, acute stress, or undernourishment, vital functions take priority. Brain, heart, circulation, blood glucose, immune defense, and temperature regulation come first. Hair growth, fertility, skin brightness, athletic recovery, and long-term tissue remodeling wait their turn.

Modern life often creates the inverse problem: not scarcity, but overload. Many people are calorie-replete and micronutrient-poor—overfed in energy, undernourished in order. Refined starch, liquid sugar, low fiber, and ultra-processed foods increase hepatic demand, disturb triglyceride handling, strain glucose regulation, and encourage visceral accumulation in susceptible metabolic terrain.

This is the paradox of industrial abundance. The liver processes excess. The pancreas answers repeated glucose exposure. The gut struggles with low fiber and additives. Mitochondria operate under oxidative pressure. Energy that could support repair is diverted toward management of the overflow.

A confused system does not recover by receiving louder messages. It recovers by receiving clearer ones.

Food Quality: The Matrix of Meaning

Modern nutrition often measures value through isolated metrics. Calories, grams, percentages, and labels can inform clinical judgment, but they do not capture the whole meaning of food.

Quality resides in structure: fiber, water, minerals, phytochemicals, intact cell walls, texture, freshness, preparation, temperature, and degree of processing. Two diets may contain the same calorie count and create entirely different internal terrain.

A day built on refined flour, liquid sugar, processed oils, and fortified snacks can create unstable appetite, weak microbial fermentation, glycemic volatility, and inflammatory friction. A day built on grains, vegetables, fruit, legumes, water, and simple preparation can support satiety, bowel regularity, microbial resilience, and steady energy.

Food quality cannot be outsourced to marketing language. Organic, gluten-free, high-protein, low-carb, fortified, natural, and plant-based can each clarify or confuse. The practical questions are more honest: Does this food retain structure? Does it require chewing? Does it contain water and fiber? Does it satisfy without overstimulation? Does the patient become clearer after eating?

The Sim-Bo reliance on brown rice, vegetables, fruits, hydration, and simple timing is not arbitrary restriction. It is the discipline of reducing noise until nourishment becomes readable again.

Water, Oxygen, and the Metabolic Medium

Water and oxygen are often omitted from nutrient conversations because they are too obvious to impress the modern mind. Yet neither metabolism nor repair proceeds without them. Water dissolves, transports, lubricates, cools, moistens, and permits chemical exchange. Oxygen accepts electrons in aerobic energy production and allows fuel to become usable work.

Mild dehydration can turn simple strain into complexity: tension headaches, dry stools, irritability, poor exercise tolerance, muscle tightness, dull thinking, and fatigue. Hydration is not mere volume. It is the fluid environment in which transport, electrical gradients, enzyme activity, and waste clearance occur.

Some biophysical research explores structured water near hydrophilic surfaces, sometimes described as exclusion-zone water. The clinical lesson is not to chase another trend. It is to remember that cells require an aqueous environment for charge, transport, and motion.

Oxygen depends on behavior. Shallow, rapid breathing reinforces sympathetic tone and reduces diaphragmatic movement. Slow diaphragmatic breathing supports autonomic regulation, rib-cage mobility, venous return, and steadier physiology. Breath is not separate from nutrition. It is part of the medium that allows nutrients to become energy.

Movement completes the circuit. Walking after meals supports circulation, glucose handling, digestive motility, and mental reset. A meal does not end when swallowing ends. It continues through circulation, uptake, mitochondrial conversion, microbial fermentation, and clearance.

The Symbiosis Within

Human metabolism is not solitary. Mitochondria, microbes, immune cells, gut lining, liver, nervous system, and endocrine organs exchange resources continuously. Health is cooperation.

Fiber-feeding microbes produce short-chain fatty acids such as butyrate, which support gut-barrier integrity, immune regulation, microbial ecology, and gut-brain conversation. Plant polyphenols and minerals feed other branches of the same network. Mitochondria require

B vitamins, magnesium, iron, copper, CoQ10-related pathways, oxygen, antioxidants, movement, sleep, and substrate availability to produce energy without excessive oxidative strain.

A low-fiber, ultra-processed diet starves microbial partners. Constant stress shifts motility. Poor sleep changes appetite. Sedentary living weakens glucose disposal. Artificial sweetness and refined starch confuse satiety. No organ fails alone; no organ heals alone.

Simple, fiber-rich, minimally processed foods restore the terms of the alliance. Dense plant fiber feeds beneficial colonies. Phytochemicals participate in antioxidant defense. Minerals support enzymes. Water and movement preserve transit. Rhythm gives the ecosystem a stable tempo.

A patient raised on refined foods may not immediately tolerate massive raw fiber. The answer is not to abandon fiber, but to introduce it with intelligence: cooked vegetables, gradual increases, hydration, chewing, and consistency. The microbiome adapts best when challenged steadily, not shocked unpredictably.

Eating as Dialogue, Not Data

Patients often ask, Exactly how much should I eat? The deeper question is, What is this meal asking my physiology to do?

Numbers have a place. Lived physiology speaks through hunger, fullness, stool quality, energy, sleep, mood, temperature, cravings, and mental clarity. Slow eating gives gastric stretch receptors and gut-derived satiety peptides—including CCK, GLP-1, and PYY—time to speak. Thorough chewing improves mechanical breakdown. Eating without screens restores attention to the plate. Gratitude is not mystical decoration; a calmer state supports parasympathetic tone, which prepares digestion to work.

Sim-Bo naturally trains this dialogue by limiting novelty and reducing culinary noise. A simple meal becomes familiar enough for subtle changes to be felt. The patient stops chasing external rules and begins reading the response: steady energy or crash, calm digestion or bloating, clear thinking or fog, restorative sleep or restlessness.

This is applied physiology. Data matters, but data without perception becomes another abstraction. The goal is measurable clarity joined to disciplined observation.

The patient who learns to observe digestion becomes less dependent on trend. Hunger separates from stimulation. Nourishment separates from heaviness. Fullness separates from inflammation. Craving separates from need.

Conclusion: Relearning the Mother Tongue

To understand nutrients is to remember that food is a language physiology already knows how to read. The exchange between the meal selected and the cells built from it is ancient, subtle, and constant. When the daily message becomes clearer—whole food, sufficient protein, fiber, minerals, water, oxygen, movement, and rest—regulation becomes easier.

Energy steadies. Digestion calms. Appetite becomes more honest. Sleep deepens. Metabolic static declines. These changes do not come from one special ingredient. They arise from a cleaner conversation.

We live in an age obsessed with digital translation, algorithms, and instant messaging, yet the most important translation remains internal. Nutrients become tissue. Breath becomes energy. Fiber becomes microbial instruction. Minerals become electrical stability. Water becomes transport. Rest becomes repair. Food, prepared and received with cadence, becomes the mother tongue of healing.

The practical conclusion is deliberately simple: eat food with structure; chew it; time it; hydrate; breathe; move; sleep; observe; repeat. The sophistication lies not in novelty, but in the steady execution of what physiology already understands.

Clinical Case Study 4

Restoring Digestive Clarity Through Whole-Food Structure

Patient: Sarah W., 38-year-old female, urban planner.

Chief Concerns: Post-prandial abdominal bloating with afternoon distention, cognitive sluggishness, fluctuating weight, poor satiety, and a strange sense of being undernourished despite a high-calorie, fortified Western diet.

Clinical Presentation

Sarah was not underfed by calorie count. She was overfed with fragments and starved of structure.

Most of her meals came from protein isolates, fortified snack products, refined grains, synthetic multivitamin gummies, sweetened beverages, and low-fiber convenience foods. On paper, she was consuming enough. In lived physiology, the pattern produced bloating, irregular digestion, weak satiety, mental dullness, and unstable energy.

She tried to solve the problem by adding more products: another protein powder, another probiotic, a stronger multivitamin, a new digestive enzyme. Each addition created hope, then the same distention and fatigue returned. The treatment strategy was therefore subtractive first. Remove the noise. Restore the matrix. Let digestion reveal the truth.

Initial Findings

Abdominal palpation showed marked tympany and tension across the umbilical and epigastric regions, consistent with gas retention and digestive stagnation.

Tongue presentation was pale and puffy with scalloped lateral edges and a thin, sticky white coating.

Pulse was slippery and weak at the right middle position, with wiry constraint at the left middle position.

Traditional Asian Medicine Assessment

Sarah's pattern reflected Spleen Qi deficiency complicated by Dampness and Liver constraint. In Five-Element language, Wood was overacting on Earth: mental pressure and internal tension were constraining digestive transformation. The pattern matched the bloating, heaviness, food sensitivity, weak satiety, and cognitive sluggishness.

The clinical priority was clear from both traditions of observation: reduce complexity, restore intact food structure, calm the nervous system, and rebuild digestive timing.

Plan and Intervention

Sarah committed to a twelve-week Sim-Bo metabolic recalibration focused on food structure rather than supplementation escalation.

Dietary simplification: Protein isolates, synthetic vitamin gummies, highly fortified snack products, sweetened beverages, and refined flours were removed so her true digestive baseline could emerge.
3 parts grains: Brown rice, millet, and sweet potatoes became recognizable carbohydrate anchors, providing steady energy, minerals, texture, and digestive pacing.
2 parts vegetables: Lightly steamed greens, carrots, squash, and other fibrous vegetables rebuilt fiber intake, stool regularity, mineral density, and microbial substrate.
1 part fruit: Whole fruit provided sweetness, hydration, polyphenols, and satiety without relying on sweetened processed products.
Meal cadence: Meals were placed at consistent times, eaten without screens, and simplified enough for Sarah to notice cause and effect in bloating, energy, stool, and appetite.
Targeted acupuncture: LR13 and LR14 were used to harmonize Liver-Spleen tension and reduce digestive constraint; ST36 and SP3 supported digestive transformation, motility, and resilience.
Emperor's Cupping Therapy®: gentle decompression over the abdominal fascia and thoracic Back-Shu region supported tissue glide, local circulation, and relaxation of the abdominal wall and paraspinal musculature.
Herbal medicine: A modified Xiao Yao San approach supported Liver-Spleen harmonization, reduced constraint, and improved digestive comfort.

For the first two weeks, observation was the main assignment. Sarah recorded meal timing, bloating intensity, stool quality, energy, and mental clarity. The point was not obsessive tracking. It was restoring cause and effect.

Twelve-Week Outcome Pattern

Abdominal bloating: Markedly reduced; afternoon distention no longer occurred daily.
Cognitive state: Clearer thinking and steadier afternoon energy by

patient report.

Digestive function: More regular bowel movements with less post-meal discomfort.

Satiety and appetite: Fewer cravings for fortified snacks and improved recognition of fullness.

Tongue presentation: Reduced puffiness and scalloping, with a cleaner coating in TAM observation.

Clinical Meaning

Sarah's case carries the central lesson of Chapter 4: nutrition is not chemistry alone. It is structure, rhythm, digestibility, and living architecture. Her improvement did not come from adding more isolated compounds. It came from removing unnecessary complexity and returning meals to a form that digestion, microbes, metabolism, and appetite could understand.

She needed fewer products and more coherence.

Transition: From Language to Building Blocks

Every functional language has an alphabet. In nutrition, that alphabet is built from molecules.

Protein is the first great building block. It builds tissue, supports immunity, repairs injury, carries growth instructions, and shapes the terrain of aging, strength, and recovery. Used with precision, it restores. Used without timing, proportion, or context, it can create strain.

From food as language, the path narrows to one of its most powerful letters.

Chapter 5

Protein: Friend or Foe?

The Cult of Protein

Walk through a modern supermarket and protein appears less like a nutrient than a religion. It is engineered into bars, cereals, shakes, powders, water, cookies, and snacks, each label promising strength, leanness, endurance, and control.

The culture has turned protein into a symbol of discipline. Athletes chase it. Dieters use it to silence appetite. Aging patients are told to increase it reflexively. Wellness brands attach the word to almost anything and sell it as virtue.

Protein deserves respect, not worship.

It is the great builder of the human frame: muscle, collagen, enzymes, antibodies, transport proteins, hormones, tendons, ligaments, and repair machinery. Without amino acids, tissue loses its capacity to renew. Yet the builder is demanding. Every gram beyond useful need must be processed, converted, cleared, or stored indirectly through energy pathways. Excess does not become automatic strength. It becomes metabolic accounting.

Protein matters enormously. Modern culture has mistaken necessary structure for unlimited advantage.

Protein marketing exploits a primal fear: the fear of becoming weak. Once that fear is activated, the patient stops asking whether the food is digestible, balanced, or necessary. The label says strength, and the nervous system obeys. A healer must break that spell. Strength is not purchased by the gram; it is earned by assimilation, movement, sleep, and the correct dose of building material.

The Builder's Paradox

Protein begins its work in the stomach. Hydrochloric acid and pepsin unfold its complex chains, breaking them into smaller peptides and amino acids. These fragments pass through the intestinal wall, enter portal circulation, and become raw material for renewal.

Skin, intestinal lining, immune proteins, red blood cells, connective tissue, and muscle are constantly turning over. Life is not a static possession; it is a disciplined process of demolition and rebuilding. Protein supplies the bricks.

But amino acids carry nitrogen, and nitrogen demands clearance. When amino acids are used for structure, the process is elegant. When they exceed need, the liver must remove the nitrogen group, convert ammonia into urea, and send that urea to the kidneys for excretion. This is normal physiology. Under chronic excess, normal physiology becomes constant labor.

The builder creates strength only when the construction site can use the material. Dumping excess bricks on a finished house does not make it stronger. It creates clutter, pressure, and cleanup.

The organism maintains an amino acid pool, not a protein warehouse. It draws from food, tissue turnover, and internal recycling. When a meal supplies enough amino acids, repair proceeds quietly. When the meal floods the pool beyond need, the surplus becomes chemical responsibility.

This is why protein must be judged by use, not by image. A patient can consume impressive numbers and still fail to build strength if digestion is weak, sleep is poor, inflammation is high, or muscle is never challenged. Protein does not create tissue by itself. It requires timing, hormones, movement, rest, and a system willing to receive the instruction.

Assimilation is the hidden gatekeeper. Stomach acid, pancreatic enzymes, bile flow, intestinal lining, microbial balance, chewing, temperature, and nervous system state all decide whether protein becomes tissue or residue. A patient with weak digestion does not need a louder protein signal. He needs a meal he can actually transform.

The Myth of More and the Nitrogen Load

Protein's inflated reputation grew out of a legitimate fear: deficiency. Severe protein deprivation weakens immunity, muscle, skin integrity, wound repair, and child development. Early nutrition science rightly treated protein as essential. Modern marketing turned essential into maximal.

The body can store carbohydrate as glycogen and fat as adipose reserve. It has no equivalent warehouse for surplus amino acids. Excess must be handled immediately. The liver deaminates. The urea cycle works. The kidneys filter. ATP is spent to manage what the tissues did not require.

This is the nitrogen load: not a dramatic emergency, but a steady metabolic demand. In the right amount, protein supports repair. In excess, it turns nourishment into administrative work.

High-protein, low-carbohydrate regimens often produce rapid early weight loss because appetite drops, glycogen-associated water is lost, and food choice narrows. The result can feel thrilling. But speed is not the same as restoration. If the pattern leaves the person dehydrated, constipated, irritable, sleepless, or heavy after meals, the diet is not creating vitality. It is extracting performance from stress chemistry.

Protein obeys the law that governs all powerful nutrients: proportion determines medicine.

Modern high-protein culture also ignores hydration. A dry, stimulant-driven patient living on protein bars, jerky, shakes, eggs, and meat while drinking coffee instead of water is not building resilience. He is asking the liver and kidneys to process dense material in a dehydrated state.

The heavier the protein, the more the meal requires moisture, fiber, minerals, movement, and digestive warmth. Without those companions, the food may nourish on paper while increasing internal strain in practice.

Acid Load and Mineral Balance

Protein metabolism leaves an acid load that must be balanced. This is commonly discussed through Potential Renal Acid Load, or PRAL. Sulfur-containing amino acids, more concentrated in many animal proteins, generate acid residues that the kidneys must help excrete. Fruits, vegetables, and many fibrous plant foods bring potassium, magnesium, organic acids, water, and minerals that reduce the net renal acid load.

Blood pH remains tightly defended; the organism does not casually become acidic. The cost lies in the effort required to maintain that balance. A diet built around large servings of protein with little plant material asks the kidneys to manage acid load with fewer buffering allies.

A Sim-Bo plate answers this with architecture. Protein is present, but it is surrounded by grains, vegetables, hydration, fiber, minerals, and color. The builders do not arrive alone. They arrive with sweepers, buffers, carriers, and regulators.

The clinical lesson is simple: never eat protein naked. Pair it with plants. Give the kidneys water, minerals, and fiber. Let the plate itself carry balance.

PRAL restores humility to plate design. It reminds us that protein never arrives alone; it arrives inside a chemical neighborhood. Fish with seaweed is one neighborhood. Meat with refined bread, fried oil, soda, and no fiber is another. The kidney experiences the difference.

Traditional plates understood this without laboratory language: beans with greens, fish with vegetables, lentils with herbs, small meat with broth and roots. The meal was never meant to be a protein monument. It was meant to be a balanced terrain.

mTOR, IGF-1, and the Growth Command

Protein is more than raw material. It is a growth command.

Amino acids, especially leucine, interact with mTOR, one of the central nutrient-sensing pathways of human physiology. mTOR tells cells that materials are available and growth can proceed. In childhood, athletics, trauma recovery, tissue repair, and frailty, this command can be valuable. Tissue needs instruction to rebuild.

The danger begins when the command never rests. Constant abundance keeps the system leaning toward growth and away from cleanup. Autophagy, the internal process of recycling damaged components, requires periods when the cell is not being told to build. The organism needs both construction and housekeeping. Protein excess favors construction long after the project is complete.

Animal-rich patterns can also influence IGF-1, a powerful growth-related hormone involved in repair, development, and cellular proliferation. IGF-1 is not an enemy. It is a signal. The problem is chronic amplification without rhythm.

Longevity is not built by suppressing growth forever. It is built by cycling growth and repair with intelligence. Build when rebuilding is needed. Clean when cleanup is due. Protein must serve that cadence, not dominate it.

Resistance training changes the meaning of protein because muscle contraction creates a legitimate call for synthesis. A sedentary system receiving constant protein hears growth without work. An active system receiving appropriate protein hears repair after effort. The same amino acids become different instructions depending on whether the need has been earned through movement.

This is the distinction between building and swelling. Building follows demand. Swelling follows excess. The clinician must learn which one is occurring.

Animal Protein, the Microbiome, and Metabolic Residue

Protein source changes the entire downstream conversation.

Animal foods arrive dense, direct, and concentrated. Plant-centered protein arrives inside a matrix of fiber, water, minerals, resistant starch, polyphenols, and microbial substrate. That packaging alters digestion, gut ecology, acid load, satiety, stool pattern, and inflammatory tone.

In certain gut environments, compounds such as choline and carnitine can be metabolized by intestinal microbes into trimethylamine, later converted in the liver into TMAO. This is terrain, not morality. The same food enters different microbial ecosystems and produces different consequences.

Industrial animal foods often bring more than amino acids: processing residues, oxidized fats, heme iron, sodium load, cooking byproducts, and the absence of fiber. These factors shape how the meal lands in the vascular system, the microbiome, and the immune environment.

Plant proteins carry a different instruction. Lentils, beans, tofu, tempeh, quinoa, millet, nuts, seeds, and grains deliver amino acids with the fibers and phytochemicals that feed microbial allies. They build without asking the gut to sacrifice its ecology.

The difference is metabolic architecture.

The colon reveals what the small intestine failed to complete. When protein residue reaches the lower bowel in excess, the microbiome does not remain neutral. It ferments what it receives. Odor, gas, stool pattern, abdominal pressure, and heaviness after high-protein meals often tell the truth long before a laboratory report does.

Fiber changes that conversation. It gives beneficial microbes their preferred fuel and reduces the dominance of putrefactive pathways. A protein meal without fiber is an instruction without punctuation. It can be understood, but it is harsher than necessary.

How Much Is Enough?

The modern protein question is usually asked in the wrong direction. People ask how high they can go. The better question is how little excess is needed to maintain strength, repair, immunity, and metabolic calm.

Formal nutrition references often begin around 0.8 grams per kilogram of body weight for healthy adults. That number is a baseline reference, not a sacred law. Needs rise with growth, pregnancy, intense training, injury, surgery, sarcopenia risk, frailty, and certain clinical conditions. Needs fall when digestive capacity, kidney function, or inflammatory strain demands restraint.

The practical eye is often wiser than the anxious calculator. A palm-sized serving of protein-rich food at a meal is usually enough to provide structure without turning the plate into a demolition site. The rest of the meal should speak in grain, vegetable, fruit, hydration, fiber, and color.

Protein sufficiency feels steady. It does not leave the patient heavy, thirsty, constipated, irritable, or sedated after eating. It supports clear energy without demanding a nap.

The Sim-Bo standard is not heroic intake. It is exact usefulness.

The Plant Advantage

Plants are not weak food. They are organized chemistry.

A plant-centered protein pattern wraps amino acids in microbial fuel, minerals, water, and antioxidants. Fiber slows digestion, feeds short-chain fatty acid production, improves stool rhythm, and strengthens the intestinal barrier. Polyphenols communicate with immune cells and microbes. Minerals help buffer the acid load and maintain electrical stability.

Culinary complexity is unnecessary. Brown rice with lentils. Millet with fermented tofu. Oats with seeds. Beans with greens. Quinoa with vegetables. Simple combinations create amino acid adequacy without turning protein into the entire identity of the meal.

When animal protein is used, it belongs as a precise instrument, not a monument. A small portion of high-quality protein can flavor a meal, support targeted repair, and satisfy tradition. It belongs in proportion.

The old prosperity symbol was abundance. The new clinical refinement is proportion.

Plant protein becomes most therapeutic when it is prepared with respect. Soaking reduces hardness. Fermentation improves tolerance. Slow cooking softens fibers. Warming spices awaken the digestive tract. A poorly prepared bean can create digestive strain; a well-prepared bean can become medicine.

Sim-Bo does not replace meat with processed imitation meat and call the problem solved. It returns to foods the organism can recognize: grains, beans, vegetables, broths, fermented preparations, seeds, fruits, and clean water.

The old fear of incomplete plant protein is often overstated in practical life. A single plant food may not contain every amino acid in ideal proportion, but a day built from grains, legumes, seeds, nuts, vegetables, and fermented foods can supply the full pattern with remarkable elegance. The Sim-Bo method does not depend on one perfect food. It depends on a repeated architecture that makes adequacy ordinary.

This architecture also changes appetite. Whole plant meals require chewing, volume, water, and time. They stretch the stomach gently and feed the microbiome slowly. The patient becomes full through structure rather than force. That is a different form of satiety from the abrupt appetite suppression created by dense protein products.

The Filtration Cost: Liver and Kidneys

The liver and kidneys do the quiet accounting for protein excess.

The liver deaminates surplus amino acids, converts ammonia into urea, and coordinates whether carbon skeletons become energy, glucose, or fat-related intermediates. The kidneys filter urea and maintain fluid, mineral, and acid-base balance. These organs are resilient, but resilience is not permission for constant overload.

A chronically high-protein pattern can increase urea production, raise filtration demand, intensify thirst, alter bowel rhythm, and increase the need for hydration and mineral balance. In patients with hypertension, insulin resistance, kidney vulnerability, gout tendency, or liver strain, the cost rises.

The early signs are often ordinary: heavy fatigue after dense meals, strong thirst, constipation, darker urine, morning puffiness, stiffness, headaches, or mental fog. These signs are not diagnoses. They are invitations to examine load, hydration, bowel rhythm, and laboratory markers with discipline.

When protein is brought back into proportion and plants return to the center of the plate, filtration demand often lightens. BUN, creatinine trends, uric acid patterns, blood pressure, stool quality, and post-meal energy can all become useful clinical mirrors.

The clinical mistake is to wait until laboratory markers become alarming before changing the pattern. The liver and kidneys are resilient because they are designed to protect life silently. Their silence is not permission to overwork them. It is an invitation to respect their reserve.

A high-protein diet can look successful on a scale while quietly increasing filtration demand. Weight may fall, appetite may be suppressed, and the patient may feel proud. But if sleep worsens, bowels slow, thirst increases, breath becomes heavy, and energy declines, the apparent success is too expensive.

Laboratory values belong in this conversation. BUN, creatinine, uric acid, urine specific gravity, albumin, liver enzymes, blood pressure, fasting glucose, and inflammatory markers can all help reveal whether the protein pattern is being used cleanly. Numbers do not replace clinical observation; they sharpen it. The best reading comes when symptoms, meals, constitution, and labs are interpreted together.

Timing, Fasting, and Repair

Protein belongs where tissue can use it.

A small, steady distribution across simple meals often works better than a single massive serving. Protein in the presence of whole grains, vegetables, and healthy fat enters more slowly, creates less urgency, and supports a calmer anabolic signal. Brown rice with sprouted lentils and steamed greens is not glamorous; it is mechanically intelligent. Each component moderates the others.

Repair also requires intervals. Constant eating prevents the system from hearing the difference between nourishment and cleanup. Gentle time boundaries around meals can restore metabolic order by allowing digestion to finish and repair processes to begin.

Fasting becomes useful only when it is rhythmic and well matched to the patient. Erratic deprivation, stimulant-driven appetite suppression, and punishment fasting create stress chemistry. The Sim-Bo approach does not glorify deprivation. It restores sequence: eat simply, digest completely, rest deeply, repair quietly.

Late-night protein is particularly demanding in patients with reflux, sluggish bile flow, poor sleep, or morning heaviness. The digestive tract should not be forced to process dense repair material when the circadian system is preparing for cleanup and neurological restoration.

The cleanest pattern is usually simple: adequate protein earlier in the day, lighter intake in the evening, digestive rest overnight, and enough movement to make the amino acids necessary. Protein should follow work, not replace it.

Protein, Hormones, and the Arc of Aging

Protein sits at the crossroads of growth and aging.

Youth requires growth. Injury requires growth. Frailty requires rebuilding. But adult longevity requires a different rhythm: enough building material to preserve muscle, immunity, connective tissue, and enzymes, with enough restraint to allow autophagy, insulin sensitivity, and inflammatory resolution.

Aging poorly is often a failure of proportion in both directions. Too little protein in later life accelerates weakness, poor wound repair, low resilience, and muscle loss. Too much dense protein without plants, movement, hydration, and digestive capacity pushes the terrain toward growth signals without adequate cleanup.

The sweet spot is neither scarcity nor excess. It is sufficiency matched to stage of life. Children, athletes, laborers, injured patients, and elders do not have the same need. A person rebuilding after illness does not need the same plate as a sedentary executive with high insulin and poor sleep.

Protein must be prescribed by context: age, muscle, work, digestion, inflammation, kidney reserve, training demand, and therapeutic goal. That is the difference between nutrition and slogan.

The aging patient needs neither protein panic nor protein neglect. Muscle is an organ of glucose regulation, balance, heat, confidence, and survival. Preserving it requires both amino acids and resistance. Food supplies the material. Movement gives the material a reason to become tissue.

Age with clean strength: enough muscle to move, enough appetite to nourish, enough restraint to clear, and enough metabolic quiet to repair.

Cultural Reverence and Misunderstanding

Dense protein foods have long carried symbolic power. Meat at a feast meant survival. Eggs meant fertility. Milk meant growth. A large portion once signaled that starvation had been defeated for the day.

Industrial abundance changed the equation. Foods that once appeared occasionally became cheap, constant, and oversized. The ancient symbolism remained, but the need changed. A serving that once marked celebration became an everyday habit.

To reduce protein excess at the modern table can feel like refusing care, strength, status, or progress. That emotional inheritance must be understood. People do not cling to excess only because of ignorance. They cling to the feeling of safety that abundance once represented.

Sim-Bo reframes the symbol. Strength is not the largest serving.

Strength is the meal that leaves the patient clear, warm, satisfied, and capable of repair. A simple bowl of brown rice, fermented tofu, vegetables, and fruit may look humble. Clinically, it can be highly refined: structure without heaviness, amino acids without excess, nourishment without noise.

Finding the Middle Path

Protein teaches proportion more sharply than any other nutrient.

Too little weakens structure. Too much creates strain. The middle path builds without congesting. It asks the patient to eat with observation rather than ideology.

Study the hour after a meal. Heavy sedation suggests excess, poor digestion, poor timing, or the wrong source. Nervous hunger suggests inadequate balance. Calm energy suggests that the meal matched the person. Rotate plant sources to widen amino acid patterns and microbial exposure. Pair protein with vegetables and whole grains. Hydrate enough to support filtration. Move the muscles that will use the amino acids.

Protein should follow work. The more a person lifts, walks, carries, heals, trains, and repairs, the more useful protein becomes. A sedentary body asking for athlete-level protein is not building strength. It is asking the liver and kidneys to manage surplus.

The final teacher is perception. When dietary noise falls, the person can feel the difference between nourishment and weight. The simplest meals begin to satisfy in a way that engineered high-protein products rarely can.

A practical protein audit is simple. For seven days, record the source, portion, timing, preparation, and feeling after each protein-rich meal. Do not record to judge yourself. Record to detect pattern. Does meat at night disturb sleep? Do lentils feel better when soaked and slow-cooked? Does cold protein powder create bloating? Does midday tofu with rice and greens leave the mind clear? The answer is usually already present in the patient's own physiology.

The master rule is proportion with feedback. A meal should build without leaving debris. It should satisfy without sedation. It should strengthen without thirst. It should leave the patient more available for life, not more occupied with digestion.

Conclusion: The Builder's Lesson

Protein is the builder. It renews tissue, repairs injury, preserves muscle, supports immunity, and gives structure to physical life. But the builder must be governed. Without proportion, the same material that restores strength can become excess work for digestion, filtration, and inflammatory regulation.

The solution is respect.

Let protein serve structure. Let plants carry the buffering, cleansing, and microbial intelligence around it. Let timing create space for repair. Let movement create a legitimate need for rebuilding. Let simplicity keep the instruction clear.

When protein returns to its rightful place, it is neither hero nor enemy. It is a faithful builder inside a well-ordered house.

Clinical Case Study 5

Reigniting Digestive Warmth Through Thermal Sim-Bo Nutrition

Patient: Jonathan R., 51-year-old male, architect.

Chief Concerns: Weight gain with visible fluid retention, chronic loose stools, morning lethargy, cold extremities, cold lower abdomen, and a sense that even "clean" food left him heavy rather than nourished.

Clinical Presentation

Jonathan's case revealed a missing dimension of nutrition: food must match digestive capacity.

For three years, he followed a modern clean-eating pattern built almost entirely around iced green smoothies, raw kale salads, refrigerated fruit, cold water, and low-calorie raw meals. The foods looked virtuous on a wellness chart. Inside his physiology, they behaved like cold rain on a weak stove.

He ate modest calories, yet gained weight through fluid retention. He consumed vitamins and greens, yet his morning energy collapsed. He ate clean by modern standards, yet his stools remained loose and unformed. The pattern was thermal mismatch.

In Traditional Asian Medicine, the Spleen and Stomach require warmth to transform food into usable nourishment. Jonathan's constant cold intake weakened the middle burner. Fluids stagnated. Dampness accumulated. Digestion slowed. Energy failed to rise in the morning.

Initial Findings

Blood Pressure: 108/72 mm Hg, with a broader pattern of low drive, coldness, and morning weakness.

Tongue: Pale, swollen, scalloped along the edges, with a slippery white coating.

Pulse: Deep, slow, and weak across multiple positions.

TAM Assessment

Spleen Yang Deficiency with Cold-Dampness: Cold, raw intake weakened transformation and transportation, allowing fluids to stagnate and stools to remain loose.

Kidney Yang Deficiency: Chronic coldness and depletion reached the deeper metabolic reserve, contributing to cold extremities and severe morning lethargy.

Treatment Principles

Remove iced, raw, and thermally cold foods during the therapeutic reset.
Warm the middle burner and rebuild digestive momentum.
Use warm grains, cooked vegetables, and pungent spices to restore internal movement.
Support fluid metabolism and reduce Cold-Damp accumulation.

Plan and Intervention

Thermal Sim-Bo structure: Raw salads, iced smoothies, refrigerated fruit meals, and cold water were removed for twelve weeks.
3 parts grains: Warm congees built from roasted buckwheat, millet, and pearl barley became the anchor, providing gentle density, stable energy, and digestive warmth.
2 parts vegetables: Roasted root vegetables and sauteed greens were prepared with ginger, cardamom, scallion, and black pepper to support warmth, aroma, and digestive activation.
1 part fruit: Fruit was lightly stewed or taken at room temperature rather than iced or refrigerated.
Fluid protocol: Cold drinks were replaced with warm water and ginger-infused tea between meals.
Acupuncture and moxibustion: Moxibustion was applied over CV12 and CV8 to warm the center and support digestive function; ST36, SP6, and BL20 were used to support transformation, fluid metabolism, and vitality.
Emperor's Cupping Therapy®: Warming decompression was applied over the mid-thoracic and lower lumbar Back-Shu regions to reduce myofascial restriction and support circulation through the posterior chain.
Botanical medicine: Li Zhong Wan was used within the TAM framework; prepared Fu Zi was used only in a clinically supervised context to support marked internal cold and Yang deficiency.

Observed Clinical Response

Fluid retention and weight: Body weight decreased by 18 pounds, with visible reduction in edema and abdominal heaviness.
Bowel pattern: Loose, watery stools became formed and more predictable.

Temperature: Cold extremities improved, and peripheral warmth became more consistent.

Tongue presentation: Swelling and scalloping decreased; coating became thinner and less watery.

Morning energy: Lethargy improved, with sharper alertness on waking and less need for stimulants.

Interpretive Note

Jonathan's case clarifies a critical lesson: nutrition is not only ingredient quality. It is temperature, preparation, timing, digestive strength, and internal climate.

Raw food can be medicine in one person and a tax in another. Cold smoothies can feel cleansing to a robust constitution and depleting to a cold, damp, exhausted one. The same food changes meaning when the terrain changes.

His recovery did not come from more restriction. It came from matching nourishment to physiology. Warmth returned. Digestion consolidated. Fluids moved. Energy rose. The meal became usable again.

Jonathan also clarifies why nutrient charts alone are insufficient. His diet was full of plants, low in calories, and outwardly clean. Yet the internal result was heaviness, coldness, fluid, and fatigue. The missing element was not morality. It was transformation.

A meal becomes medicine only when the patient can digest it.

This also explains why protein advice fails when it is separated from temperature and constitution. Jonathan did not need a higher protein target. He needed the capacity to cook the protein internally. Once warmth and timing returned, moderate protein became useful again.

Transition: From Structure to Source

Protein has taught the first law of structural nutrition: a building material becomes medicine only when quantity, timing, source, digestion, and need are aligned.

Source is the final test. Amino acids can arrive wrapped in fiber, water, minerals, and microbial food. They can also arrive concentrated, industrialized, oxidized, and stripped of the plant matrix that once buffered their force.

The story now narrows from protein itself to the modern mythology of animal protein: the food most often equated with strength, status, and recovery, yet also the form most capable of becoming metabolic strain when misunderstood.

Chapter 6

The Truth About Animal Protein

The Great Divide

Few subjects in nutrition create more heat than animal protein. Meat is treated as strength. Dairy is treated as growth. Eggs are treated as completeness. Across much of human history, animal-derived food carried the prestige of rarity. It appeared after a successful hunt, during seasonal abundance, at ceremonial tables, or in periods of recovery when dense nourishment was genuinely needed.

Industrial abundance changed the meaning of that food. What once functioned as an occasional restorative became a daily default. Scarcity gave animal protein prestige; repetition gave it consequences. The same food that can rebuild depleted tissue when used carefully can strain metabolism when it becomes the center of every meal.

The truth about animal protein is not a moral drama. It is a question of density, dose, matrix, preparation, frequency, and terrain. Animal protein is a concentrated biological instrument. In the right context, it supplies repair. In chronic excess, it adds load: nitrogen waste, acid residue, heme iron, saturated fat context, microbial metabolites, and growth signals that must be processed by the liver, kidneys, vessels, gut, and immune system.

The Sim-Bo position is therefore neither worship nor fear. It is proportion. Plant foods form the daily architecture. Animal foods, when used, belong in small, deliberate amounts, chosen with care and prepared with restraint. The body does not reward dietary ideology. It responds to the chemistry of what arrives, how often it arrives, and whether the internal terrain has room to handle it.

How Protein Arrives

At the level of amino acids, animal and plant proteins share a basic biochemical language. Digestion eventually reduces them into smaller peptides and amino acids that can be absorbed and used for tissue repair, enzymes, immune proteins, transport molecules, hormones, and structural maintenance. But food never enters physiology as amino acids alone. It enters as a package.

Animal protein arrives inside a dense matrix. With red meat, that matrix often includes heme iron, saturated fat, cholesterol, collagen, purines, carnitine, choline, and compounds formed through cooking. With dairy, it brings casein, whey, calcium, lactose in some forms, growth-associated signaling, and a hormonal imprint shaped by the biology of mammalian milk. With eggs, it brings choline-rich yolk, sulfur-containing amino acids, cholesterol, fat-soluble nutrients, and remarkable density in a small volume.

Density is not a flaw by itself. Density is power. But power must be timed and measured. A depleted patient, an undernourished elder, an athlete in repair, or a person recovering from severe tissue loss may temporarily need more concentrated building material. The same concentrated material, eaten daily in large portions by a sedentary, inflamed, sleep-deprived adult, can become another demand placed on already overworked systems.

Plant protein arrives differently. Whole legumes, grains, seeds, nuts, mushrooms, and fermented soy bring amino acids inside a broader field of fiber, water, minerals, resistant starch, polyphenols, and microbial substrate. Their amino acids are delivered more slowly, with less sudden nitrogen pressure and more support for bowel regularity and microbial metabolism. The difference is not simply animal versus plant. The difference is environment. Protein behaves according to the company it keeps.

Heme Iron, Fat Context, and Oxidative Pressure

Animal foods contain nutrients of real value. Heme iron is efficiently absorbed. B12 is concentrated in animal sources. Certain forms of zinc, selenium, creatine, carnosine, taurine, and fat-soluble nutrients can be clinically useful. The problem begins when useful density becomes chronic overload.

Heme iron illustrates this principle. In deficiency, it can restore oxygen-carrying capacity and strength. In excess, especially inside a diet already high in oxidative stress and low in antioxidants, it can act as a pro-oxidant. The same mineral that supports hemoglobin can participate in reactions that irritate lipids, vessels, and tissue if the system has no counterbalancing plant matrix.

Industrial animal foods also carry a fat context. The issue is not merely saturated fat in isolation, but the larger pattern in which dense animal foods are consumed: low fiber, refined starch, high heat cooking, processed sauces, alcohol, late meals, sedentary life, and poor sleep. In that environment, animal protein becomes part of a heavier metabolic architecture. The vessel lining, liver, gallbladder, gut microbiome, and immune system all participate in the consequence.

A small portion of gently prepared fish or pasture-raised egg inside a plant-rich meal is not equivalent to a large grilled steak eaten late at night with refined starch, alcohol, and no vegetables. Nutrition is not a courtroom where foods are declared innocent or guilty. It is a living chemistry in which dose, company, timing, and preparation determine meaning.

Growth Commands: IGF-1 and mTOR

Protein does more than build tissue. It gives growth instructions.

Amino acids, insulin, energy availability, exercise, and growth factors all influence the mTOR pathway, a central regulator of protein synthesis, cellular growth, repair, and autophagy. IGF-1 participates in growth, tissue development, and repair. In childhood, injury recovery, frailty, or severe depletion, these signals can be necessary and protective. Growth must be timed. Constant growth signaling is the concern.

Mature physiology must alternate between building and cleaning. The organism needs phases of construction and phases of maintenance. Animal protein, especially when consumed in large daily amounts, tends to speak loudly in the language of building. That command can be useful after strain or tissue loss. It becomes costly when the internal environment is already overstimulated, inflamed, and deprived of rest.

Constant abundance blurs the ancient alternation between feast and repair. The system is told to build while it still needs to clean. Autophagy, mitochondrial renewal, immune calibration, and digestive rest all require quieter periods. A life of continuous dense protein intake keeps the signal tilted toward construction. The Sim-Bo method restores the missing half of the cycle: simplicity, plant dominance, digestive rest, and enough quiet for repair to resume.

Plant proteins tend to deliver building blocks with a gentler command. They still nourish structure. They still provide amino acids. But in whole-food form they arrive with fiber, minerals, water, and phytonutrients that slow the meal, feed the microbiome, and reduce the sharpness of the growth message. This is why plant-dominant patterns can support long-term maintenance without forcing a constant state of metabolic acceleration.

Acid Load and Mineral Balance

Animal protein also carries an acid load. This is not a slogan about making the blood alkaline. Blood pH remains tightly defended. The question is the work required to defend it.

Sulfur-containing amino acids such as methionine and cysteine produce acid residues during metabolism. The kidneys must excrete that acid load while maintaining mineral and electrolyte balance. In a young, resilient system with strong renal reserve and abundant plant minerals, this work is usually handled quietly. Under chronic excess, sedentary living, dehydration, high sodium intake, low vegetable intake, and metabolic syndrome, the demand becomes heavier.

Plant-dominant meals change the equation. Potassium, magnesium, fiber, and organic acids from vegetables and fruits help support mineral balance and reduce the net acid load placed on renal handling. The point is not to chase alkaline myths. The point is to stop asking the kidneys to manage dense protein, low hydration, high salt, refined starch, and minimal plants at the same time.

The Sim-Bo plate is protective because its architecture is naturally buffered: grains for steady energy, vegetables for minerals and fiber, fruit for water and phytochemical intelligence, and protein held in deliberate proportion. The kidneys do not need heroic detoxification rituals. They need sane inputs, hydration, mineral support, and long periods without excess.

Heat, Cooking, and Inflammatory Residue

Preparation changes protein. High heat gives flavor, aroma, browning, and cultural satisfaction, but it also creates chemical residues. Grilling, charring, frying, and repeated high-temperature cooking can generate advanced glycation end products, heterocyclic amines, polycyclic aromatic hydrocarbons, oxidized lipids, and other compounds that add strain to the immune and detoxification systems.

The same meat prepared in different ways can have different physiological impact. A small portion slowly stewed with vegetables and broth is not the same as a charred portion seared at high heat and eaten with refined carbohydrates. One is softened by water, time, and plant minerals. The other concentrates heat stress and oxidative residue.

Traditional cuisines understood this without laboratory language. Meat was often sliced thin, simmered, stretched through broth, paired with greens, fermented vegetables, rice, herbs, seaweed, bitter plants, or mineral-rich soups. The preparation itself reduced the impact. Modern industrial eating removed the restraint. It enlarged the portion, intensified the heat, added refined starch and alcohol, and turned a rare ingredient into daily bulk.

Cooking is part of medicine. Gentle heat, moisture, smaller portions, and abundant plant pairing transform the metabolic meaning of animal food. Heavy heat and heavy quantity turn density into irritation.

The Gut Connection: TMA, TMAO, and Endotoxin

The gut decides much of the final story.

Carnitine and choline from red meat and eggs can be metabolized by certain gut microbes into trimethylamine, or TMA. The liver converts TMA into TMAO. This compound has become a major focus in cardiovascular and metabolic research because it connects animal-food patterns, microbial ecology, liver metabolism, and vascular risk.

The practical lesson is clear: the same food produces different downstream chemistry depending on the microbiome that receives it. A fiber-rich gut with diverse microbial partners behaves differently from a dysbiotic gut shaped by low fiber, antibiotics, alcohol, processed food, and chronic stress. Animal protein inside a resilient microbial ecosystem is handled differently than animal protein dropped into a stagnant intestinal terrain.

Plant proteins bring their own microbial instruction. Beans, lentils, grains, seeds, and vegetables deliver fermentable fibers that support short-chain fatty acid production, including butyrate. These metabolites help maintain the intestinal barrier, regulate immune tone, and support metabolic communication between gut, liver, brain, and immune system. The microbes do not simply digest food. They interpret it.

This is one of the deepest reasons Sim-Bo favors plant dominance. It is not only about amino acids. It is about the microbial civilization that daily food builds. A plant-centered pattern cultivates partners. A meat-heavy, low-fiber pattern cultivates residue.

Ecological Efficiency and the Return to the Human System

Human nutrition cannot be separated from ecology. This is not moral performance. It is biological continuity.

Industrial animal protein requires large inputs of feed, water, land, transportation, refrigeration, antibiotics in many production systems, waste management, and energy. Those inputs do not disappear. They return through soil depletion, polluted water, air quality, environmental residues, microplastics, stress chemistry in the food chain, and the cumulative load of industrial production. The human organism does not live outside the planet that feeds it.

Plant-dominant eating is efficient because it shortens the chain. When amino acids come through grains, beans, lentils, tofu, vegetables, nuts, and seeds, the energy path is simpler. The meal carries less ecological drag and often less metabolic residue. The same principle governs both soil and tissue: fewer unnecessary conversions, less waste, more direct nourishment.

Choosing plants most of the time is therefore not deprivation. It is alignment. It respects the internal terrain and the external field that sustains it.

Liver, Kidneys, and the Cost of Excess

The liver and kidneys bear the silent cost of chronic excess.

Amino acids cannot be stored in the way glycogen and fat can. When intake exceeds immediate structural need, the nitrogen group must be removed. The liver converts ammonia into urea, and the kidneys excrete it. This is normal physiology. Under occasional demand, the system handles it. Under daily excess, the work becomes a tax.

The high-protein modern pattern often arrives with other pressures: dehydration, caffeine, alcohol, late-night eating, high sodium, low vegetables, poor sleep, stress hormones, and sedentary circulation. In that total environment, nitrogen clearance becomes only one part of a larger filtration challenge. Dark urine, persistent thirst, morning puffiness, heavy fatigue after meals, lower-back heaviness, and recurrent joint irritation are not random inconveniences. They are early language from a system doing too much cleanup.

The answer is not panic. The answer is rotation and rest. Protein-heavy days must be balanced by plant-dominant days. Dense meals must be followed by lighter meals. The kidneys and liver require hydration, minerals, fiber, movement, sleep, and time away from constant dense intake. Like fertile soil, metabolism recovers when it is not planted with the same demanding crop every day.

This is why Sim-Bo places brown rice, vegetables, fruits, legumes, tofu, mushrooms, seaweeds, broths, and simple hydration at the center of recovery. These foods do not shout. They clear. They move. They mineralize. They feed the microbiome. They give the filtration organs less to argue with.

Moderation and Adaptation

Humans are adaptive omnivores. That statement carries both freedom and responsibility.

An adaptive organism can use different foods under different conditions. It can survive scarcity, endure seasonal change, and rebuild after physical stress. But survival capacity is not the same as daily ideal. The fact that human beings can digest animal protein does not make it the rightful center of every plate.

Ancestral eating patterns were shaped by effort, weather, geography, and availability. Dense animal food was often intermittent. Plants, roots, grains, greens, sea vegetables, legumes, fruits, herbs, and fermented foods carried the daily cadence. Modern abundance inverted that relationship. Animal foods became inexpensive, constant, oversized, and detached from the effort once required to obtain them.

Restoring proportion is the clinical task. A protective baseline is simple: let plant foods dominate most meals, and let animal protein, if used, appear with restraint. Two plant-centered meals for every meal that contains animal food is a practical starting point for many patients. For some, a longer plant-dominant reset may be necessary. For others, carefully chosen animal food may remain occasional, intentional, and clinically useful.

Quality matters. Regeneratively raised, grass-finished meat; low-mercury wild fish; truly pastured eggs; and traditional fermented dairy are not the same as industrial meat, processed cheese, and factory-farmed bulk protein. Preparation matters as much as source. Gentle cooking, broth, steaming, poaching, and stewing reduce stress on the meal. The portion must serve the plate, not dominate it.

The Sim-Bo Standard

The Sim-Bo philosophy turns this science into daily practice.

Simple and Boring does not mean joyless. It means legible. It means the digestive system knows what is coming. It means the liver and kidneys can predict the workload. It means the microbiome receives fiber with consistency. It means appetite is no longer manipulated by spectacle.

For patients moving away from meat-heavy eating, the first step is portion reduction, not identity warfare. Cut the animal portion in half. Replace the missing volume with mushrooms, lentils, adzuki beans, fermented tofu, seaweed, greens, or mineral-rich vegetable broth. Keep the meal warm. Keep it slow. Keep it plain enough that the aftermath can be felt clearly.

Within weeks, many patients report lighter digestion, steadier energy, clearer morning appetite, fewer cravings, improved stool regularity, and less post-meal heaviness. The effect does not come from a single special food. It comes from reduced friction. The system stops spending so much energy on dense protein clearance and begins allocating energy toward repair, sleep, circulation, mood, and clarity.

This is the central intelligence of Sim-Bo: remove the dramatic inputs, and the quiet systems begin speaking again.

Culture, Reverence, and Purpose-Driven Vitality

Food is memory. Meat at a family table may signify love, sacrifice, wealth, celebration, survival, ancestry, or hospitality. A clinical recommendation that ignores this emotional architecture will fail, even if the physiology is correct.

Healing therefore requires respect without surrendering precision. Familiar foods can remain meaningful without remaining daily. A high-quality animal meal can mark gratitude, ceremony, recovery, or connection. It loses its sacredness when it becomes automatic bulk.

Reverence changes eating. When a food is rare, chosen carefully, prepared slowly, and eaten with gratitude, the nervous system receives the meal differently. Breath slows. Chewing improves. Attention returns. The parasympathetic state supports digestion, bile flow, enzyme secretion, and satiety. Celebration can nourish when it is deliberate. Rushed excess cannot.

The purpose of dietary discipline is not to become pure. It is to become available for life. We moderate density so that energy can serve work, family, patients, leadership, study, faith, art, and demanding service. Food is not the destination. It is the architecture that allows purpose to move through the body with less resistance.

The Middle Way

The modern argument between carnivore certainty and vegan certainty misses the deeper lesson. The human system thrives on proportion and suffers in extremity.

Animal protein teaches respect for power. Plant foods teach respect for rhythm. The mature plate contains humility: enough structure to repair, enough fiber to clear, enough mineral density to buffer, enough water to move, enough restraint to allow the organs to rest.

The signs of excess are often quiet: heavy fatigue after meals, thirst that does not resolve, morning stiffness, darker urine, sluggish bowels, irritability, joint heat, skin congestion, or a dull pressure in the low back and legs. These are not moral failures. They are messages. The remedy is usually simple before it becomes complicated: lighten the protein load, increase plant volume, hydrate intelligently, walk after meals, and restore timing.

Balance the plate, and the physiology often follows. The body does not need constant dietary luxury. It needs consistent respect.

Conclusion: Returning to the Original Blueprint

Animal protein is a powerful instrument in functional nutrition. Used with precision, it can rebuild. Used as daily bulk, it adds residue. The difference lies in relationship: portion, frequency, source, preparation, season, constitution, and recovery time.

The original human blueprint was not built around constant density. It was built around cycles: effort and rest, scarcity and nourishment, building and cleaning, celebration and simplicity. Industrial abundance distorted those cycles by making the rare constant and the dense ordinary.

To live with less need for rescue, we must restore proportion. Dense foods must be handled with discipline. Plant foods must become the daily foundation. Filtration organs must be given rest. The gut must be fed fiber. The immune system must hear fewer signals of irritation. The meal must become legible again.

When the relationship with animal protein becomes precise, the old debate loses its power. The question is no longer whether meat is good or bad. The question is whether today's meal supports repair, clarity, movement, sleep, and purpose—or whether it adds another layer of work to a system already doing too much.

Clinical Case Study 6

Restoring Lower Burner Clarity in Gout and Renal Strain

Patient: Richard B., 45-year-old male, corporate litigator.

Chief concerns: Recurrent gout flares, chronic joint stiffness, dark and scanty urine, lower-leg edema, heavy post-meal fatigue, and reliance on pain-relieving medication during acute episodes. Medication status remained under the supervision of the appropriate prescribing clinician.

Clinical Presentation

Richard lived on a high-pressure executive schedule and a diet built around steakhouse dinners, aged cheeses, processed meats, alcohol, late meals, and long hours of sitting. He viewed animal protein as strength and restraint as weakness. His meals were dense, acidic, salty, and fiber-poor. His body answered with gout.

The pattern was unmistakable. Dense animal protein increased purine and nitrogen demand. Late eating and alcohol strained liver rhythm. Low hydration concentrated urine. Sedentary work weakened lymphatic movement. Stress narrowed recovery. The lower body became the storage site for the unresolved chemistry of excess: heat, swelling, stiffness, edema, and recurrent acute pain.

Initial Findings

Blood pressure: 142/90 mm Hg, consistent with elevated cardiovascular and renal strain in the clinical picture.

Tongue: red with a thick, sticky, dark yellow coating at the root, reflecting Damp-Heat accumulation in the Lower Burner pattern.

Pulse: rapid, slippery, and full at the proximal positions.

Primary TAM pattern: Damp-Heat sinking into the Lower Burner, complicated by food excess, stress constraint, poor fluid transformation, and joint obstruction.

Treatment Principles

Reduce the animal-protein load and remove industrial meat and aged dairy from the daily pattern.

Support urinary flow and fluid transformation through plant-dominant Sim-Bo meals.

Use mineral-rich vegetables, adzuki beans, barley, hydration, and fiber to reduce acid load and support clearance.

Release lumbar and lower-body myofascial restriction to support circulation, comfort, and drainage.

Calm inflammatory recurrence while rebuilding a sustainable dietary structure.

Plan and Intervention

Richard committed to a twelve-week plant-dominant Sim-Bo protocol. The treatment did not frame meat as a forbidden identity. It removed the daily excess that kept his system under strain.

Sim-Bo dietary prescription: Pearl barley, brown rice, and adzuki beans formed the grain foundation. Steamed greens, bitter vegetables, celery, cucumber, daikon, seaweed, and mineral-rich broths supplied fiber, potassium, magnesium, and fluid support. Sprouted lentils and fermented organic tofu replaced daily meat as the primary protein sources.

Animal-food reset: Industrial meat, processed meats, aged cheese, and late-night steakhouse meals were removed during the therapeutic phase. Alcohol was suspended. Meal timing shifted earlier to protect sleep and reduce nocturnal digestive load.

Acupuncture: SP9 and KI3 supported fluid transformation and Kidney-Spleen coordination; ST36 supported digestive resilience; LR3 supported constraint release; local points were selected as needed for joint pain and lower-leg stagnation.

Emperor's Cupping Therapy®: Stationary and sliding cupping were applied along the lower back, sacral region, and posterior chain to reduce myofascial restriction, support local circulation, and ease the tissue tension associated with lower-body congestion.

Botanical medicine: Si Miao San was used within the TAM framework to clear Damp-Heat, support joint comfort, and promote more regular urinary flow. The prescription was individualized and monitored clinically.

Follow-Up Clinical Response

Gout flares: Acute flares decreased during the follow-up period, with no major flare reported in the final month of care.

Joint stiffness: Morning stiffness became milder and shorter in duration by patient report.

Urine pattern: Urine became clearer and more regular as hydration, plant intake, and meal timing improved.

Lower-leg edema: Swelling visibly decreased, especially in the morning.
Post-meal energy: Heavy fatigue after protein-rich meals was replaced by steadier afternoon energy.
Blood pressure: Readings improved during follow-up, with medication decisions remaining under the appropriate prescribing clinician.
Tongue and pulse: The root coating thinned, redness softened, and pulse quality became less slippery and full within TAM observation.

Clinical Takeaway

Richard's case demonstrates the core lesson of this chapter: protein builds structure, but chronic density creates residue. His problem was not a single steak, a single cheese plate, or a single celebration. It was repetition without recovery. His filtration organs, joints, gut, and vessels had been asked to process the same heavy message day after day.

The plant-dominant Sim-Bo reset changed the message. Fiber returned. Hydration improved. Meal timing steadied. Dense animal foods stopped dominating the plate. Acupuncture, cupping, and botanical medicine supported circulation, fluid transformation, and inflammatory settling. As the daily load decreased, the lower-body heat and swelling began to release.

The lesson is simple: when the river is stagnant, the answer is not more density. The answer is flow.

Transition: From Structure to Energy

Protein builds structure. Fat and carbohydrate move the structure through life.

A house can be carefully built and still remain cold, dark, and silent without energy. The same is true of physiology. Amino acids provide scaffolding, enzymes, transporters, and repair material, but motion, thought, warmth, mood, and cellular work require fuel. That fuel comes primarily through fat and carbohydrate.

For most of human history, energy entered slowly. Fats were bound inside whole foods. Sugars were held inside fruit, roots, grains, and fiber. The metabolic flame burned with steadiness because the fuel was naturally paced. Modern industry changed the fuel before it reached the mouth: oils were refined, seeds were extracted under heat and pressure, grains were stripped, sugars were concentrated, and texture was engineered to bypass satiety.

The next threshold is energy itself. Structure has been clarified. Now the question becomes combustion: whether fat and sugar burn cleanly into vitality or leave oxidative smoke behind. From the truth about animal protein, we turn toward the volatile chemistry of fuel.

Chapter 7

Fat, Sugar, and the Inflammatory Cycle

The Dual Nature of Energy

Energy is one of life's great gifts. It is also one of its great hazards.

Every cell depends on ATP to think, contract, detoxify, repair, and survive. Yet energy production is never free. Whenever nutrients are converted into usable power, metabolism leaves a residue: oxidized lipids, excess glucose, reactive oxygen species, and inflammatory debris that must be cleared before they begin to injure tissue.

Fat and carbohydrate are the two primary fuels of human metabolism. In a well-regulated system, they work with elegant separation. Glucose provides rapid power when movement, cognition, or stress demands immediate output. Fat provides slower endurance during rest, fasting, sleep, and sustained work. Health depends on the ability to shift between them without distress.

Modern life has disturbed that partnership. Constant snacking, hidden sugars, fried industrial oils, late-night eating, and sedentary routines keep the bloodstream crowded with fuel that is not being used. The result is metabolic congestion: glucose rises, insulin stays elevated, fat oxidation weakens, mitochondria strain, and inflammatory chemistry gathers in the background long before a formal diagnosis appears.

This is why energy management sits at the center of chronic disease. A patient may eat enough calories and still feel starved for usable power. Another may restrict calories and still remain metabolically congested. The deciding factor is not intake alone; it is whether fuel enters at the right speed, meets real physical demand, and leaves behind waste the system can clear.

Fat and sugar become inflammatory when they lose timing. Sugar becomes destructive when it arrives too quickly and too often. Fat becomes problematic when it is oxidized, overheated, or trapped in tissues that are not using it. The clinical question is not which fuel is evil. The question is whether the organism still knows when to burn each one.

To understand the inflammatory cycle, we must understand how these two fuels become either clean energy or biochemical smoke.

Ancient Appetite and Engineered Craving

In the ancestral world, concentrated sweetness and rich fat were rare. Wild honey appeared briefly. Ripe fruit followed seasons. Dense animal fat, nuts, seeds, and other energy-rich foods required effort to find, gather, hunt, or protect. The nervous system learned to value these foods because they meant endurance through scarcity, warmth through cold, fertility, and survival.

Dopamine rewarded the discovery of dense energy. It taught the organism to remember sweetness and fat with intensity. That ancient reward system was not a flaw. It was a survival map.

The modern food environment broke the map. A supermarket aisle now offers more concentrated sweetness and fat than an ancestral village might have seen in weeks. Scarcity vanished, but the old circuitry remained. The nervous system still celebrates sweet and fatty foods as rare survival treasure, even when they are available every hour of the day.

The modern food industry understands this circuitry with precision. It does not merely sell food; it sells anticipation. The sound of a package opening, the color of a label, the smell of fried starch, and the cold sweetness of a drink all become cues before digestion has even begun. Appetite is triggered upstream of hunger.

Leptin, CCK, GLP-1, PYY, gastric stretch, and vagal feedback all participate in the conversation of satiety. Hyper-palatable food overwhelms the tempo of that conversation. It arrives fast, asks little chewing, and rewards the brain before the gut has time to speak. The result is not appetite freedom. It is appetite captivity.

Hyper-palatable foods exploit the mismatch between ancient appetite and industrial abundance. They combine refined sugar, processed starch, industrial fat, salt, and engineered flavor in ratios that outrun ordinary satiety. Pleasure arrives faster than regulation. Hunger becomes less a physical need than a neurochemical echo, a learned demand for stimulation.

The inflammatory cycle often begins here: not with a failure of willpower, but with ancient appetite trapped inside industrial abundance.

Sugar: Swift Fuel and Glycation

Glucose is a rapid fuel. The brain, red blood cells, and working muscle depend on it. In its intact form - whole fruit, unrefined grains, legumes, and root vegetables - carbohydrate arrives with fiber, water, minerals, resistant starch, polyphenols, and digestive pacing. The matrix slows absorption and gives metabolism time to respond.

Refined sugar behaves differently. A sweetened beverage or pastry can deliver glucose quickly, without the structural brakes that normally guide absorption. Blood sugar rises. Insulin responds. Energy may surge briefly, then fall. That fall is perceived by the nervous system as instability. The result is fatigue, irritability, cravings, and another search for fast fuel.

Liquid sugar is especially disruptive because it bypasses the natural labor of eating. There is little chewing, little fiber, little volume, and little delay. It delivers energy as speed rather than nourishment. The liver receives the load without the gradual pacing that whole food normally provides.

Repeated often enough, the pattern teaches metabolism to live in swings rather than steady waves. Insulin remains busy. Muscle cells become less responsive. The liver is asked to process excess. The pancreas works harder to maintain order. Over time, glucose regulation becomes less flexible.

Excess circulating sugar also reacts with proteins and lipids through glycation, forming advanced glycation end-products, or AGEs. These compounds stiffen collagen, burden arterial elasticity, irritate nerves, and contribute to the slow hardening of tissue that many people mistake for ordinary aging. Sugar's damage is not only caloric. It is structural.

Glycation also teaches an important lesson about time. Damage does not need drama to become serious. A small daily excess, repeated across years, can stiffen tissue more powerfully than a single obvious injury. The inflammatory cycle is built less by catastrophe than by repetition.

The tongue experiences sweetness for seconds. The vascular wall may remember it for decades.

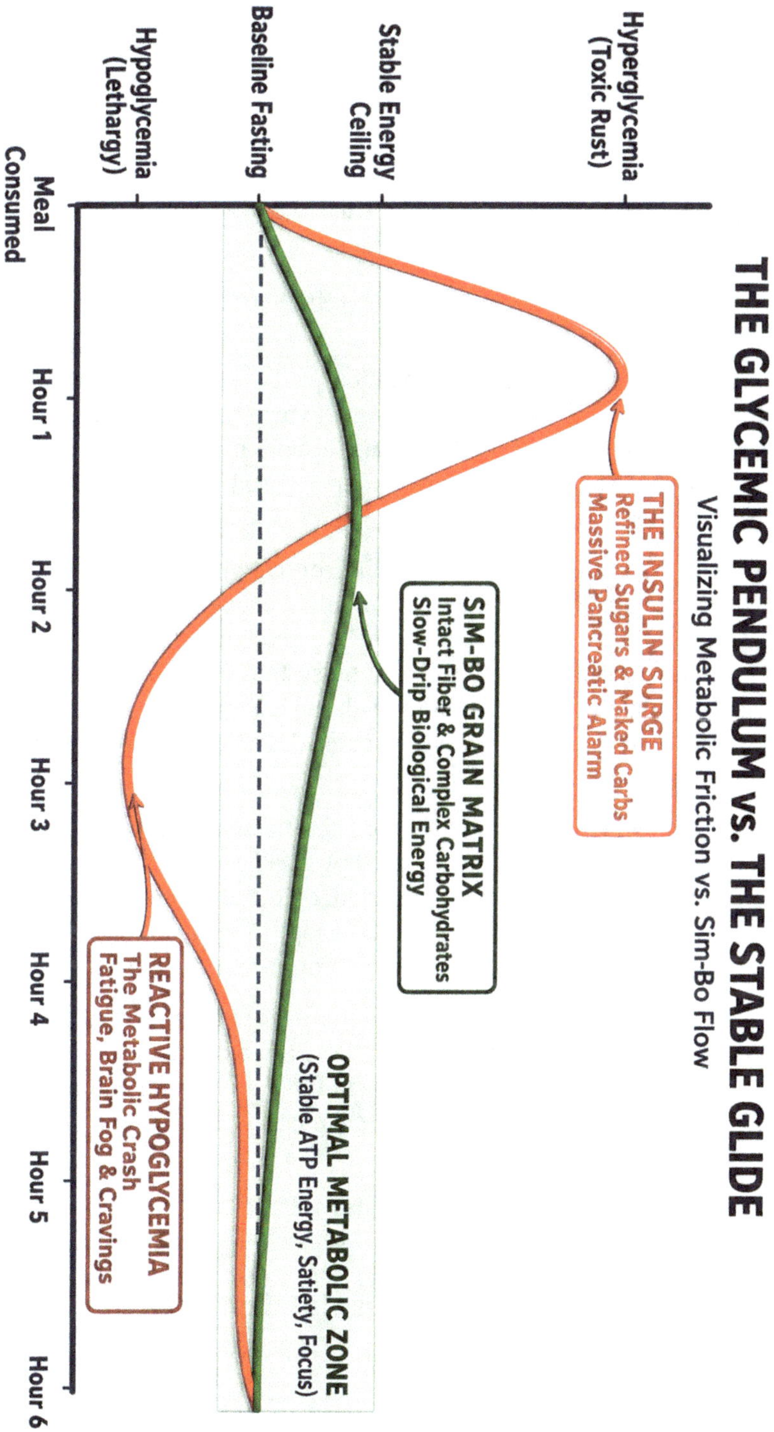

Figure 2. The glycemic pendulum vs. the steady glide.

Fat: Endurance Fuel and the Lipid Paradox

Fat is concentrated endurance. It carries more energy per gram than carbohydrate and supports membranes, bile flow, hormone production, neurological tissue, and long-burning fuel availability. A healthy metabolism can use fat quietly and efficiently, especially between meals, during low-intensity movement, overnight, and in periods of digestive rest.

The crisis is not fat itself. The crisis is quality, processing, timing, and metabolic setting.

Whole-food fats - olives, avocados, nuts, seeds, and traditional minimally processed oils - arrive with texture, minerals, polyphenols, and satiety. They help slow the meal, support membrane fluidity, and contribute to a steadier energetic cadence. Used in proper proportion, they bring calm to the plate.

Refined industrial oils behave differently when extracted, stored, repeatedly heated, and embedded in ultra-processed foods. Oxidized lipids can damage membranes, intensify oxidative stress, and create inflammatory residues that the immune system must handle. The issue is not one isolated fatty acid standing alone; it is the industrial context in which unstable fats are produced, cooked, consumed, and combined with refined starch and sugar.

Bile flow, gallbladder function, pancreatic secretion, and microbial tolerance all shape how fat is handled. A small amount of intact fat can stabilize a meal. A large amount of fried, oxidized fat eaten late at night can overload digestion and disturb sleep. The same macronutrient carries a different instruction depending on preparation and setting.

Traditional food cultures respected this distinction intuitively. Fat was used to carry flavor, warmth, and satiety, not to saturate every bite of every meal. Modern processing changed fat from a slow companion into an invisible excess hidden inside chips, pastries, sauces, dressings, and restaurant oils.

Fat can warm the house. It can also fill the room with smoke. The difference is not ideology. It is source, preparation, dose, and timing.

The Partnership of Fuels: Metabolic Flexibility

Metabolic flexibility is the ability to shift between glucose and fat without distress. After a meal, glucose can be used and stored appropriately. Between meals, fat oxidation resumes. During activity, muscle draws fuel. During sleep, repair and stored energy use quietly continue.

This partnership is partly governed by the competition between glucose and fatty-acid oxidation, often described through the Randle cycle. When both fuels arrive in constant excess - especially refined carbohydrate paired with processed fat - mitochondria receive more substrate than the moment requires. Insulin remains elevated, fat release slows, and the system drifts toward glucose dependence while stored fuel accumulates.

A flexible metabolism is quiet. It does not panic when a meal is delayed. It does not crash after lunch. It can move from fed to fasting, from rest to activity, from glucose to stored fuel, without forcing the mind into irritability or the hands into another snack.

Muscle is central to this flexibility. It is not merely tissue for appearance or athletic performance. Muscle is a metabolic sink, a glucose reservoir, an endocrine organ, and one of the strongest protectors against the collision between sugar and fat. Without muscular demand, fuel has nowhere useful to go.

The metabolic problem is not eating carbohydrate. It is eating refined carbohydrate too often, with too little fiber, too little movement, too much processed fat, and too little space between meals. The problem is not eating fat. It is consuming oxidized or industrially processed fat in a system already overloaded with glucose, stress chemistry, and inactivity.

When fat oxidation sits idle, ectopic lipid can accumulate in the liver and skeletal muscle. That accumulation interferes with insulin response and reduces metabolic flexibility. Sugar raises the insulin demand; elevated insulin restrains fat mobilization; unburned fat contributes to insulin resistance; insulin resistance intensifies inflammation. The loop is elegant in design and destructive in excess.

The Future of Metabolic Medicine

The future of metabolic medicine will not be satisfied with glucose numbers alone. It will look deeper: mitochondrial efficiency, ectopic fat, muscle glucose uptake, lipid oxidation, meal timing, sleep architecture, and the inflammatory terrain surrounding insulin response.

The old model treated metabolism as a number problem: lower glucose, lower weight, lower cholesterol. The deeper model treats metabolism as a flow problem: where does fuel enter, where does it go, how long does it remain, and what residue does it leave behind?

In that model, the plate, the walk, the sleep cycle, the stress response, and the mitochondria belong to one system. A glucose reading is no longer an isolated score. It is a shadow cast by timing, tissue demand, liver regulation, sleep depth, and inflammatory tone.

Medication will remain necessary for many patients, especially when blood sugar, vascular risk, or organ stress requires immediate control. But the next clinical frontier will be the restoration of fuel flexibility: teaching metabolism to burn what it stores, use what it absorbs, and rest when no fuel is needed.

True metabolic repair will not be measured only by a lower number on a lab report. It will be felt as steady appetite, clear cognition, warmer circulation, deeper sleep, easier movement, and the quiet return of energy that no stimulant can manufacture.

The Oxidative Storm

Every molecule of glucose or fat used for energy must pass through mitochondrial pathways. When fuel supply matches demand, electrons move cleanly through the respiratory chain and ATP production proceeds with relative order. When fuel floods the system while physical demand remains low, the engine backs up.

Escaping electrons react with oxygen and form reactive oxygen species. In small amounts, these molecules help adaptation. They tell the cell that work has occurred and repair should begin. In chronic excess, they injure mitochondrial DNA, oxidize lipids, damage proteins, and trigger inflammatory pathways.

Oxidative stress is not automatically pathological. Life uses small oxidative pulses to strengthen adaptation. Exercise creates oxidative signals, then stimulates antioxidant defense. Fasting creates metabolic pressure, then activates cleanup. The poison is not stress itself; the poison is stress without recovery.

This distinction matters clinically. Patients often try to solve oxidative stress by swallowing more antioxidants while continuing to overload the system with excess fuel, poor sleep, alcohol, refined oils, and emotional urgency. Supplemental defense cannot compensate for a daily pattern that keeps generating smoke.

Whole foods bring built-in protection: polyphenols, vitamin C, carotenoids, minerals, fiber, and microbial metabolites that help buffer oxidation. Ultra-processed diets deliver energy with far less defense. The result is not merely weight gain. It is oxidative debt.

The immune system interprets unresolved oxidative damage as

danger. Cytokines rise. White blood cells mobilize. Repair chemistry becomes defense chemistry. The fuel that should have sustained life becomes another source of alarm.

The Emotional Chemistry of Craving

Craving is not a moral defect. It is chemistry asking for stability.

When blood sugar drops quickly after a refined-carbohydrate surge, the nervous system reads the fall as threat. The HPA axis activates. Cortisol rises. Adrenaline sharpens urgency. The organism seeks fast, dense fuel because the ancient brain still believes that sudden energy loss means danger.

In a world of wild fruit and seasonal honey, that signal had logic. In a world of vending machines, sweetened coffee drinks, and packaged snacks, the same signal becomes a loop. Relief arrives quickly, then fades. Another drop follows. The nervous system learns that sugar is not only food; it is a temporary feeling of control.

Cravings also carry memory. A person may reach for sugar at 3 p.m. not because the tissue needs sucrose, but because the nervous system remembers that sweetness once softened pressure. Food becomes emotional punctuation: a pause, a reward, a substitute for breath, a momentary boundary in an overstimulated day.

Chronic stress, poor sleep, emotional depletion, and lack of purpose intensify the loop. Many people are not addicted to sweetness alone. They are attached to the short-lived autonomic comfort sweetness provides.

The Sim-Bo answer is not humiliation. It is replacement of chaos with predictability. When breakfast, lunch, movement, hydration, and sleep become steady, the craving loses its stage. The nervous system stops negotiating with emergency chemistry.

Breaking the cycle requires more than restriction. It requires stable meals, adequate fiber, calm eating, purposeful work, emotional steadiness, sleep, and a life that no longer demands sugar as medication for the nervous system.

Restoring Fuel Flexibility

Fuel flexibility returns through cadence, not force.

- Eat at consistent times so insulin rises and falls in predictable waves.
- Create clean space between meals so fat oxidation can return to the metabolic stage.
- Walk after meals when clinically appropriate; contracting muscle

can move glucose into tissue through pathways that reduce the demand on insulin.

Protect deep sleep so overnight fuel use, hormonal recovery, and neurological repair can proceed.

Build each plate with intact grains, vegetables, modest fat, adequate protein, and hydration rather than isolated stimulation.

The first goal is not dietary perfection. The first goal is timing the organism can trust. A regular meal pattern trains insulin, bile, pancreatic enzymes, hunger hormones, and microbial fermentation to expect a consistent workload. Predictability lowers the need for emergency compensation.

The second goal is clean contrast: eating and not eating, movement and rest, daylight and darkness. Constant grazing erases contrast. Late screens erase contrast. Sedentary work erases contrast. Sim-Bo restores the edges that metabolism needs in order to know what state it is in.

Under these conditions, appetite becomes more honest. Morning energy does not depend as heavily on stimulants. Afternoon fatigue softens. Cravings lose urgency. The metabolic flame steadies because the system is no longer forced to process conflicting instructions all day.

The Anti-Inflammatory Plate

A restorative plate is not assembled through obsession. It is built through structure.

A base of unrefined grains, such as brown rice, millet, or quinoa, provides a slower glucose curve and a dependable energetic foundation.

A generous volume of vegetables supplies fiber, minerals, antioxidants, bitterness, texture, and microbial fuel.

A precise portion of whole-food fat, such as avocado, olives, nuts, seeds, or cold-pressed traditional oil, slows the meal and supports membrane stability.

Clean, digestible plant-centered protein, such as sprouted lentils, fermented tofu, tempeh, or beans, supports repair without overwhelming filtration.

Water or unsweetened herbal tea preserves hydration without adding artificial sweetness or stimulant noise.

The plate should also be emotionally simple. A patient should not need a calculator, an app, or a complicated hierarchy of forbidden foods to eat a healing meal. The eyes should understand it. The hands should be able to prepare it. The gut should recognize it.

Brown rice, vegetables, legumes, fruit, water, and modest fat do not impress the modern palate at first because they are not engineered to overwhelm it. Their power is quieter. They restore satiety by removing the constant argument between appetite and stimulation.

Configured this way, the meal produces a rolling hill rather than a jagged spike. Insulin responds without panic. Mitochondria receive fuel they can use. Digestion experiences order rather than collision. The Sim-Bo plate is not exotic. It is simply legible.

Movement: The Forgotten Regulator

No nutrient works in isolation. Movement determines how fuel behaves after it is swallowed.

Skeletal muscle is a major reservoir for glucose disposal. When muscle contracts, GLUT4 transporters move toward the cell surface and help bring glucose into tissue, including through insulin-independent pathways. A short walk after meals can improve post-meal glucose handling because working muscle gives fuel a destination.

This is why post-meal walking is one of the simplest metabolic interventions available. It does not require punishment, equipment, or athletic identity. It simply asks muscle to participate in the meal. The plate gives fuel; the walk gives that fuel a place to go.

In a sedentary patient, food becomes a burden more easily because the largest glucose-disposal organ is underused. In an active patient, the same meal can be handled with greater grace. Movement changes the meaning of the meal.

Movement also releases myokines, improves circulation, assists lymphatic flow, supports mitochondrial turnover, and changes mood through physical completion. The meal is not finished when eating stops. It continues through movement, uptake, oxidation, storage, repair, and clearance.

Sedentary living leaves fuel without use. The bloodstream carries energy that muscles are not asking for. The immune system reads the residue as imbalance. Movement is therefore not an aesthetic afterthought. It is the punctuation that completes the sentence of nutrition.

The Peaceful Metabolism

When sugar and fat return to partnership, hunger becomes quieter. Cognitive energy holds longer. Sleep deepens. The nervous system stops chasing emergency fuel and begins to trust the day.

Peaceful metabolism is not sedation. It is readiness without alarm. The mind is clear, but not frantic. Hunger appears, but does not command. Energy rises, but does not spike. Sleep arrives because the system has completed its work for the day.

This is the clinical difference between stimulation and vitality. Stimulation borrows energy from tomorrow. Vitality is generated from order today.

Patients following the Sim-Bo structure often describe a practical clarity: fewer crashes, steadier appetite, lighter digestion, and a less frantic relationship with food. Objective markers may follow the same direction: triglycerides trend downward, fasting glucose becomes steadier, insulin response improves, and inflammatory markers may soften as the overall metabolic load decreases.

This shift is not punishment and not deprivation. It is the relief of order. The system is no longer being asked to burn too much, too often, without movement, without rest, and without cleanup.

Conclusion: Steady Heat, Long Life

Fire teaches two lessons: it must burn to sustain life, and it must be contained to prevent destruction.

Fat and sugar are elemental fuels. They are not enemies. They are teachers. They show exactly whether daily life is ordered or chaotic, whether meals are built for nourishment or stimulation, whether energy is being used or merely stored, whether pleasure is supported by structure or left to become compulsion.

The modern world teaches appetite to chase intensity. Sim-Bo teaches metabolism to value steadiness. That difference changes everything: how a patient wakes, how they think after lunch, how they sleep, how they move, and how they experience hunger.

Steady heat is not dramatic. It does not announce itself like a stimulant. It becomes visible in a calmer face, steadier mood, less swelling, easier digestion, clearer thought, and the absence of constant negotiation with cravings.

A life with less dependence on rescue requires mastery of this inner heat. Feed it with intact food. Give it movement. Allow it to rest. Protect the hours when repair occurs. Eat with enough simplicity that metabolism can understand the message.

When oxidative smoke clears, health reveals itself as steady energy, clear appetite, warm circulation, sound sleep, and the quiet confidence of a system burning clean.

Clinical Case Study 7: Breaking the Insulin Pendulum

Restoring Fuel Cadence in Central Adiposity, Cognitive Fatigue, and Sugar Craving

Patient: Emily S., 45-year-old female, Executive Director.

Chief Concerns: Mid-afternoon cognitive fatigue, persistent central adiposity despite repeated dieting, strong sugar cravings, post-meal heaviness, and a sense of systemic stagnation.

Clinical Presentation

Emily illustrates a common modern pattern: a patient eating "healthy" convenience foods while living in constant glycemic instability. Her daily routine depended on sweetened yogurt, granola bars, fruit smoothies, coffee, long meetings, and long sedentary work blocks. None of these choices looked extreme in isolation. Together, they created an insulin pendulum.

She had tried multiple diets built around restriction, but restriction had only made her more reactive. Skipping meals intensified cravings. Low-calorie snacks kept her unsatisfied. Smoothies felt virtuous but often delivered rapid sugar without enough chewing or fiber. Her program looked disciplined from the outside, yet it lacked metabolic architecture.

The clinical focus was not blame. It was sequencing: slow the fuel, restore structure, give the liver and muscle a predictable rhythm, and teach the nervous system that energy would arrive without crisis.

Refined and liquid carbohydrates entered quickly. Insulin rose sharply. Energy lifted briefly, then fell. The afternoon crash brought cravings, more quick fuel, and another cycle. Triglycerides rose, central weight persisted, and cognitive endurance became unreliable. The clinical task was not to starve her; it was to restore cadence.

Initial Findings

Fasting triglycerides: 210 mg/dL, consistent with a significant lipid-metabolism concern requiring lifestyle correction and medical monitoring as appropriate.

Tongue: Pale and puffy with scalloped edges and a slippery central

coating, consistent with Spleen Qi deficiency and Damp-Phlegm accumulation within the Traditional Asian Medicine framework.

Pulse: Slippery and weak at the right middle position, suggesting digestive depletion complicated by damp accumulation.

Pattern: Spleen Qi deficiency with Damp-Phlegm accumulation, with a secondary inflammatory heat pattern associated with metabolic stagnation.

Treatment Principles

Flatten the insulin curve by removing refined sugars, fruit juices, and naked carbohydrates.

Use intact grains and fibrous vegetables as the glycemic anchor.

Support Spleen Qi and improve metabolic transformation.

Reduce Damp-Phlegm accumulation through food structure, movement, acupuncture, cupping, and botanical support.

Replace calorie-counting anxiety with predictable meals and post-meal movement.

Plan and Intervention

Emily committed to a twelve-week Sim Bo metabolic reset.

The early phase emphasized repetition. Emily ate simple meals at consistent times so her digestive system could anticipate its work. She stopped treating hunger as an emergency and began treating it as information.

The therapeutic logic was simple: reduce the speed of glucose entry, increase fiber exposure, protect hydration, move after meals, and use traditional therapies to support digestion, circulation, and autonomic settling.

The Sim-Bo dietary prescription used brown rice and quinoa as slow-release carbohydrate anchors, paired with large servings of lightly steamed vegetables such as broccoli, bok choy, daikon radish, and leafy greens.

Processed sugars, fruit juices, refined flours, sweetened yogurts, and granola bars were removed. Whole fruit was retained in controlled portions and paired with fiber-rich meals rather than consumed as liquid sugar.

Meals were timed consistently. Post-meal walking was prescribed to give circulating glucose an immediate muscular destination.

Acupuncture focused on ST36, SP9, CV12, and related points to support digestive transformation, reduce damp accumulation, and stabilize cravings.

Emperor's Cupping Therapy® was applied along the abdominal and mid-thoracic regions to reduce myofascial restriction, support local circulation, and assist relaxation of the digestive region.

Ping Wei San was modified with Shan Zha within the Traditional Asian Medicine framework to support food transformation, damp resolution, and lipid-metabolism patterns.

Clinical Response at Twelve Weeks

Fasting triglycerides improved from 210 mg/dL to 95 mg/dL.

Mid-afternoon cognitive crashing was replaced by steadier mental endurance through the workday.

Central adiposity decreased, with a 16-pound reduction noted during the follow-up period.

Sugar cravings markedly decreased, and the patient reported a more stable relationship with food.

Tongue presentation improved, with reduced puffiness, less scalloping, and a cleaner coating.

Case Meaning

Emily's case illustrates the central law of this chapter: energy crashes and central weight gain are not simply failures of discipline. They often reflect poor fuel timing, rapid carbohydrate delivery, insufficient fiber, sedentary work patterns, and a nervous system trained to seek quick relief.

Her improvement did not require novelty. It required subtraction: fewer liquid sugars, fewer sweetened convenience foods, fewer frantic corrections, fewer long sedentary gaps after meals. In that space, ordinary physiology had room to reassert itself.

Emily did not need to defeat appetite. She needed to stop provoking it.

Once the glycemic pendulum quieted, her metabolism did not need more stimulation. It needed order. Intact grains provided steady fuel. Vegetables delivered fiber and minerals. Movement gave glucose a destination. Acupuncture, cupping, and botanical medicine supported the regulatory framework. Her cravings softened because the emergency chemistry softened.

The Sim-Bo lesson is direct: when the fuels stop colliding, physiology can stop fighting the meal.

Transition: From Science to Simplicity

Fat, sugar, insulin, mitochondria, oxidative stress, and craving all point toward the same conclusion: complex metabolic science eventually returns to a simple demand for order.

Balance cannot survive by accident in a culture built on hyper-consumption. It must be protected by repeated, ordinary choices: plain meals, clean timing, intact foods, movement after eating, sleep at night, and less stimulation than the modern appetite wants.

This is the final lesson of Part II's first movement. Protein, animal foods, fat, and sugar all become clearer when complexity is removed. The molecular details matter, but their practical expression is humble: eat food the system can read, at times it can trust, in a life that gives fuel a purpose.

The next movement is not more complication. It is the philosophy that makes compliance possible: radical simplicity.

Simplicity is not a retreat from science. It is the practical form science takes when the body has been heard. The path now narrows from molecular complexity into the disciplined quiet of the Sim-Bo way.

Part III

The Sim-Bo Diet™: Simplicity as Healing

Part III begins where modern health culture usually refuses to go: into less. After the history of chronic inflammation, the cost of convenience, and the language of nutrients, the path now narrows into practice. Sim-Bo does not multiply rules. It removes interference.

The philosophy is plain: when food becomes recognizable, timing becomes steady, and the mind stops chasing novelty, physiology receives a message it can trust. The 3:2:1 Formula grows from that message. Complex grains, fibrous vegetables, and whole fruit become more than ingredients; they become the daily architecture of calm regulation.

This is not restriction. It is clarity. It is the disciplined geometry of enough.

Chapter 8

The Philosophy of Simplicity

The Medicine of Less: The Power of Via Negativa

Healing begins when life becomes quiet enough for physiology to listen.

Modern commercial culture teaches recovery through addition: more tests, more supplements, more devices, more data, more protocols, more stimulation. The market loves addition because addition can be sold. Sim-Bo begins with a different law. The first medicine is not another input. The first medicine is subtraction.

Via negativa is the art of improvement through removal. Remove the food that confuses digestion. Remove the schedule that leaves no recovery. Remove the digital noise that keeps the nervous system braced. Remove the constant comparison that turns ordinary life into a contest. What remains is not emptiness. What remains is space for regulation.

Simplicity is not deprivation. It is restoration. A river clears when its flow is no longer blocked. A forest renews after dormancy. Soil recovers when it is no longer forced to produce without season. Human physiology obeys the same pattern. When inputs arrive without pause, metabolism clogs, heats, and strains. When the environment becomes simpler, the system cools, clears, and repairs.

The medicine of less is not passive. It requires discipline. It asks a sharper question than modern wellness usually asks: What can be removed today so that healing no longer has to fight through noise?

The Birth of Sim-Bo

The name Sim-Bo did not come from a branding exercise. It came from the consultation room.

I first called the method the Simple Diet. The aim was direct: remove dietary confusion and return the patient to a clean baseline. Brown rice, steamed greens, fruit, hydration, regular meals, early sleep, steady movement. Nothing exotic. Nothing performative. Nothing designed to impress the ego.

The complaint came quickly and repeatedly. Patients looked at the plan and sighed: 'Dr. Choi, this is so boring.'

They were correct. The plan was boring by design. A nervous system trained for hyper-palatable food, caffeine, urgency, social comparison, and constant digital stimulation does not need more excitement. It needs trustworthy repetition. Boredom is not the failure of Sim-Bo. Boredom is the therapeutic environment.

Simple became the clinical intention. Boring became the patient's honest diagnosis of the method. Together, they became Sim-Bo: Simple and Boring.

The deeper truth is this: when food becomes boring, life can become vibrant again. The digestive system stops defending itself against every meal. The autonomic nervous system stops scanning every day for danger. Appetite becomes more honest. Sleep becomes easier to enter. Energy returns not as stimulation, but as steadiness.

The Clinical Meaning of Boredom

Boredom has been insulted by modern culture because boredom cannot be easily sold. It has no packaging, no subscription, no upgrade, and no dramatic before-and-after identity. Yet in the clinic, boredom often marks the first arrival of safety.

A patient accustomed to stimulation usually mistakes calm for emptiness. The first week of simple food can feel strangely quiet. Meals no longer create emotional fireworks. Snacks no longer interrupt discomfort. The nervous system, no longer distracted by taste intensity and novelty, begins to reveal what was underneath: fatigue, grief, tension, restlessness, or genuine hunger.

This is why the boring phase must not be abandoned too quickly. The discomfort is diagnostic. It shows how strongly appetite had been entangled with entertainment, anxiety relief, reward, and identity. When the patient stays with simplicity long enough, the same quiet that once felt empty becomes restorative. Food returns to its proper role: nourishment, not anesthesia.

Biochemical calm rarely feels dramatic at the beginning. It feels like less noise. Later, it becomes deeper sleep, steadier bowels, softer cravings, clearer thinking, and a more trustworthy appetite.

The Illusion of Complexity and the Trap of Optimization

Modern wellness sells complexity because complexity looks sophisticated. It sells powders, monitors, peptide cycles, fasting apps, macro spreadsheets, sleep scores, glucose curves, and supplement stacks. Each tool can have a place. None can replace the foundation.

Patients often arrive exhausted from managing their own health. They bring bags of capsules, wearable data, conflicting diet rules, and a nervous system trained to monitor itself with suspicion. Their glucose may be tracked, their sleep may be scored, and their supplements may be organized by hour. Yet the daily foundation is usually unstable: irregular meals, late screens, inconsistent sleep, rushed eating, emotional overload, and no quiet.

The pursuit of health becomes another stressor. The mind becomes a surveillance system. The patient no longer lives in the body; the patient manages the body from above, like a machine under inspection.

Sim-Bo breaks that spell. It returns the patient from optimization to participation. A plain meal eaten at a consistent time gives the gut, pancreas, liver, microbiome, and nervous system fewer variables to interpret. The organism no longer spends its energy decoding novelty. It can use that energy for repair.

Complexity drains attention. Simplicity returns it.

Simplicity as a Clinical Baseline

A complicated patient does not always need a complicated first step. The first step is often a clean baseline.

In practice, the baseline is not a punishment. It is a diagnostic clearing. When the diet is crowded with bars, powders, sauces, snacks, coffee, restaurant food, late meals, alcohol, supplements, and erratic fasting, no clinician can clearly read the response. Was the bloating caused by the protein powder, the emulsifier, the cold smoothie, the late-night meal, the stress, the caffeine, the raw salad, or the combination? Complexity hides the cause.

A Sim-Bo baseline removes the argument. Brown rice. Cooked vegetables. Fruit. Water. Warmth. Time. Breath. Repetition. Once the pattern is simplified, the patient's own physiology becomes easier to observe. Energy after meals, stool quality, sleep depth, mood, temperature, cravings, and pain all become more legible.

This is the clinical genius of the ordinary. It does not claim to solve every problem in one stroke. It reveals the terrain. And once the terrain is visible, treatment becomes more precise.

Predictability and the Physiology of Calm

Predictability is not merely psychological comfort. It is physiology.

The hypothalamus, autonomic nervous system, endocrine glands, digestive tract, and immune system all respond to timing. Regular meals prepare digestive secretion. Regular darkness prepares melatonin. Regular waking prepares cortisol's morning rise. Repeated daily structure tells the nervous system that the environment is safe enough for repair.

The vagus nerve sits at the center of this conversation. It carries sensory information from the organs to the brain and sends regulatory instructions back down into the heart, lungs, stomach, liver, spleen, and intestines. When life becomes predictable, vagal tone strengthens. Breath deepens. Gastric motility improves. Heart rhythm settles. The immune response becomes less defensive.

The cholinergic anti-inflammatory pathway gives this ancient intuition a modern language. Vagal activity can influence inflammatory macrophages through acetylcholine-mediated signaling. In simpler terms, calm is not only a mood. Calm is an immune instruction.

This is why a humble bowl of brown rice and vegetables, eaten daily at a steady hour, can become more clinically meaningful than another isolated supplement. The food matters, but the cadence matters as well. The meal is not only nourishment. It is a repeated message: the environment is stable; the emergency is over.

The Ego, Dopamine, and the Ordinary

The ordinary has become invisible because the modern ego is trained to worship novelty.

It wants personalization, dramatic change, imported superfoods, punishing cleanses, unusual ingredients, visible effort, and public proof. It wants a diet that feels like identity. Sim-Bo offers none of that. It offers a quiet bowl, a steady hour, a clean plate, and the courage to repeat what works.

Dopamine is not an enemy. It is the chemistry of pursuit. It helps us seek, learn, explore, and act. The problem begins when every meal, every screen, every purchase, and every social interaction is designed to spike novelty. The nervous system begins to confuse stimulation with vitality.

Metabolic healing hides in the opposite direction. Deliberate repetition builds trust. Trust allows the immune system to stop bracing. The deepest repair rarely comes through spectacle. It comes through the daily ordinariness of cooking, chewing, walking, breathing, sleeping, and waking at the same human pace.

A simple life requires psychological strength. It requires the ability to be content when the culture tells you contentment is failure. It requires the courage to become uninteresting to the market and deeply legible to your own physiology.

The Three Layers of Simplicity

Sim-Bo simplicity has three layers: food, time, and thought.

Food simplicity reduces unnecessary variables. Meals centered on brown rice, vegetables, fruit, hydration, and modest supportive proteins create a pattern the digestive system can recognize. Fewer ingredients do not mean fewer nutrients. They mean fewer distractions. Whole foods bring water, fiber, minerals, phytochemicals, texture, and digestive pacing in one coherent matrix.

Time simplicity restores biological timing. Eating, waking, moving, resting, and sleeping at consistent hours stabilizes the clocks that govern glucose handling, digestive secretion, liver function, gut motility, temperature, and repair. Circadian order is not decorative. It is one of the master regulators of metabolism.

Thought simplicity reduces internal noise. Chronic worry, comparison, unfinished digital loops, social performance, and multitasking keep the nervous system in guarded readiness. Journaling, silent meals, prayer, breathwork, walking outdoors, and deliberate pauses clear enough space for the mind to stop manufacturing emergency.

Each layer supports the others. Plain food makes appetite honest. Consistent timing makes digestion predictable. A quieter mind allows the meal to be received. Together, they form a therapeutic framework stronger than any single tactic.

Repetition Without Monotony

Repetition is often misunderstood as stagnation. In clinical practice, repetition is the method by which unstable systems regain trust.

A musician repeats scales not because music is small, but because freedom requires structure. A martial artist repeats basic forms not because movement lacks imagination, but because precision must become embodied before spontaneity becomes safe. A patient repeats simple meals for the same reason: the digestive tract, endocrine system, and nervous network need a stable phrase before they can improvise again.

Monotony is mechanical repetition without attention. Sim-Bo is different. It is deliberate repetition with observation. The same bowl of rice and vegetables becomes a daily diagnostic instrument. Was energy steady after the meal? Did the stomach feel warm or heavy? Did the bowel pattern change? Was sleep deeper? Did cravings soften? Did mood become more even? These observations are nearly impossible when each day brings a different diet, a different supplement stack, a different fasting window, and a different stimulant.

The modern palate confuses excitement with nourishment. It wants every meal to entertain. Recovery asks another question: can this meal restore order without demanding performance from digestion? The answer is often yes, and that yes is quiet.

Repetition does not imprison the patient. It creates a clean laboratory of daily life. Once the system stabilizes, variety can return with intelligence. Until then, consistency is not a lack of sophistication. It is the precondition for discernment.

Subtraction and Autophagy

Healing through subtraction is not vague spirituality. It is visible in cellular housekeeping.

When intake is continuous, stimulation is constant, and sleep is shallow, the organism remains busy processing the present. Repair is postponed. Cleanup is delayed. Autophagy, the process by which cells recycle damaged organelles and misfolded proteins, depends on periods of lowered demand. It requires intervals when physiology is not constantly being asked to digest, defend, adapt, and respond.

Sim-Bo subtraction creates those intervals. It removes the processed snack, the late-night screen, the unnecessary supplement, the punishing workout, the second cup of stimulation, the fear-driven health rule. Each removal releases energy back to regulation.

The question is simple and severe: What is no longer serving repair?

Remove the multi-ingredient foods that leave digestion confused.
Remove the overpacked schedule that leaves no parasympathetic entry point.
Remove the internal narrative that keeps the shoulders raised and the jaw clenched.
Remove the health practices that look disciplined but deepen exhaustion.

Subtraction is not absence. It is the creation of room.

The Science of Predictability

Simplicity is measurable neuroendocrinology.

Every organ performs more efficiently when the next environmental event is not a surprise. The pancreas responds more cleanly to a meal it can anticipate. The gallbladder and stomach prepare more effectively when mealtimes are stable. The brain coordinates alertness and sleep through repeated light-dark cues. The gut microbiome adapts to regular fiber, texture, and timing.

Erratic habits force constant recalculation. Shifting meal times, irregular sleep, grazing, stimulant cycles, and late digital exposure create a state of metabolic uncertainty. The system burns energy preparing for too many possibilities. Regulation becomes expensive.

Regularity lowers the cost of living. Cortisol can rise in the morning instead of leaking across the entire day. Insulin can respond to meals instead of managing endless intake. Melatonin can rise at dusk instead of competing with screens. Digestion can enter its work without urgency.

This is homeostasis in motion: not a frozen balance, but a dynamic order that flows because daily cues are trustworthy.

Simple Is Not Easy

Simple is often harder than complex because it removes the drama that once gave the patient identity. It is easier to buy another supplement than to repeat an early bedtime. It is easier to begin a new protocol than to eat a plain breakfast for thirty days. It is easier to chase a theory than to sit at a quiet table and observe what actually happens after a meal.

Complexity gives the ego a feeling of advancement. Simplicity asks the ego to become useful. It asks the patient to stop performing health and start practicing it. It removes the theater and leaves the work.

This is why Sim-Bo is not casual minimalism. It is disciplined minimalism. The plate may look plain, but the choice behind it is demanding: refuse unnecessary novelty, refuse the false prestige of complexity, and return to what the system can actually use.

The Comfort of Boredom

Modern culture treats boredom as a defect. Sim-Bo treats it as a door.

Boredom is the absence of emergency. It is the interval in which the nervous system stops reaching for another hit of novelty. In that interval, memory consolidates, attention widens, emotional material surfaces, and the Default Mode Network has room to operate. Creativity, reflection, grief, and integration all require space that entertainment constantly interrupts.

The boring meal creates a similar lull in digestion. Brown rice, fruit, and vegetables deliver steady carbohydrate, fiber, water, minerals, and phytonutrients without the assault of industrial salt, sugar, and unstable fats. After repeated exposure, the palate recalibrates. Subtle flavor returns: the nutty warmth of grain, the mineral sweetness of root vegetables, the clean brightness of fruit, the quiet fragrance of steam.

What first appears monotonous becomes meditative. The meal no longer exists to entertain the mouth. It exists to restore clarity. Simplicity does not numb life. It removes the static that had been covering it.

Social Resistance and the Leadership of Contentment

The greatest obstacle to simplicity is rarely hunger. It is social pressure.

A culture built on variety, speed, and display mistrusts a disciplined routine. Friends may question restraint. Marketing will whisper that something is being missed. Social media will parade novelty as proof of success. In that atmosphere, eating a plain bowl of rice and vegetables becomes an act of quiet leadership.

People who master simplicity often develop a steadiness others notice before they notice any physical change. Their energy becomes less dramatic and more reliable. Their speech slows. Their decisions become cleaner. They stop needing constant stimulation to feel alive.

Contentment is not passivity. It is strength without spectacle. It is the ability to receive enough, repeat enough, and stop when the system has been nourished. This is cultural leadership because it refuses the central command of the market: consume more to become more.

Enoughness as a Clinical State

Enoughness is not merely a moral idea. It has physiology. The person who believes nothing is enough eats differently, works differently, trains differently, spends differently, and sleeps differently. The nervous system interprets the world as a place of shortage even when the table is full.

When enough becomes believable, the chemistry changes. The meal can end. The evening can close. The breath can deepen. The patient no longer needs constant stimulation to prove aliveness. This is where simplicity becomes emotional medicine: it teaches the system that survival does not require perpetual acquisition.

Contentment is therefore not the opposite of ambition. It is the ground from which clean ambition can rise. A person driven by panic burns energy before the work begins. A person rooted in enough can act with steadier force.

Simplicity and the Mind

The same principle that governs digestion governs thought: what enters must be processed.

A mind fed on sensational news, conflict, notification loops, and constant performance pressure becomes inflamed in its own way. Attention fragments. Sleep becomes lighter. Irritability rises. Executive function weakens. The brain does not live outside the physiology it directs.

Simplifying informational intake restores coherence. One uninterrupted hour without screens can feel uncomfortable at first because the nervous system is detoxifying from novelty. Walking outside without headphones lets breath, movement, sound, and vision synchronize again. Eating without a screen returns attention to chewing, aroma, warmth, satiety, and gratitude.

These are not small lifestyle decorations. They are neurophysiological interventions. They reduce sensory load so the parasympathetic system can lead. When the mind receives fewer artificial emergencies, the entire organism has fewer reasons to defend.

The Art of the Ordinary

Strong cultures have always turned ordinary acts into ritual: tea, rice, bread, soup, shared labor, seasonal meals, morning light, evening prayer, quiet walking. These rituals were not decorative. They taught the nervous system where it belonged in time.

The ordinary becomes medicine when it is performed with attention. Washing rice. Cutting vegetables. Heating water. Sitting at the table. Breathing before the first bite. Chewing until the food becomes part of you. These acts restore the dignity of nourishment.

Gratitude is not an accessory to digestion. A grateful state softens the face, lowers defensive tone, deepens the breath, and prepares the stomach to receive. The meal becomes more than fuel. It becomes a declaration that enough exists in this moment.

The person who can feel enough has already begun to heal.

The Discipline of Enough

Modern culture teaches appetite to distrust sufficiency. Enough food is made to feel inadequate. Enough rest is made to feel lazy. Enough silence is made to feel lonely. Enough ordinary life is made to feel like failure.

This psychological scarcity is a metabolic event. The person who never feels enough rarely digests enough, sleeps enough, pauses enough, or breathes enough. The nervous system interprets perpetual wanting as unfinished threat. Desire itself becomes a form of sympathetic stimulation.

Sim-Bo trains enoughness through repeated contact with completion. A plain meal is prepared. It is eaten slowly. The plate empties. Hunger settles. Nothing dramatic happens, and that is the medicine. The absence of drama teaches the system that survival does not require chase.

Enoughness does not kill ambition. It protects it from exhaustion. A person who is not constantly negotiating cravings, novelty, comparison, and fatigue has more power for purposeful work. Simplicity does not make life smaller. It gathers scattered energy into one direction.

The discipline of enough is not passive. It is a refusal to let the marketplace define the size of desire.

The Quiet Revolution

Sim-Bo is revolutionary because it asks for nothing extraordinary.

It does not demand rare ingredients, elaborate tracking, expensive equipment, or heroic suffering. It asks for repetition. It asks for enough humility to eat simple food without needing applause. It asks for enough discipline to protect sleep, enough honesty to remove noise, and enough courage to stop worshiping complexity.

It replaces the illusion of control with trust earned through consistency. It replaces variety without nourishment with repetition that repairs. It replaces excitement with endurance, performance with presence, and frantic intervention with clear daily order.

Simplicity heals because energy stops chasing novelty and returns to structure. The nervous system, no longer forced to interpret constant change, settles into safety. In safety, inflammation softens. In safety, digestion improves. In safety, joy returns in quieter and more durable forms.

To live simply is not to live small. It is to stop fighting nature's original design.

Conclusion: The Beginning of Healing

Simplicity is not the final destination of healing. It is the starting line.

When internal and external life become quiet enough, perception sharpens. True hunger separates from craving. Physical fatigue separates from emotional depletion. Purposeful action separates from frantic motion. The patient begins to hear the difference between stimulation and vitality.

This clarity is medicine because it restores choice. A person cannot change what remains hidden beneath noise. Once the noise falls away, the next act becomes obvious: eat simply, move steadily, sleep on time, breathe before reacting, and protect the environment in which repair occurs.

The Measure of Progress

Progress in Sim-Bo is measured differently from progress in modern optimization culture.

The first signs are often quiet: fewer cravings, less urgency around food, a warmer abdomen after meals, deeper evening fatigue, more natural morning hunger, slower speech, easier bowel movement, calmer reactions, and a return of interest in ordinary tasks. These changes may seem small to the impatient mind. Clinically, they reveal that regulation is returning.

A patient trained by dramatic programs may overlook these early signs because they are not theatrical. There is no extreme cleanse, no punishing challenge, no identity to announce. Yet the quiet signs matter more. A calmer appetite means the reward system is softening. A warmer digestion means parasympathetic tone is improving. Easier sleep means the day is no longer ending in emergency chemistry. The ordinary markers are the true markers.

Sim-Bo teaches the patient to respect subtle improvement before demanding dramatic transformation. Health usually returns as a cadence before it appears as a number.

In philosophy, healing begins. In repeated practice, healing becomes durable.

Clinical Case Study 8: The Medicine of Subtraction

Reducing Additive Stress to Restore Energy, Warmth, and Autonomic Stability

Patient: Karen M., 48-year-old female, public relations executive.

Chief concerns: profound morning fatigue, non-restorative sleep, sudden weight gain around the hips and thighs, chronic cold hands and feet, emotional overdrive, and a heavy, leaden sensation despite constant effort to remain healthy.

Clinical Presentation

Karen had built her life around pressure disguised as discipline. She practiced intense HIIT workouts, erratic fasting windows, constant productivity tracking, late-night work, and a rotating list of supplements meant to push more energy out of an exhausted system.

Her problem was not laziness. It was the opposite. She was doing too much to a system that needed fewer demands. The apparent health practices had become additive stressors: more intensity, more restriction, more surveillance, more urgency. Her symptoms were not random. They were survival responses from an organism asking for safety.

The clinical priority was subtraction: remove the practices that were increasing sympathetic load, rebuild a stable morning anchor, warm the digestive center, restore gentle movement, and give the nervous system a pattern it could trust.

The first two weeks were the hardest because removal exposed withdrawal from urgency. Without intense workouts, she felt guilty. Without fasting, she feared losing control. Without late-night productivity, she felt unproductive. These reactions were part of the treatment. They showed how deeply performance had become fused with self-worth.

The clinical work therefore required more than changing meals. It required changing the meaning of rest. Rest had to become active medicine, not failure. Warm breakfast had to become reassurance, not indulgence. Gentle walking had to become strength training for the autonomic nervous system. Slowly, her daily choices stopped communicating threat and began communicating trust.

Initial Findings

Blood pressure: 95/60 mm Hg, consistent with a depleted, low-reserve presentation in the broader clinical picture.

Tongue: pale, flabby, swollen, scalloped, and wet in appearance.

Pulse: deep, thin, and forceless, with notable weakness at the proximal positions.

Traditional Asian Medicine pattern: Kidney Yang and Spleen Qi deficiency, with coldness, fluid retention, digestive weakness, and mental overdrive.

Treatment Principles

Remove high-friction exercise and erratic fasting.
Rebuild a warm morning meal anchor.
Support Kidney Yang and Spleen Qi through warming food, moxibustion, and botanical medicine.
Shift the autonomic pattern from performance pressure toward parasympathetic recovery.
Release protective myofascial guarding through careful cupping and acupuncture support.

Plan and Intervention

Karen committed to a twelve-week Sim-Bo recovery protocol built around less input, warmer nourishment, and steadier timing.

The Sim-Bo dietary prescription became the warming anchor. Her erratic fasting routine was stopped. A grounding meal was placed within thirty minutes of waking so the nervous system no longer began the day in perceived scarcity.

3 parts grains: slow-cooked oats, sweet rice, and warm grain porridge to support steady energy and digestive warmth.
2 parts vegetables: roasted root vegetables and cooked greens to provide minerals, fiber, and grounding texture.
1 part fruit: gently warmed fruit or stewed fruit in the morning or early afternoon, used for sweetness without overstimulation.
Supportive protein: small amounts of slow-cooked broth or easily digested protein were used strategically rather than as a heavy centerpiece.

Autonomic reset required removing the practices that looked healthy but acted like stress. HIIT was replaced with restorative Qi Gong, gentle walking, and outdoor light exposure. Coherent diaphragmatic breathing was prescribed twice daily to train the shift from urgency to recovery.

Targeted acupuncture and moxibustion focused on CV4, CV6, ST36, SP6, HT7, and Kidney-supportive points to warm the center, rebuild reserve, and settle mental agitation. Emperor's Cupping Therapy® was applied along the lumbar and thoracic regions to reduce myofascial guarding, support local circulation, and help the posterior chain release its chronic protective tone.

Jin Gui Shen Qi Wan was used within the Traditional Asian Medicine pattern to warm Kidney Yang, support fluid metabolism, improve cold extremities, and strengthen the depleted presentation. The herbal strategy was not stimulation; it was restoration.

Twelve-Week Follow-Up

Morning energy improved from prolonged difficulty waking to waking naturally with steadier alertness.

Resting blood pressure improved from 95/60 mm Hg to 115/75 mm Hg during follow-up.

Cold hands, cold feet, and deep chills markedly improved, with warmer peripheral circulation by patient report.

Weight decreased by 12 lbs., with visible reduction in lower-body fluid retention and heaviness.

Tongue presentation showed improved color, reduced swelling, and less pronounced scalloping.

Anxious mental racing decreased as exercise intensity, fasting pressure, and schedule overload were removed.

Clinical Pattern

Karen's case illustrates the central law of Chapter 8: healing often begins when the exhausted system is no longer asked to prove itself.

She had tried to outwork depletion. The clinical solution was not more stimulation, more tracking, or more heroic discipline. It was warmth, rhythm, food she could digest, movement she could recover from, and a daily pattern that no longer treated her nervous system as an enemy to be conquered.

The future of high-performance medicine will distinguish fitness from depletion. The same workout that builds resilience in one patient can deepen collapse in another. The same fasting window that sharpens one metabolism can exhaust another. True clinical judgment recognizes the difference.

The medicine was subtraction. Remove the excessive demand, and regulation returned.

The same principle applied to her professional life. Karen did not need to abandon ambition. She needed to stop confusing emergency speed with excellence. Once her schedule contained fewer unnecessary accelerants, the quality of her work improved because her attention was no longer being purchased with exhaustion.

Her family noticed the change before she fully trusted it. She spoke more slowly. She ate breakfast sitting down. She stopped apologizing for rest. These small behaviors were not decorative; they were the visible evidence that her internal terrain had begun to believe in safety again.

Karen also illustrates a difficult truth for driven patients: discipline can injure when it is divorced from listening. Her workouts required discipline. Her fasting required discipline. Her supplementation required discipline. Her schedule required discipline. The problem was not weakness; it was discipline aimed in the wrong direction.

The clinical pivot occurred when discipline became protective rather than punitive. She used discipline to stop, not to push. She used discipline to sleep, eat warm food, breathe slowly, and walk gently. She used discipline to decline intensity. That shift changed the entire message entering her nervous system.

In exhausted patients, restraint is often the highest form of strength.

Transition: From Philosophy to Structure

Simplicity becomes medicine when it reaches the plate.

A philosophy can calm the mind, but structured food trains the day. Sim-Bo takes the principle of less and gives it geometry: three parts whole grain, two parts fibrous vegetables, one part fruit. The ratio is not a trick. It is a repeatable form of metabolic order.

Three. Two. One. Grain, vegetable, fruit. Steady fuel, cleansing fiber, living sweetness. The formula turns simplicity from an idea into a daily practice the digestive system can anticipate and the nervous system can trust.

In philosophy, healing begins. In structure, it becomes repeatable.

Chapter 9

The 3:2:1 Formula for Healing

The Birth of a Simple Formula

In every serious discipline, mastery begins with structure. Musicians begin with scales. Architects learn proportion before ornament. Healers learn to observe timing, appetite, temperature, pulse, tongue, stool, sleep, and the quiet cadence of recovery. Nutrition is no different. A therapeutic diet must be simple enough to remember, stable enough to repeat, and flexible enough to survive ordinary life.

The 3:2:1 Formula was created from that clinical necessity.

The ratio is direct: three parts complex grain, two parts fibrous vegetables, one part whole fruit. No obsessive calorie counting. No anxious weighing of every gram. No digital algorithm standing between the patient and the plate. The structure itself becomes the teacher. The grain anchors energy. The vegetables move and regulate. The fruit refreshes and completes.

The genius of the formula is repetition. When meals arrive in a recognizable proportion day after day, the nervous system reads predictability. Digestion anticipates its work. Appetite becomes easier to interpret. The microbiome receives a steadier supply of fiber. Energy becomes less erratic. The plate stops acting like a daily experiment and becomes a rehearsal for metabolic order.

Sim-Bo is not complexity disguised as wellness. It is proportion made visible.

The Geometry of Nourishment

Human metabolism was shaped by whole food, seasonal availability, physical work, and repeated patterns. It was not shaped by constant snacking, isolated powders, sweetened drinks, refined oils, and meals designed for entertainment rather than nourishment.

Traditional food cultures were rarely built around mathematical tracking, yet many carried a quiet geometric intelligence. The sustaining center of the meal came from intact grains, roots, beans, tubers, or other complex carbohydrates. Vegetables and herbs supplied fiber, minerals, bitterness, color, and microbial nourishment. Fruit appeared as sweetness in its natural architecture: water, fiber, minerals, acids, pigments, and fragrance. Dense proteins and extracted fats were used with restraint, often as accent, seasoning, celebration, or targeted rebuilding food.

This arrangement supplied what modern eating often lacks: slow fuel, mineral density, bowel movement, microbial substrate, hydration, and sensory completion. The meal had structure. It contained energy without chaos, sweetness without liquid sugar, and fullness without chemical overstimulation.

The industrial diet inverted this geometry. Refined flour replaced intact grain. Seed oils and animal-fat density expanded. Protein became the center of the plate. Vegetables became decoration. Fruit was converted into juice, syrup, flavoring, or dessert. The result was not only excess calories. It was a collapse of order.

The 3:2:1 Formula restores that order through a plate the eye can understand.

> Three parts grain anchor sustained energy and digestive steadiness.
> Two parts vegetables provide fiber, minerals, color, and regulatory chemistry.
> One part fruit completes the meal pattern with water, sweetness, antioxidants, and gentle refreshment.

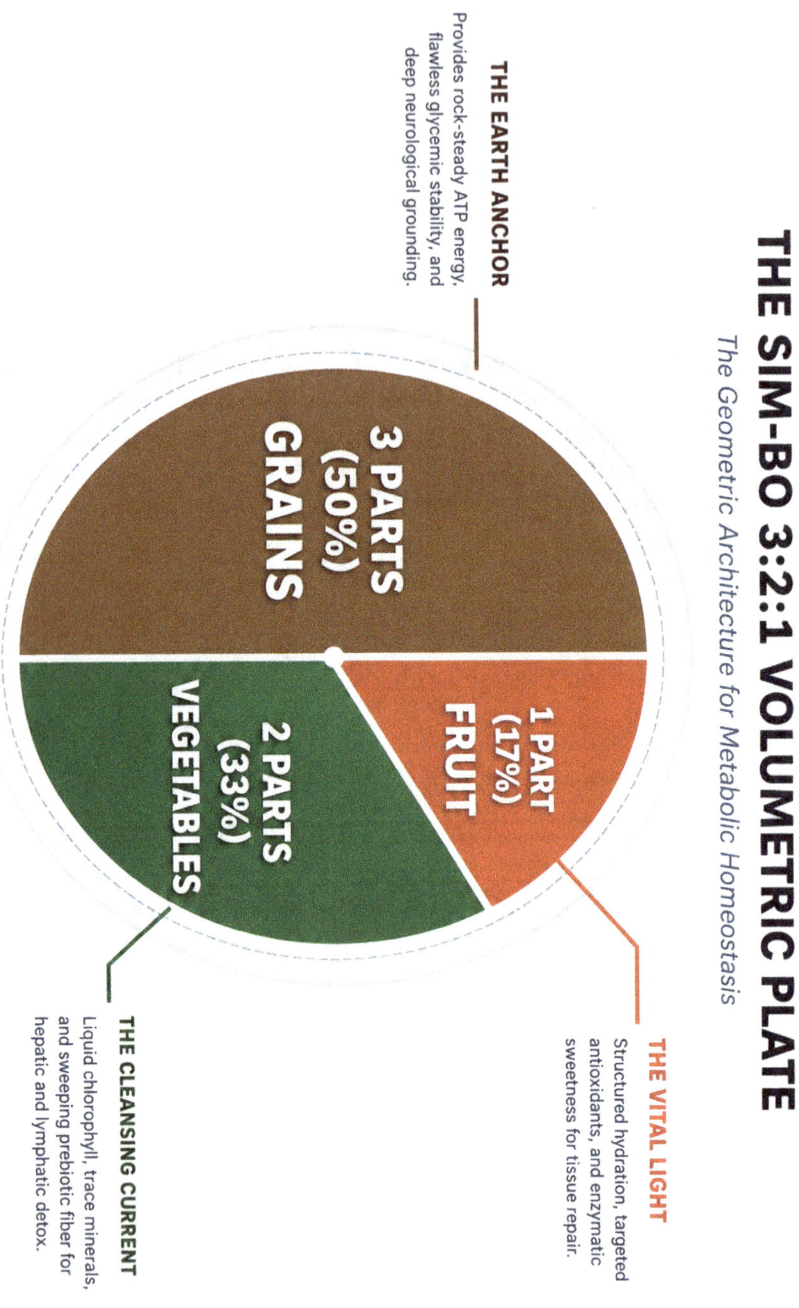

Figure 3. The Sim-Bo™ 3:2:1 volumetric plate.

Together, these three elements form a practical architecture of metabolic peace. The formula is not a prison. It is a compass.

The Future of Ratio-Based Nutrition

Clinical nutrition is beginning to outgrow the tyranny of isolated numbers. Calories matter. Protein matters. Carbohydrate and fat matter. But the larger question is architecture: how a meal is arranged, how quickly it enters circulation, how the microbiome receives it, how appetite interprets it, and how consistently the pattern is repeated.

The future of nutritional medicine will not be won by counting harder. It will be won by designing meals that the human system can read. Ratio, timing, preparation, texture, and repetition will matter as much as grams. The plate will be treated less like a ledger and more like a living instruction.

Why Proportion Works Better Than Calculation

Calculation keeps the mind busy. Proportion trains the eye. A patient can forget a number, lose a food scale, misread a label, or become anxious over a tracking app. But the eye remembers the plate. Once the ratio is learned, every meal becomes self-correcting.

This matters clinically because many patients arrive already exhausted by health information. They know too much and practice too little. They have counted grams, chased macros, purchased supplements, and downloaded food apps, yet still cannot build a plate that leaves them calm three hours later. The 3:2:1 Formula returns intelligence to the hand, the bowl, and the table.

The formula is also generous enough to respect appetite. Some days the bowl is larger. Some days it is smaller. The ratio remains. Healing does not require the personality of an accountant. It requires the discipline of a practitioner: observe, repeat, refine.

When proportion replaces calculation, food stops becoming a math problem and returns to its original role as daily architecture.

Three Parts Grain: The Ground of Energy

Intact, unrefined grains are the ground of the Sim-Bo plate. Brown rice, millet, barley, intact oats, amaranth, quinoa, and other whole grains deliver complex carbohydrate inside a physical structure that slows absorption and supports steadier energy.

A grain is not merely starch. It is architecture. Bran, germ, fiber, minerals, resistant starch, natural oils, and plant proteins arrive together. When prepared properly, this architecture offers a slow curve of glucose rather than the sharp entry of refined flour or liquid sugar.

The brain receives fuel. Skeletal muscle receives energy. The digestive tract receives bulk and rhythm.

In the Sim-Bo philosophy, grain is never a garnish. It is the foundation that allows the rest of the meal to settle. A warm bowl of brown rice, millet, or barley is humble, but humility is not weakness. The most stabilizing foods are often the least theatrical.

The grain base also has a psychological effect. It quiets the restless search for stimulation. Patients accustomed to caffeine, snacks, and refined sweets often discover that cravings soften when the morning and midday meal contain enough slow carbohydrate to anchor the day.

The Healing Grain Principle

Cook with patience. Long, steady cooking softens structure, improves tolerance, and draws out natural sweetness without added sugar.

Chew until the grain becomes soft and fluid. Digestion begins in the mouth. Chewing awakens saliva, slows the meal, and gives the vagus nerve a signal of safety.

Rotate with the seasons and constitution. Millet, barley, rice, oats, buckwheat, or other grains carry different textures, thermal qualities, and digestive effects. The practitioner learns to match the grain to the person, not merely the recipe.

When the grain base is steady, the meal stops demanding drama. It becomes ground beneath the day.

This is why grain must be prepared with respect. Undercooked grain can feel heavy and resistant. Overly refined grain can enter too quickly and fail to satisfy. Properly cooked grain occupies the middle path: soft enough to digest, intact enough to sustain, plain enough to calm the senses.

In many depleted patients, the return to warm grain is the return to center. The meal no longer pulls the system upward into stimulation or downward into heaviness. It simply holds. That holding quality is one reason brown rice receives its own full chapter after this formula is established.

Two Parts Vegetables: The Cleansing Current

If grain is ground, vegetables are movement. They bring color, fiber, mineral intelligence, bitterness, water, and the subtle chemistry that plants develop to survive wind, sun, pests, drought, and soil stress. Those same compounds help human physiology regulate oxidative pressure and inflammatory tone.

In the 3:2:1 ratio, vegetables occupy the largest visible territory of the plate. This is not decorative abundance. It is functional volume. Vegetables slow the meal, increase chewing, feed microbes, support bowel movement, and bring broad-spectrum micronutrients into the daily pattern.

Their colors carry different forms of protection.

> Deep green vegetables - kale, spinach, bok choy, collards, watercress - supply magnesium, folate, vitamin K, chlorophyll-rich pigments, and phytonutrients that support vascular health, liver pathways, and antioxidant defense.
> Orange and yellow vegetables - carrots, squash, pumpkin, sweet potato, yellow peppers - deliver carotenoids that support epithelial surfaces, mucosal integrity, skin, eyes, and immune resilience.
> Purple and red vegetables - beets, red cabbage, radicchio, purple carrots - provide anthocyanins, betalains, nitrates, and polyphenols that support endothelial function, nitric-oxide activity, circulation, and protection against oxidative strain.
> White vegetables - garlic, onion, daikon, cauliflower, turnip, cabbage cores - bring sulfur compounds, glucosinolates, pungency, and respiratory-clearing strength.
> Black and deep-purple plant foods - eggplant skin, black garlic, purple sweet potato, black mushrooms, sea vegetables - concentrate dark pigments, mineral-rich polysaccharides, and microbiome-supportive compounds.

Preparation matters. Gentle steaming, slow simmering, quick stir-frying, light fermentation, and seasonal raw foods all create different digestive effects. Raw vegetables may be excellent for a strong, warm constitution, yet cooling and taxing for a depleted patient. Cooked vegetables may be less glamorous, but they often carry medicine more gently.

Vegetables are the internal brushes of the Sim-Bo plate. They do not perform a dramatic cleanse; they provide the daily fiber, minerals, moisture, and plant intelligence that allow waste to move, microbes to feed, and the blood chemistry to soften.

The patient should learn to see vegetables not as a side dish but as the moving field of the plate. Their fibers carry waste forward. Their minerals buffer the meal. Their bitterness awakens digestion. Their color teaches the eye that nourishment has spectrum, not merely volume.

For weak digestion, the first step is often not more raw intensity. It is better preparation. Soft steaming, soup, congee vegetables, and gentle seasoning can make plant medicine absorbable. The goal is not to win a contest of rawness. The goal is to deliver vegetable intelligence in a form the patient can actually receive.

One Part Fruit: The Sweet Balance

Fruit completes the triad. It is sweetness held inside restraint. In its whole form, fruit arrives with water, soluble fiber, organic acids, fragrance, minerals, and pigments. It teaches pleasure without chaos.

Fruit belongs in Sim-Bo because healing cannot be built only on discipline. The nervous system also needs refreshment. A small portion of whole fruit, placed wisely, can cool irritability, support hydration, satisfy the desire for sweetness, and bring brightness to a simple plate.

The difference between whole fruit and fruit juice is the difference between architecture and extraction. Whole fruit requires chewing, carries fiber, slows entry, and gives satiety signals time to arise. Juice strips sweetness away from structure. What was once a living package becomes a rapid sugar stream.

Fruit is best used fresh, whole, and unprocessed. For many patients it works beautifully as a light morning element, a mid-afternoon refreshment, or a small companion to a grain-based meal. Heavy evening fruit, especially in sensitive digestion, may disturb sleep or ferment uncomfortably. Placement matters.

- Dark berries and grapes provide polyphenols and pigments that support vascular and antioxidant resilience.
- Apples and pears offer pectin and gentle fiber that can steady bowel movement and soothe digestion.
- Citrus brings acidity, aroma, vitamin C, and brightness that awakens appetite and supports tissue repair.
- Bananas and plantains offer potassium-rich grounding, especially when used with clinical judgment and proper timing.

Fruit is not a reward for virtue. It is part of the design. It reminds the patient that sweetness can live inside order.

Fruit also trains restraint. Because it is pleasant, patients are tempted to turn it into a main event. Sim-Bo keeps it in its proper place: enough to refresh, not enough to dominate. The one-part measure protects sweetness from becoming another stimulant.

This is the deeper education of the formula. It does not forbid pleasure. It gives pleasure a boundary. Within that boundary, sweetness becomes restorative rather than destabilizing.

The Hidden Fourth Element: Water and Warmth

Water is not counted in the visible 3:2:1 ratio, yet it quietly makes the entire formula possible. It dissolves nutrients, moves blood volume, supports lymphatic flow, regulates temperature, protects mucosal surfaces, and assists the kidneys in clearing metabolic by-products.

Many patients misread thirst as fatigue, hunger, or craving. A dry system asks for stimulation because it cannot move chemistry efficiently. Caffeine, sugar, and salty snacks then become poor substitutes for the basic fluid environment required for metabolism.

Hydration should be steady, not violent. Large amounts of water forced into the stomach during meals can dilute digestive concentration and create heaviness. Small, regular intake between meals is often more useful. Warm or room-temperature water is frequently better tolerated than ice-cold water, especially in patients with weak digestion, bloating, cold abdomen, or loose stool.

Herbal teas can extend hydration into therapeutic rhythm: ginger for warmth, mint for lightness, roasted barley for earthiness, jujube for gentle sweetness, chrysanthemum for heat, and other simple infusions matched to constitution.

Water conducts the 3:2:1 orchestra. Warmth gives it tempo.

Warmth is equally important. A cold meal may be clean on paper yet difficult for a depleted digestive system to transform. Warmth relaxes. Warmth opens. Warmth gives the stomach permission to receive. In clinical practice, the difference between a cold salad and a warm bowl can be the difference between bloating and comfort.

The formula therefore lives not only in ratio, but in temperature, texture, and pace. A cold, rushed 3:2:1 meal will not have the same effect as a warm, chewed, unhurried one. The architecture is the beginning. The manner of eating completes it.

How 3:2:1 Rebalances Metabolism and the Stress Axis

The 3:2:1 pattern does more than simplify shopping. It trains metabolism through repeated clarity.

Each meal provides a recognizable sequence: slow carbohydrate from grain, fiber and minerals from vegetables, light sweetness and hydration from fruit. The nervous system stops treating every meal as a surprise. The pancreas receives fewer shocks. The liver meets a steadier workload. The microbiome receives a more dependable stream of fermentable fiber.

When this structure is practiced consistently:

Blood sugar rises in a gentler curve because intact grains and vegetables slow the entry of glucose.
Fiber delays gastric emptying, supports bowel regularity, and nourishes microbes that produce short-chain fatty acids.
Fruit supplies sweetness within a whole-food matrix rather than as isolated liquid sugar.
Chewing and predictable timing support vagal tone, digestive secretion, and a calmer stress response.
Meal simplicity reduces decision fatigue and lowers the emotional charge around food.

Over time, the digestive tract begins to expect order. Patients often report steadier appetite, less bloating, fewer cravings, clearer morning energy, and a calmer relationship to meals. These changes are not magic. They are the result of removing conflicting inputs and repeating a pattern the system can interpret.

The hypothalamus, adrenal system, thyroid rhythm, reproductive axis, and digestive tract are all sensitive to timing and perceived safety. A chaotic life keeps them guessing. A stable plate becomes one of the daily signals that the environment is no longer an emergency.

This is where the formula becomes more than food. It becomes environmental medicine. The patient is no longer asking, What should I eat next? The patient begins to ask, What pattern can my physiology trust? That question changes everything.

A trustworthy pattern reduces the need for compensation. Less compensation means more reserve. Reserve is the quiet foundation of resilience: the ability to recover after stress, digest without distress, sleep without struggle, and think without constant stimulant support.

The Flow of the Day: Circadian Nutrition

The 3:2:1 formula is not only a ratio. It is a daily cadence.

Digestion follows light, temperature, movement, and rest. The liver, gut, pancreas, and microbiome all carry clocks. A meal eaten at noon is not processed in the same internal atmosphere as the same meal eaten late at night under stress. Timing is part of nutrition.

Morning: The Primer. Begin with warmth and steadiness. Soft grain porridge, congee, or brown rice with a small portion of fruit can anchor blood sugar and wake digestion gently.
Midday: The Peak. This is the strongest time for the most substantial

3:2:1 meal: generous grain, abundant vegetables, and a measured fruit element or fermented side, depending on the person.
Evening: The Taper. As darkness approaches, the meal should become lighter. Steamed vegetables and a smaller grain portion are often better tolerated than heavy protein, sugar, fried foods, or late fruit.

This solar logic is not superstition. It is behavioral respect for circadian order. When dinner is smaller and earlier, sleep receives less competition from digestion. When lunch is substantial, daytime activity can use the energy. When breakfast is warm and simple, the morning begins with steadiness rather than stimulation.

Timing teaches the organs to prepare. The meal becomes expected, and expectation reduces strain.

Adapting the Formula to Modern Life

A formula that cannot survive travel, work, family, and social meals is not a healing system. It is a fantasy. The 3:2:1 structure is durable because it can be seen with the eye and adapted without losing its center.

For demanding mornings: prepare grains and root vegetables in advance. Reheat them gently with water, broth, or tea. The goal is warmth, softness, and reliability before the day accelerates.
For social meals: keep the plate geometry quietly in mind. Choose the available grain or starch, expand the vegetables, and keep dense protein or rich foods as a smaller accent.
For transition from a meat-heavy pattern: reduce the portion before demanding total elimination. Replace part of the animal protein with beans, lentils, mushrooms, fermented soy, or other tolerated plant foods.
For cultural flexibility: every cuisine can express the pattern. Rice with greens and pear. Farro with vegetables and figs. Corn, beans, peppers, and papaya. Barley, cabbage, mushrooms, and apple. The formula respects culture while restoring proportion.

The ratio is not a restrictive rule. It is a way of seeing. Once the eye understands the structure, the patient can find it almost anywhere.

When the Formula Becomes Instinct

At first, the 3:2:1 plate is deliberate. The patient constructs it consciously: grain, vegetable, fruit; ground, movement, refreshment. After repetition, the eye begins to recognize imbalance immediately. A plate with too much dense protein feels visually heavy. A plate with no vegetable field feels inert. A meal built around dessert feels unstable before it is even eaten.

This is the restoration of instinct. Modern eating trains appetite to follow stimulation. Sim-Bo retrains appetite to recognize proportion. The palate becomes less impressed by intensity and more sensitive to steadiness. Plain food begins to taste complete because the nervous system is no longer screaming for novelty.

The formula succeeds when the patient no longer needs to force it. The structure becomes native. A good meal starts to look obvious.

The Emotional Effect of Order and the Stamina for Purpose

There is a quiet peace that only predictability can give.

When meals follow the same architecture, the mind no longer spends energy negotiating every bite. Decision fatigue decreases. Cravings become less theatrical. Hunger becomes easier to distinguish from boredom, stress, loneliness, and exhaustion.

This emotional effect is not separate from physiology. Stable meals support stable glucose. Stable glucose supports steadier mood. Adequate fiber and mineral intake support microbial and neurotransmitter pathways. Slow chewing creates time for satiety. Consistency becomes psychological medicine because it reduces the number of choices the nervous system must defend against.

Sim-Bo is not designed to produce a small life. It is designed to give the patient enough stamina to live a consequential one. A person who is always reacting to food, fatigue, cravings, and digestive distress has little reserve for leadership, service, scholarship, parenting, prayer, creativity, or mission. Order gives energy back to purpose.

The point is not dietary perfection. The point is usable life.

The Six-Week Autonomic Reset

Six weeks is long enough for repetition to become a new internal expectation. It is also short enough for a patient to practice with seriousness rather than vague intention.

During this forty-two-day reset:

Build most meals from the 3:2:1 ratio every day.
Drink warm water or simple herbal tea between meals rather than constantly sipping through digestion.
Remove hyper-processed snacks, liquid sugar, refined sweets, and unstable fried foods.

Keep meal timing within a stable window so digestion can anticipate its work.

Protect sleep as part of the formula, not as an optional wellness accessory.

Walk gently after meals when appropriate, especially after the largest meal of the day.

By the second week, many patients notice calmer digestion, clearer skin, steadier appetite, or less emotional urgency around food. By the fourth week, the pattern often begins to feel easier. By the sixth week, the formula no longer feels like an imposed rule; it begins to feel like the natural shape of a meal.

The reset works because repetition lowers internal negotiation. Physiology learns the schedule. Appetite learns the boundary. The mind learns that simplicity will not deprive it. The plate becomes familiar enough to be trusted.

Signs of Assimilation

A formula is only useful if it changes lived experience. The earliest signs are often quiet: less urgency for coffee, fewer late-night cravings, warmer digestion, better stool formation, and less anxiety around food choices. These changes matter because they show that the meal is no longer provoking the system.

Later signs are steadier: clearer skin, improved joint comfort, less morning heaviness, calmer mood, and more reliable energy between meals. Laboratory markers may also improve when the inflammatory load declines, but the first laboratory is daily life itself. The patient begins to wake, eat, work, and sleep with less internal resistance.

The 3:2:1 formula should be judged by this standard: does life become easier to inhabit? If the answer is yes, the pattern is doing its work.

The Sim-Bo Plate as Cellular Meditation

Every meal is an opportunity to train attention.

Before eating, look at the plate: the grain, the vegetables, the fruit, the steam, the color, the shape, the fragrance. This pause is not decoration. It tells the nervous system to shift from pursuit to reception.

Chew slowly enough for the food to change. Let solid become soft. Let the mouth begin the work the stomach should not have to finish alone. Stop when satisfied rather than when mechanically full. The meal becomes complete not when the plate is empty, but when the system has received enough.

Gratitude is not sentimental language. It is an organizing state. A calm mind changes posture, breath, saliva, gastric tone, and the pace of eating. The Sim-Bo plate becomes meditation because it asks the patient to return attention to the most basic act of survival: receiving nourishment with presence.

The modern habit is frantic haste. The healing habit is deliberate attention.

The Social Life of 3:2:1

A healing formula must also survive the table of other people. Food is never only chemistry. It is family, celebration, culture, memory, hospitality, grief, and belonging. Sim-Bo does not erase that reality; it gives the patient a quiet center inside it.

At a shared meal, the formula can remain invisible. Choose the grain or starch that is closest to whole. Increase the vegetables. Let fruit or a simple plant element provide completion. Keep rich foods as accent rather than center. The practitioner does not need to announce discipline. The plate announces it silently.

This is mature dietary practice. It does not require drama, argument, or superiority. It requires clarity. The patient learns to participate socially without surrendering the geometry that keeps physiology calm.

Conclusion: Eating as Alignment

The 3:2:1 Formula is more than a nutritional strategy. It is a daily pattern of alignment.

Three parts grain root the meal in steady energy.
Two parts vegetables move, mineralize, and regulate.
One part fruit refreshes the pattern with water, sweetness, and color.

Together, they restore proportion without extremism. A simple meal repeated with care can rebuild appetite, digestion, mood, energy, and trust in ordinary food. The ego may dismiss it as too plain. Physiology recognizes it as relief.

The formula teaches that healing often begins when the meal stops performing and starts supporting. Pattern is medicine. Proportion is language. Repetition is trust.

Clinical Case Study 9: Restoring the Biological Border Through the 3:2:1 Formula

Patient: Clara L., 34-year-old female, industrial architect.

Chief concerns: symmetrical joint inflammation, chronic cystic acne, brain fog, erratic digestion, painful bloating, and episodes of rapid transit. She had been told that long-term immune-directed medication might eventually be considered if symptoms continued to escalate.

Clinical Presentation

Clara's professional life revolved around structural integrity. She understood load, stress points, boundary failure, and the danger of tiny fractures in a system meant to hold. Her internal architecture showed the same principle. Years of irregular meals, refined carbohydrates, gluten-heavy convenience foods, industrial oils, and sugar had created a pattern of digestive volatility and immune overactivation.

Her problem was not a lack of willpower. It was a loss of structure. Meals arrived without proportion. Sleep arrived without cadence. Stress was constant. The gut reacted, the skin reflected it, and the joints became the visible territory of a deeper inflammatory pattern.

Her architectural training made the explanation immediate. A building fails when its borders cannot hold pressure. A digestive system also fails when its border is inflamed, overexposed, and constantly challenged by incompatible inputs. Clara needed fewer assaults and better structure.

Initial Findings

hs-CRP: 5.2 mg/L at baseline, consistent with elevated inflammatory burden.

Tongue: dusky and swollen with red petechiae and a greasy yellow root coating.

Pulse: slippery and rapid, especially in the right middle position.

Traditional Asian Medicine assessment: Spleen Qi deficiency complicated by Damp-Heat and Blood-level heat, with Liver constraint aggravating digestion under occupational stress.

The treatment principle was to restore the border: calm the gut, reduce inflammatory friction, rebuild digestive timing, clear heat, and give the immune system fewer reasons to remain on guard.

Plan and Intervention

3:2:1 Dietary Structure: Clara committed to a strict twelve-week Sim-Bo pattern centered on warm grains, cooked vegetables, low-glycemic whole fruit, stable meal timing, and removal of the foods that most consistently aggravated her digestion and skin.
Three Parts Grain: Slow-cooked millet and white-rice congee were used at the beginning because they were soft, warm, and easy to tolerate. The goal was not culinary excitement; it was mucosal calm and digestive predictability.
Two Parts Vegetables: Lightly steamed zucchini, bok choy, carrots, sweet potato, and other gentle vegetables supplied fiber, minerals, and a soothing texture while avoiding excessive raw volume during the early phase.
One Part Fruit: Low-glycemic fruit was used away from the heaviest digestive periods to provide sweetness, hydration, and antioxidant support without provoking bloating.
Protein Support: Slow-simmered broth was used strategically for collagen-rich support and digestive tolerance. It was not treated as the centerpiece of the meal.
Acupuncture: ST36 and SP6 were used to support digestive resilience and Spleen Qi; LI11 and SP10 were selected to clear heat and regulate inflammatory skin and joint patterns.
Emperor's Cupping Therapy®: sliding decompression along the posterior Bladder meridian supported tissue glide, circulation, and lymphatic movement.
Herbal Medicine: Shen Ling Bai Zhu San was used within the Traditional Asian Medicine framework to strengthen Spleen Qi, transform Dampness, and support more stable digestion.

Measured and Reported Changes

Inflammatory Marker: hs-CRP improved from 5.2 mg/L to 0.8 mg/L during the follow-up period.
Joint Symptoms: Symmetrical joint inflammation markedly decreased, with improved comfort and function by patient report.
Dermatological Status: Cystic acne cleared substantially, with no active deep lesions reported at the twelve-week visit.
Digestive Function: Bloating, pain, and rapid-transit episodes decreased; bowel rhythm became more predictable.
Cognitive State: Brain fog lifted significantly, and Clara reported steadier focus during long design sessions.
Tongue Presentation: The tongue became less swollen, color improved, and the coating became thinner and cleaner.

Reflection on the Case

Clara's case illustrates the central law of Chapter 9: structure heals by reducing noise. Her immune system did not need more novelty. It needed a stable border, a stable meal, and a stable daily cadence.

The 3:2:1 formula gave her physiology a geometry it could trust. Grain softened the energy curve. Vegetables restored movement and mineral density. Fruit returned sweetness without chaos. Timing gave digestion a boundary. Acupuncture, cupping, and botanical support helped the system settle into that new order.

The lesson is not that every inflammatory case follows one identical path. The lesson is that many dysregulated systems recover when the daily architecture stops provoking them. Clara did not heal through complexity. She healed through proportion.

Transition: From Structure to Substance

The rhythm of eating has found its shape. Now the formula must become food.

Every philosophy needs a physical anchor. For Sim-Bo, that anchor begins with a humble grain: brown rice. It is simple enough to be overlooked, steady enough to be trusted, and complete enough to become the daily ground beneath the entire method.

Within its bran, germ, starch, minerals, and fiber lies the next lesson of Sim-Bo: the ordinary can carry extraordinary intelligence when left whole, prepared with patience, and eaten with respect.

Healing rarely begins with exotic rarity. It begins with reverence for the ordinary.

Chapter 10

Brown Rice: The Healing Grain

The Humble Grain and the Architecture of Grounding

If simplicity had a flavor, it would taste like warm brown rice: quiet, nutty, steady, and quietly grounding.

Brown rice carries the entire Sim-Bo philosophy inside one ordinary grain. It is modest enough to be eaten every day and complete enough to anchor a therapeutic plate. It does not seduce the palate with intensity. It teaches the nervous system a more important lesson: nourishment does not need drama to be powerful.

Across Asian food traditions, monastic kitchens, rural households, and long-working communities, rice has served as daily ground. Brown rice, kept intact with its bran and germ, preserves more of the original architecture of the seed. In the Sim-Bo 3:2:1 formula, it represents the defining 3: the base that steadies the meal, gives warmth to digestion, and provides the slow energy on which vegetables and fruit can do their finer work.

The importance of brown rice is not exotic. Its power is ordinary repetition. A bowl eaten once is food. A bowl prepared well, chewed patiently, and repeated with discipline becomes cadence. It gives the day a nutritional floor. It tells metabolism that fuel will arrive predictably, that digestion can settle into its work, and that appetite does not need to chase stimulation every few hours.

This is why brown rice deserves its place at the center of the Sim-Bo table. It is not a magical grain. It is something more useful: a reliable grain. Reliability, repeated long enough, becomes medicine in the practical sense of the word.

The modern palate often mistakes power for intensity. Brown rice corrects that misunderstanding. Its strength is not in a dramatic biochemical spike, but in the way it lowers the need for drama altogether. It gives enough sweetness to calm craving, enough texture to engage chewing, enough starch to sustain thought, and enough fiber to keep the digestive current moving.

The Grain Anatomy: Where Structure Holds Intelligence

A single kernel of brown rice is not a blank starch pellet. It is a structured seed. Its anatomy matters because food structure determines how nourishment is received.

The Bran - The Protector: The fibrous outer layer contains insoluble fiber, B vitamins, minerals, and antioxidant compounds. It slows the meal, gives the intestine texture to work against, and supports bowel movement through natural bulk.

The Germ - The Living Core: The germ is the embryo of the seed. It carries vitamin E, small amounts of natural oils, minerals, and growth potential. It is one reason intact grains feel more nourishing than polished starches.

The Endosperm - The Fuel: The starchy center supplies carbohydrate energy. In brown rice, that fuel remains accompanied by bran and germ, which moderate its pace and make it part of a larger nutritional architecture.

When rice is polished into white rice, the bran and germ are removed. What remains is useful starch, but much of the buffering structure has been lost. White rice can still have a place in certain digestive states or cultural settings, but it does not carry the same mineral density, fiber load, or slow-release structure as the intact grain.

Brown rice teaches proportion through its own anatomy. Fuel without structure becomes speed. Structure without fuel becomes emptiness. The intact seed holds both: energy and restraint, sweetness and fiber, carbohydrate and mineral, warmth and patience.

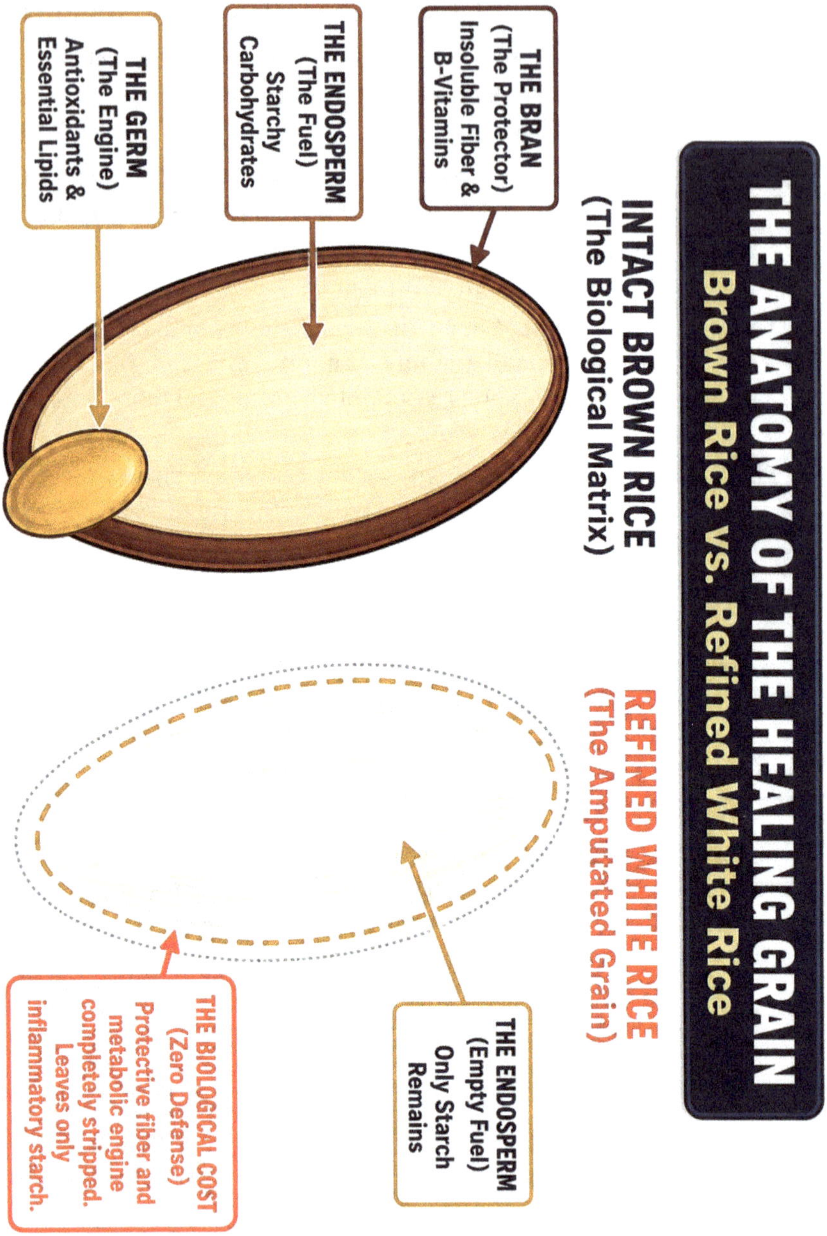

Figure 4. The anatomy of whole vs. refined grain.

Energy That Listens: The Glycemic Cadence

Refined grain moves quickly. Brown rice moves with cadence.

Its fiber, intact texture, and natural grain structure slow chewing, gastric emptying, and enzymatic access to starch. Glucose enters circulation in a steadier arc, and insulin can answer without panic. This does not make brown rice magical or universally appropriate in unlimited amounts. It makes it legible. It delivers energy with pacing.

That pacing changes the lived experience of a meal. The mind does not surge and crash. Afternoon cravings soften. Hunger becomes easier to interpret. The person feels fed rather than stimulated. In clinical life, that distinction is enormous. Stimulation asks for repetition. Nourishment allows rest.

This steady fuel explains why grain-centered meals have long supported meditation, manual work, study, and daily endurance. Deep practice requires alertness without agitation and fullness without heaviness. Properly cooked brown rice provides that middle ground: grounded energy, not nervous excitation.

In the language of Asian medicine, this is the meeting of qi and shen: physical energy steady enough to support a quiet mind. In modern terms, it is the simple elegance of a carbohydrate arriving with its own brake system.

Fiber, Bile, and Intestinal Renewal

Brown rice does not cleanse by force. It cleanses by structure.

The fiber in intact grain increases stool bulk, supports transit, and helps the bowel maintain a regular mechanical rhythm. Soluble components can interact with bile acids in the intestine, encouraging the system to use cholesterol in bile production and excretion. Insoluble fiber adds texture and movement, giving the colon a signal to keep its current flowing.

This is not a substitute for clinical lipid care when medication is required. It is the daily terrain on which lipid metabolism, bile flow, stool elimination, and microbial fermentation take place. No supplement can replace the physical contact between intact fiber and the intestinal lumen.

As the gut receives steady whole-grain fiber, the microbial ecology has a more predictable substrate. Fiber-feeding bacteria can produce short-chain fatty acids, including butyrate, which support colon-cell nourishment, barrier integrity, and immune regulation. The language here is important: brown rice supports the conditions for microbial balance. It does not instantly repair every intestinal barrier or halt every inflammatory disorder. It gives the gut something coherent to work with.

Many patients experience the change first as simplicity: less bloating, easier stool formation, reduced urgency, and a sense that the abdomen has stopped arguing with every meal. That is not theatrical detoxification. It is digestive order returning.

Minerals and Micronutrients: Earth's Quiet Blueprint

Brown rice is not valuable only because it contains carbohydrate. Its deeper value lies in the mineral and micronutrient pattern that travels with the grain.

Magnesium supports neuromuscular relaxation, vascular tone, and hundreds of enzymatic reactions. Manganese participates in antioxidant enzyme systems. B vitamins help convert carbohydrate into usable energy. Phosphorus contributes to energy transfer. Potassium supports fluid and electrical balance. None of these nutrients needs theatrical exaggeration. Their importance is greater than that. They are quiet governors of daily physiology.

This is why intact food matters. The grain does not deliver a single isolated compound. It delivers a mineral pattern inside a chewable structure, accompanied by fiber, water from cooking, texture, warmth, and satiety. The meal arrives as architecture, not fragments.

When a patient lives on refined starches, dry baked goods, sweetened beverages, and fortified processed foods, the arithmetic may appear acceptable. The deeper pattern is weak. Calories arrive without enough texture, minerals, microbial substrate, or digestive pacing. Brown rice restores a different order: slow fuel with mineral intelligence.

Protein with Proportion

Brown rice contains a modest amount of plant protein. That modesty is part of its wisdom.

The purpose of brown rice is not to behave like meat, protein powder, or a fortified bar. Its amino acids arrive gently, paired with fiber and starch, as part of a sustaining grain. When combined across the day with legumes, lentils, fermented soy foods, seeds, nuts, and vegetables, it contributes to a broader plant-protein pattern that supports repair without turning every meal into a heavy filtration event.

This is gentle completeness. Sim-Bo does not seek maximal stimulation from a single food. It seeks proportion across the plate and repetition across the week. Brown rice supplies the ground. Beans, lentils, tofu, vegetables, and seeds complete the surrounding architecture.

Protein is essential. Excess is not automatically strength. Brown rice reminds the patient that daily maintenance does not require domination by one nutrient. It requires a meal whose parts cooperate.

Texture, Warmth, and Digestive Kindness

Texture is clinical.

In the Sim-Bo kitchen, brown rice is never treated as a dry, punishing food. It is soaked, rinsed, cooked slowly, and served warm. The goal is tenderness with structure: grains expanded, hydrated, and soft enough for the digestive tract to receive without resistance.

Warm, well-cooked grain gives the stomach a different instruction than cold, dry, undercooked, or rushed food. It invites chewing. It slows the meal. It carries water into the digestive process. It reduces the need to chase flavor with salt, oil, and stimulation. Proper cooking converts austerity into comfort.

Soaking and thorough rinsing also express respect for the grain and the patient. They improve texture, help remove surface residues, and may reduce some mineral-binding effects of phytates. For people who eat brown rice frequently, sourcing matters as well. Rotating grains, rinsing carefully, cooking with adequate water, and choosing reliable sources are not acts of fear; they are acts of mastery.

The act of eating should not be a contest between willpower and digestion. A therapeutic grain must comfort the system it is meant to nourish. Brown rice teaches kindness through heat, water, patience, and chewing.

What Modern Nutrition Confirms

Modern nutrition gives language to what traditional kitchens learned through repetition: intact grains behave differently from stripped starches.

Brown rice and other whole grains provide fiber, resistant starch, vitamins, minerals, and antioxidant compounds such as phenolics and gamma-oryzanol. These features can support steadier glucose response, bowel regularity, lipid metabolism, microbial fermentation, and vascular health when they replace refined grain products within a broader whole-food pattern.

The key phrase is broader pattern. Brown rice cannot rescue a diet built on fried oils, sweetened beverages, sleepless nights, and chronic stress. It is not a pharmaceutical object. It is a structural anchor. Its effect becomes most meaningful when paired with vegetables, fruit, hydration, walking, regular sleep, and the calm repetition of the Sim-Bo method.

This is the difference between isolated nutrition and architectural nutrition. A nutrient acts. A pattern teaches. Brown rice teaches metabolism through repetition: slow energy, enough fiber, enough texture, enough warmth, enough restraint.

The Daily Practice of Rice and Parasympathetic Tone

In Sim-Bo, rice is not only eaten. It is practiced.

The practice begins before cooking. Measure the grain. Rinse until the water clears. Soak when time allows. Cook slowly. Let the aroma fill the kitchen. Serve it warm. Sit down. Chew. Do not treat the meal as background noise while the mind continues working.

This sequence matters because the nervous system reads ritual. Predictable preparation lowers urgency. Warm food signals safety. Slow chewing activates the first phase of digestion. The meal becomes a daily training in parasympathetic tone.

Patients often describe feeling anchored after switching from dry, processed starches to warm brown rice. The change is not only macronutrient chemistry. It is the felt experience of a meal that has boundaries. It begins, it nourishes, and it ends. It does not demand another hit of sweetness twenty minutes later.

A rushed person eats to silence hunger. A regulated person eats to enter relationship with nourishment. Brown rice, prepared with patience, trains that relationship.

Cultural Reverence and the Biology of Gratitude

Cultures that revered rice understood something modern eating has nearly lost: food is not merely consumption. It is continuity.

In Korea, rice has long been tied to the language of care and wellbeing. In Japan, rice cultivation has carried ceremonial meaning and communal discipline. In India and across many agrarian cultures, grain has symbolized survival, offering, and gratitude. These traditions did not need laboratory language to know that a meal eaten with reverence enters differently than a meal swallowed in agitation.

Gratitude does not need to be sentimental to be physiological. A calm state supports breath depth, vagal tone, salivation, gastric readiness, and digestive ease. Reverence slows the hand. It lengthens chewing. It turns the meal from an extraction of calories into a moment of order.

Brown rice is humble enough to receive this reverence without becoming theater. It asks for nothing exotic. It asks for water, heat, time, and attention. The patient who learns to give those four things to a grain often begins giving them back to life.

The Grain and the Gut: The Microbiome Command Center

The gut microbiome thrives on consistency.

Modern eating overwhelms microbial ecology with erratic inputs: sweeteners, emulsifiers, refined starch, alcohol, irregular timing, low fiber, and constant novelty. Brown rice moves in the opposite direction. It provides a steady substrate that beneficial organisms can adapt to, ferment, and incorporate into a more stable internal terrain.

Resistant starch and whole-grain fiber support fermentation. The short-chain fatty acids produced through that fermentation help maintain colon health and immune communication. The result is not a single dramatic event. It is gradual ecological training. Microbes respond to what is repeatedly fed.

This is why Sim-Bo does not chase endless superfoods. The microbiome does not need a new exotic command every morning. It needs reliable terrain: grain, vegetables, fruit, hydration, timing, and rest. Brown rice offers the ground on which that terrain can become steady.

The Spirit of Sufficiency

There is power in doing one simple thing well.

Modern appetite is trained to distrust sufficiency. It seeks novelty, intensity, customization, and constant upgrade. Brown rice refuses that game. It is not rare. It is not flashy. It does not promise instant transformation. It teaches the harder virtue: enough.

A warm bowl of rice, eaten slowly, says that nourishment can be quiet. It says that a meal does not need to entertain every emotional wound. It says that the nervous system can stop negotiating with stimulation and return to ordinary satisfaction.

This spirit of sufficiency is central to Sim-Bo. The goal is not to shrink life into blandness. The goal is to make food simple enough that actual life can become vivid again. When the plate stops shouting, the mind begins to hear.

The Three Clinical Jobs of Brown Rice

In the Sim-Bo system, brown rice performs three clinical jobs at once: it steadies energy, gives the bowel structure, and lowers the decision load of the meal.

First, it steadies energy. Many modern patients live between stimulation and collapse: coffee, sweet snack, crash, more coffee, late meal, poor sleep. Brown rice interrupts that pattern by providing slow fuel that does not need to shout. The patient begins to feel the difference between being stimulated and being nourished.

Second, it gives the bowel structure. The intestine is not only a chemical tube; it is a muscular, microbial, and neurological organ that responds to texture. A smooth drink, a processed bar, or a refined pastry disappears too quickly to teach the bowel much. A warm bowl of intact grain asks the system to participate: chew, secrete, churn, ferment, move, and eliminate.

Third, it lowers decision load. Healing often fails not because the patient lacks information, but because there are too many choices. Brown rice removes the argument. It becomes the reliable center around which vegetables, fruit, herbs, and small supportive additions can rotate. The plate stops being a negotiation and becomes a practice.

These three jobs explain why an ordinary grain can have an extraordinary clinical role. It is not extraordinary because it is rare. It is extraordinary because it is repeatable.

Quality, Sourcing, and Preparation

A food used daily must be chosen with discipline. Brown rice is grounding, but daily use requires care: proper sourcing, careful rinsing, adequate cooking water, and intelligent rotation when the patient needs variety.

The Sim-Bo method does not ask the patient to worship a single grain blindly. It asks the patient to learn the difference between a therapeutic anchor and a careless habit. Choose rice from reliable sources. Rinse it well. Soak it when time allows. Cook it fully. Store it properly. Do not leave cooked grains sitting for long hours at unsafe temperatures. A simple food still deserves exact handling.

This attention is not fear. It is culinary medicine. Every step changes the final instruction: the soaking softens, the rinsing clears, the simmering hydrates, the resting finishes, and the chewing completes what heat began. A hurried bowl of undercooked rice is not the same medicine as a warm, expanded grain prepared with care.

Some patients digest brown rice beautifully from the first week. Others need a transitional phase: more water, longer cooking, smaller portions, or a temporary blend with millet, barley, soft oats, or white rice during acute digestive weakness. Authority in clinical nutrition does not mean forcing one rule onto every constitution. It means holding the principle steady while adjusting the texture, timing, and amount so the patient can actually heal.

Common Mistakes with a Healing Grain

Brown rice fails when it is treated like punishment.

The first mistake is dryness. Dry rice demands too much from a depleted digestive tract. It sits heavily, absorbs fluid, and becomes hard work. Therapeutic rice should be moist, warm, and tender. The grain must be whole, but it must not be harsh.

The second mistake is excess. Because brown rice is the base of the Sim-Bo plate, some patients assume more is always better. The 3 in the 3:2:1 formula is a proportion, not permission to overload. Too much grain, even whole grain, can still create heaviness when movement is low, sleep is poor, or insulin sensitivity is compromised. The plate must remain balanced with vegetables, fruit, hydration, and walking.

The third mistake is loneliness on the plate. Brown rice was never meant to stand alone as a dry mountain. It belongs with vegetables, mineral broth, fermented elements when tolerated, gentle oils when needed, herbs, and seasonal fruit at the right time. The grain provides ground; the rest of the plate provides movement, color, moisture, and lift.

The fourth mistake is emotional impatience. Many patients expect the grain to entertain them. Brown rice will not do that. It offers a different gift: the recalibration of appetite. After several weeks, the palate begins to detect its quiet sweetness. Cravings that once demanded intensity begin to loosen. The patient discovers that boredom was not the absence of pleasure; it was the doorway into subtler pleasure.

The Brown Rice Bowl as a Clinical Instrument

A properly prepared Sim-Bo rice bowl is a clinical instrument because it standardizes the meal.

In a chaotic diet, every meal is a new experiment. The clinician cannot easily identify what caused bloating, fatigue, reflux, cravings, or sleep disruption because the inputs change constantly. Brown rice brings the baseline into focus. When the grain anchor is steady, reactions become easier to read. Vegetables can be rotated. Fruit timing can be adjusted. Protein can be tested. Hydration can be observed. The meal becomes diagnostic without becoming obsessive.

This is one reason patients often feel relief when the food becomes simple. The relief is not only biochemical. It is cognitive. Fewer decisions. Fewer ingredients. Fewer arguments with appetite. Fewer chances for the nervous system to brace against the unknown. The rice bowl becomes a daily place of return.

For the practitioner, this matters. Brown rice gives a controlled foundation on which other interventions can be evaluated. Acupuncture, cupping, herbs, breath, walking, and sleep timing all work more clearly when the dietary background is not chaotic. Sim-Bo does not flatten individuality; it removes the noise that hides individuality.

Brown Rice and the 3:2:1 Plate

Brown rice reaches its full therapeutic meaning only when it remains inside proportion. A grain can anchor the meal; it should not swallow the meal. Sim-Bo is never the worship of one ingredient. It is the mastery of relationship.

In the 3:2:1 Formula, brown rice supplies the largest grounding share of complex energy. Vegetables bring movement, minerals, color, and regulatory chemistry. Fruit completes the pattern with water, brightness, fragrance, and gentle sweetness. The grain holds. The vegetables move. The fruit lifts. The three parts prevent one another from becoming excessive.

This is why a rice-only practice is not the full Sim-Bo method. A bowl of rice alone can be clinically useful for short digestive resets, but the daily architecture needs the cleansing current of vegetables and the lightness of fruit. It also needs water, chewing, walking, sleep, and timing. The grain speaks best when the rest of life answers in the same language of steadiness.

Many patients fail when they imitate fragments of traditional food cultures without preserving the whole pattern. They eat rice without walking, fruit without timing, vegetables without warmth, and protein without proportion. Brown rice works best when the entire day supports it: morning light, regular meals, quiet chewing, and enough physical movement to use the energy it provides.

The practical plate is simple: warm rice as ground, cooked vegetables as movement, fruit as light, water as medium, and attention as the final ingredient. The formula is plain enough for a child to see and disciplined enough for a clinician to trust.

Common Mistakes With the Healing Grain

The healing grain can be mishandled. When brown rice fails a patient, the problem is often not the rice itself. It is preparation, proportion, timing, or digestive readiness.

Serving it dry and hard: Undercooked brown rice can aggravate bloating in depleted patients. During the therapeutic phase, the grain should be fully hydrated and tender.

Eating it cold without awareness: Some patients tolerate cooled grain well, but many stressed or cold digestive patterns respond better to warmth. Warmth is part of the instruction.

Drowning it in stimulation: Excess oil, salt, hot sauce, sweet sauce, or heavy toppings can turn the grain into a carrier for cravings rather than an anchor for regulation.

Treating it as unlimited: Brown rice is stabilizing, not limitless. The plate still requires vegetables, fruit, water, and proportion.

Using it without chewing: The mouth must participate. Rice swallowed too quickly becomes a digestive load rather than a calming food.

A therapeutic staple must be used with intelligence. Brown rice does not ask to dominate the meal. It asks to ground it.

Brown Rice and the Nervous System

One of the most striking clinical shifts after a return to warm whole grain is not only digestive. It is neurological. Patients often describe fewer cravings, less afternoon panic, reduced dependence on stimulants, and a steadier mood. The mechanism is not mystical. The nervous system is highly sensitive to glucose volatility, mineral availability, gut irritation, and the emotional state in which food is received.

A refined breakfast can throw the day into pursuit: spike, crash, caffeine, craving, irritation, another snack, another correction. Brown rice interrupts that pursuit. It offers fuel that arrives with less drama. It gives the morning a ground.

Chewing warm rice also slows behavior. It is difficult to eat properly prepared brown rice with the same unconscious speed as a sweetened drink or a processed snack. The texture requires contact. The mouth participates. The breath slows. The meal becomes less like stimulation and more like settlement.

This is why brown rice often works quietly on emotional reactivity. The grain does not sedate the mind. It removes unnecessary disturbance. Calm is not imposed from the outside; it appears when internal swings become steadier.

The Discipline of Repetition

Modern appetite worships variety. Healing often begins with sameness.

Repetition is not failure of imagination. It is the way physiology learns safety. The pancreas learns the curve. The stomach learns the texture. The microbiome learns the fiber. The mind learns that the next meal does not need to be negotiated. A repeated bowl of brown rice becomes an agreement between patient and physiology.

At first, repetition may feel like boredom. Then the palate changes. Subtle sweetness appears. The fragrance of the grain becomes reassuring. The absence of overstimulation begins to feel like relief. What once seemed too plain becomes the taste of stability.

This is the deeper secret of the healing grain. It does not create transformation by force. It creates the conditions in which recovery can repeat itself.

Clinical Uses of the Brown Rice Anchor

The brown rice anchor is not used the same way in every patient. Its value lies in adaptability inside a disciplined framework.

For unstable appetite: Brown rice provides a predictable morning or midday base that reduces the hunt for stimulant foods and sweet corrections later in the day.

For digestive depletion: The grain is cooked wetter, softer, and warmer, often closer to porridge or congee, so the digestive system receives nourishment with less effort.

For metabolic sluggishness: The portion remains measured and is paired with a generous volume of vegetables, followed by walking, so the fuel is used rather than stored.

For emotional agitation: The meal is kept plain and repeated at the same hour, allowing the nervous system to associate food with safety rather than novelty.

For patients transitioning away from processed starches: Brown rice replaces bread, crackers, cereal, pastries, and snack foods without forcing the person into hunger or deprivation.

This is the clinician's task: not to prescribe rice as a slogan, but to choose the texture, portion, timing, and pairing that match the patient's terrain. The same grain can ground one person, overfill another, or stabilize a third. Mastery lives in proportion.

Sim-Bo therefore treats brown rice as a foundation, not a commandment. The foundation is strong because it can carry adjustment: wetter or drier, larger or smaller, morning or midday, paired with greens or roots, supported by beans or kept very plain. The grain remains simple; the application remains precise.

Conclusion: The Seed of Simplicity

A single grain of brown rice contains the lesson of the entire path: wholeness, patience, proportion, and return.

Its bran teaches structure. Its germ teaches continuity. Its endosperm teaches fuel. Its cooking teaches time. Its chewing teaches presence. Its repetition teaches trust.

In an age of processed abundance, brown rice is not an escape into the past. It is a deliberate restoration of order. It reminds us that health is not built by chasing endless novelty, but by returning to the few daily practices that physiology can understand and trust.

The seed is small. The discipline is large. Grain by grain, meal by meal, day by day, the Sim-Bo path rebuilds the ground beneath healing.

Clinical Case Study 10

Restoring Grounding Through Brown Rice

Patient: Margaret H., 62-year-old female, retired academic.

Chief concerns: Morning stiffness, thinning hair, dry skin, low mood, low appetite, post-meal fatigue, and progressive loss of strength. Her conventional laboratory results had been described as acceptable for age, yet she felt as if her physical reserve was steadily narrowing.

Clinical Presentation

Margaret illustrates the cost of living for years on refined, dry carbohydrates: crackers, toast, pastries, sweetened coffee, and packaged grain products that filled the stomach without rebuilding the terrain. Her meals were technically sufficient in calories, but poor in structure. She was fed by starch, yet deprived of the intact grain matrix that slows glucose, delivers minerals, and gives the bowel fiber to work with.

Her presentation carried the marks of depletion: dry skin, brittle hair, morning stiffness, poor muscular tone, shallow sleep, and a quiet depression that did not feel emotional in origin as much as constitutional. She described herself as "drying out from the inside."

Within the Traditional Asian Medicine framework, her tongue and pulse suggested Kidney Yin and Jing depletion complicated by Spleen Qi weakness. In practical nutritional language, she lacked warm, mineral-rich, structured food capable of providing steady fuel and digestive confidence.

Initial Findings

hs-CRP: 3.1 mg/L, consistent with low-grade inflammatory burden.

Tongue: Thin and dry, with scattered cracks and reduced moisture.

Pulse: Deep, thready, and weak across multiple positions.

Functional pattern: Low reserve, dry tissue signs, poor morning mobility, and weak digestive transformation.

Treatment Direction

The clinical priority was grounding. Margaret did not need another stimulating protocol. She needed warmth, mineral density, digestive rhythm, and a reliable carbohydrate anchor that could replace dry refined products without shocking her appetite or digestion.

Dietary reset: Dry baked goods, refined grain products, sweetened drinks, and late-night starch snacks were removed.

Brown rice anchor: Soaked, rinsed, slow-cooked brown rice became the daily grain foundation, paired with vegetables, fruit, hydration, and consistent meal timing.

Acupuncture: KI3, CV4, BL23, ST36, and SP6 were used to support Kidney-Spleen patterns, digestive resilience, and constitutional reserve.

Cupping therapy: Gentle decompression was applied along the lumbar and sacral regions to reduce myofascial restriction, support local circulation, and ease morning stiffness.

Botanical support: Liu Wei Di Huang Wan was used within the Traditional Asian Medicine framework to nourish Yin, support fluid regulation, and address signs of dryness and constitutional depletion.

Clinical Progress Over Twelve Weeks

Inflammatory marker: hs-CRP improved from 3.1 mg/L to 0.6 mg/L during the follow-up period.

Morning stiffness: The deep, grinding sensation on waking markedly decreased, and movement became easier within the first hour of the day.

Physical vitality: She reported steadier energy, improved appetite, and greater confidence walking and climbing stairs.

Digestive pattern: Post-meal heaviness decreased; bowel rhythm became more regular with fewer dry stools.

Skin and hair: Dryness softened by patient report, and hair shedding slowed during the course of care.

Tongue presentation: Moisture improved and cracking appeared less pronounced within TAM observation.

Clinical Insight

Margaret did not improve because brown rice acted as a supernatural remedy. She improved because her daily foundation changed. Refined fragments were replaced by intact structure. Dry starch was replaced by warm grain. Erratic eating was replaced by cadence. The digestive system received a pattern it could trust.

Her case demonstrates Chapter 10's core lesson: carbohydrate quality is not a minor detail. The structure of the grain determines the structure of the message. When fuel arrives with fiber, minerals, warmth, water, and repetition, metabolism receives instruction instead of confusion.

Brown rice restored ground. From that ground, the rest of her healing had a place to stand.

The deeper lesson is practical. A depleted patient often does not need a more elaborate plan; she needs a food she can repeat without fear, digest without strain, and trust without constant calculation. For Margaret, brown rice became that food. It did not replace the rest of care. It organized the rest of care.

Transition: From Earth to Light

Every healing system needs both ground and brightness. Brown rice anchors the Sim-Bo plate with warmth, weight, steadiness, and endurance. It gives the digestive tract something dependable and gives metabolism a floor beneath its feet.

But healing cannot remain only in the earth element. Once the system is grounded, it must also be refreshed. The plasma must move. The lymph must lighten. The mind must lift. Color, fragrance, water, and sweetness must enter without chaos.

This is where fruit arrives.

If brown rice is earth, fruit is light made edible. It carries water, color, aroma, and quick renewal. It teaches that sweetness does not need to become addiction when it remains whole, seasonal, and properly timed.

The path begins in the soil. It rises toward the orchard.

Chapter 11

Fruits: Nature's Targeted Medicine

The Sweetness of Healing

The first medicine any human being tastes is sweetness.

Before language, before preference, before discipline, sweetness tells the nervous system that life is safe enough to receive. Breast milk carries that first message through fat, lactose, warmth, rhythm, and contact. Ripe fruit carries a later version of the same intelligence through water, fiber, color, aroma, mineral order, acidity, and natural sugar held inside living structure.

Modern industry corrupted sweetness by tearing it away from its orchard. Cane sugar was crystallized. Corn syrup was concentrated. Fruit flavor was imitated without fruit architecture. What once arrived with fiber, water, potassium, organic acids, polyphenols, and chewing became a naked signal of pleasure without restraint.

The Sim-Bo view restores sweetness to its rightful place. Fruit is not candy. It is not decoration. It is the light element of the therapeutic plate: bright, hydrating, colorful, cleansing in tempo, and emotionally satisfying without the violence of refined sugar. Brown rice grounds the meal. Vegetables move the current. Fruit lifts, refreshes, and completes.

This is the distinction that matters. Refined sugar excites. Whole fruit communicates. One shouts through the bloodstream. The other speaks through matrix, color, texture, fragrance, and season. One leaves appetite louder than before. The other teaches the palate that pleasure can have an ending.

Color as Clinical Intelligence

Fruit announces its medicine through color.

Red, orange, yellow, green, blue, purple, and white are not aesthetic accidents. They are visible signatures of phytochemicals created by plants to survive sun, wind, oxidation, microbes, insects, drought, and time. When eaten intact, those pigments become part of human resilience.

- Red fruits - strawberries, cherries, pomegranates, red grapes - carry anthocyanins, ellagic acid, lycopene-related pigments, and vascular-supportive polyphenols. They belong to circulation, endothelial flexibility, and the red river of blood.

- Orange and yellow fruits - citrus, mango, papaya, persimmon, apricot - bring carotenoids, flavonoids, vitamin C complexes, and aromatic acids. They belong to mucosal resilience, skin integrity, connective tissue, and immune tone.
- Green fruits - kiwi, green apple, lime, honeydew, avocado when used botanically as fruit - offer organic acids, chlorophyll-associated compounds, potassium, and refreshing sharpness. They belong to bile flow, digestive movement, and the clean edge of appetite.
- Blue and purple fruits - blueberries, blackberries, black grapes, plums - concentrate dark-spectrum polyphenols. They belong to the brain, microcirculation, oxidative defense, and the protection of delicate tissue under stress.
- White and pale fruits - Asian pear, banana, coconut flesh, lychee, white peach - provide moisture, potassium, pectin, and soothing texture. They belong to the stomach, lungs, hydration, and recovery from dryness.

A bowl of fruit is more than a beautiful plate. It is a spectrum of plant intelligence. The colors do not need to be counted with anxiety. They need to be eaten with attention. In clinical practice, the instruction can be simple: eat color, and let the counting mind rest.

The deeper principle is not variety for novelty's sake. It is diversity with coherence. A patient does not need an exotic superfruit from another continent to heal. A local berry, a ripe pear, a seasonal citrus, a simple apple prepared well - these can carry more value than a shelf full of imported powders.

Fruit as Hydration with Structure

Fruit hydrates differently from plain water because it arrives with structure.

Inside a living fruit, water is held with soluble fiber, pectins, organic acids, potassium, magnesium, trace minerals, and plant compounds. This matrix slows release, supports bowel movement, helps regulate electrolyte balance, and gives digestion something intelligent to work with. Bulk water is essential; fruit adds texture, minerals, and metabolic companionship.

Coffee, alcohol, salty packaged foods, chronic stress, and dry processed snacks leave many patients living in a state of low-grade internal dryness. Their mouths may not feel thirsty, but their stool is hard, skin is dull, muscles cramp, urine is concentrated, and afternoon fatigue arrives with strange force. Fruit often corrects this pattern more gracefully than another stimulant or another supplement.

Melons, citrus, pears, grapes, kiwi, and berries are especially useful when heat, exertion, constipation, skin irritation, or thick appetite patterns dominate. In Traditional Asian Medicine, many fruits are understood as cooling, moistening, and fluid-restoring. In modern nutritional language, they provide water, potassium, fiber, acids, and antioxidant compounds in a form digestion recognizes.

Fruit is not a replacement for hydration discipline. It is hydration with intelligence. It moistens without heaviness, refreshes without caffeine, and cools without forcing the system into collapse.

Fiber: The Orchard's Moderator

The modern fear of fruit usually begins with sugar. That fear dissolves when the whole structure is understood.

Fruit sugar is not delivered alone. In intact fruit, glucose and fructose arrive inside cell walls, surrounded by soluble fiber, insoluble fiber, water, acids, minerals, and polyphenols. Chewing slows the process. Fiber slows gastric emptying. Pectin forms a viscous gel. Microbes ferment what human enzymes cannot digest. The bloodstream receives sweetness through a moderated gate.

Commercial juice breaks that gate. Sweetened dried fruit concentrates the signal. Syrups and fruit-flavored products erase the orchard while keeping the seduction. The clinical issue is not fruit. The issue is fruit stripped of its architecture.

Soluble fiber stabilizes the meal by thickening intestinal contents and slowing absorption. Insoluble fiber adds volume, mechanical movement, and stool structure. Together, they support regular elimination, bind bile acids, feed microbial fermentation, and reduce the pressure toward artificial sweetness.

Many patients who fear fruit are not reacting to fruit itself. They are reacting to years of liquid sugar, processed snacks, stress eating, and digestive instability. When whole fruit is reintroduced in a simple pattern - usually one or two types at a time, eaten away from heavy meals - the system often receives it with surprising calm.

Fruit, Liver Flow, and the Morning Current

The liver works in silence.

It processes hormones, bile, alcohol, medications, environmental compounds, bacterial by-products, amino acid residues, and the ordinary chemistry of life. It does not need punishment. It needs less congestion and better support.

Whole fruit provides several forms of that support: vitamin C complexes, flavonoids, organic acids, water, potassium, soluble fiber, and polyphenols. Citrus peel compounds, apple pectin, berry anthocyanins, grape polyphenols, and pear moisture each contribute a different kind of assistance to the digestive-liver axis.

The old ritual of warm water with lemon in the morning survives because it is simple and physiologically sensible. Warmth softens the stomach. Sourness wakes the mouth. Aroma signals freshness. The ritual does not need mystical exaggeration. It is useful because it is gentle, repeatable, and easy to integrate into a clean morning cadence.

Grapefruit deserves special respect. It is metabolically active and can interact with several medications by affecting drug metabolism. In a book about reducing dependence on unnecessary rescue, this point is not a timid warning; it is clinical intelligence. Powerful foods must be used with precision.

The morning is the natural window for fruit because the system is moving from overnight repair into daytime activity. A light fruit meal, or fruit followed later by warm grain, can help complete the night-to-day transition without dragging the stomach immediately into heaviness.

Timing: When Sweetness Becomes Clear

Fruit is simple, but timing gives it elegance.

In the Sim-Bo cadence, fruit is usually best eaten alone, in the morning, or between major meals. For sensitive digestion, it is often better twenty minutes before a heavier meal than immediately after dense starch, oil, or animal protein. This is not superstition. It is digestive sequencing.

Fruit moves quickly. Heavy meals move slowly. When a fast, watery food is placed on top of a dense, fatty, protein-heavy meal, some patients experience bloating, gas, pressure, reflux tendency, or fermentation discomfort. The solution is not fear. The solution is order.

Late-night fruit requires judgment. Small amounts of stewed pear or warm apple may be useful for dryness, constipation, or lung irritation. Large portions of cold, very sweet tropical fruit at night can disturb sleep in patients with unstable glucose, weak digestion, or cold abdominal patterns. Timing determines whether fruit acts as refreshment or interference.

Simplicity applies here with force. One or two fruits at a sitting are usually more therapeutic than a chaotic fruit salad. The digestive system reads uniformity more easily. A bowl of berries, a ripe pear, a small plate of citrus, a banana after exertion - each has a clean message.

Antioxidants and Oxidative Rust

Every living cell must burn oxygen to create energy. This process leaves behind reactive molecules. In small amounts, those molecules participate in adaptation. In excess, they become oxidative rust.

Stress, pollution, poor sleep, inflammation, ultraviolet light, high blood sugar, alcohol, and processed oils all increase that rust. DNA, mitochondria, collagen, blood vessels, fascia, skin, and cell membranes all pay the price when oxidative pressure exceeds repair capacity.

Fruit is one of nature's most elegant answers to this problem. The pigments in berries, cherries, grapes, citrus, kiwi, pomegranate, and plums deliver polyphenols, carotenoids, flavonoids, and vitamin C complexes in a food matrix built for synergy. They do not arrive as isolated laboratory fragments. They arrive with fiber, water, acids, texture, fragrance, and satiety.

This is why whole fruit differs from a high-dose antioxidant pill. The pill isolates. The fruit orchestrates. The pill may deliver a compound. The fruit delivers a pattern.

Daily fruit consumption is not dramatic. Its strength is steady maintenance. A handful of berries, a pear, a citrus fruit, or a sliced apple does not announce itself like a drug. It quietly contributes to the ongoing work of protecting vessels, collagen, neurons, fascia, skin, and the gut lining from the ordinary friction of life.

The Emotional Signature of Natural Sweetness

Sweetness is emotional before it is intellectual.

The taste of ripe fruit touches memory, safety, childhood, summer, celebration, and relief. Refined sugar exploits that pathway. Whole fruit completes it.

Artificial sweeteners and refined sweets stimulate expectation without delivering the full architecture of nourishment. They create the sensation of reward while bypassing the fiber, minerals, water, and digestive completion that tell the system the experience is finished.

Craving remains open. The loop asks to be repeated.

Fruit has an ending. Its fiber slows the pleasure. Its water refreshes. Its acids brighten the palate. Its minerals settle the system. Its chewing requirement restores participation. After a ripe pear or a bowl of berries, the nervous system receives not only sweetness, but completion.

This is why fruit can become emotional hygiene in the Sim-Bo method. It replaces frantic craving with clean pleasure. It teaches that sweetness does not need to become addiction, and restraint does not need to become punishment. Pleasure and order can live in the same bowl.

Seasonal Fruit and Environmental Timing

Fruit is the most seasonal of the Sim-Bo triad.

In spring and summer, watery fruits answer heat, sweating, sunlight, movement, and outward expansion. Melons, berries, citrus, stone fruits, and grapes cool and refresh. They belong to long days, heat, perspiration, and active life.

In autumn, apples, pears, persimmons, and late grapes carry a different instruction. They are less explosive, more grounding, and better suited to dryness, lung sensitivity, and the descent toward cooler weather. In winter, fruit often works best warmed, baked, stewed, or paired with ginger, cinnamon, or a small amount of cooked grain. The same fruit that refreshes in July may chill digestion in January if eaten cold and excessive.

Seasonal eating reduces argument with the environment. It allows the outer climate and inner terrain to cooperate. Sim-Bo does not demand rigid rules detached from place. It asks the patient to observe: Is the day hot or cold? Is digestion strong or weak? Is the tongue dry or damp? Is the patient depleted, overheated, constipated, swollen, agitated, or dull?

Fruit trains this observation beautifully. Its cycles are visible. Its colors change. Its texture ripens and declines. It reminds the modern eater that nourishment is not abstract information floating outside time. It is seasonal intelligence.

The Morning Cleansing Cycle

Morning fruit works because it respects the direction of the day.

After sleep, the system is moving from repair toward movement. The mouth is dry, the liver has processed the night, the colon is ready to empty, and the nervous system needs gentle light rather than heavy force. Fruit answers that state with water, fiber, acidity, color, and brightness.

A breakfast of fresh fruit alone, or fruit followed later by warm brown rice, is not a cleanse in the theatrical sense. It is a lighter opening. It allows elimination to continue before the stomach is asked to handle dense protein, oil, and heavy combinations.

For patients with sluggish bowels, dry skin, sugar cravings, dull morning appetite, or afternoon crashes, a disciplined morning fruit practice can restore a clean digestive beginning. The effect is not produced by deprivation. It is produced by sequence.

The morning rule is simple: begin with light before weight. Let freshness enter before density. Let the day open before the digestive system is asked to carry a load.

For some patients, this practice becomes the first honest appetite lesson of the day. They discover whether they are truly hungry, thirsty, anxious, constipated, depleted, or simply reaching for coffee out of habit. Fruit exposes the difference because it is clean enough to be read.

The Fructose Myth

Modern dieting has taught many people to fear fruit because it contains fructose. This fear confuses molecule with matrix.

Fructose in soda, syrup, sweetened beverages, candy, and industrial desserts is concentrated, fast, fiberless, and easy to overconsume. Fructose in whole fruit arrives with chewing, water, pectin, minerals, acids, and satiety. The metabolic experience is different because the architecture is different.

Whole fruit does not behave like high-fructose corn syrup. A whole orange is not orange soda. A bowl of berries is not a pastry. An apple is not a candy bar with vitamins attached. Fruit must be judged in its natural form.

The danger begins when fruit is juiced, dried with added sugar, blended into oversized liquid meals, coated, canned in syrup, or eaten in large quantities without attention to constitution and timing. In those forms, fruit begins to lose the discipline that makes it medicinal.

For patients with advanced glucose dysregulation, severe insulin resistance, or active digestive instability, fruit selection and timing matter. Berries, kiwi, citrus, pears, and apples often serve better than large portions of tropical fruit. The principle is not fear. It is precision.

Fruit and the Microbiome

Fruit also speaks to the intestinal ecosystem.

The colon is not a waste pipe. It is a fermentation chamber, an immune training ground, and a metabolic partner. When whole fruit reaches the lower digestive tract, its pectin, resistant starch fragments, polyphenols, and soluble fibers become substrate for microbial work. Beneficial organisms transform these residues into short-chain fatty acids and other metabolites that influence gut-barrier integrity, inflammatory tone, bowel movement, and appetite regulation.

This is one reason whole fruit behaves so differently from refined sweets. Refined sugar feeds speed. Whole fruit feeds ecology. The first creates a fast reward and leaves little behind for the microbial community. The second leaves structure, color, fiber, and fermentable material. It gives the lower gut something to do.

Polyphenols are especially important here. Many are only partially absorbed in the small intestine. They travel onward, where microbes transform them into smaller compounds with different activity. The fruit is therefore not finished when it is swallowed. Its meaning continues to unfold through digestion, fermentation, and microbial interpretation.

Patients with bloating, irregular stool, skin irritation, sugar cravings, and mood fluctuation often need this microbial conversation restored slowly. Too much fruit too quickly can overwhelm a reactive gut. Too little leaves the terrain dry and underfed. The Sim-Bo practitioner uses gradual exposure: one fruit, one window, one response at a time.

Juiced, Dried, Blended, and Whole

The form of fruit determines its effect.

Whole fruit requires teeth, saliva, time, and attention. It announces itself through aroma before it enters the stomach. It asks for chewing. It creates volume. It gives the nervous system time to register satisfaction.

Juice removes much of that intelligence. Dried fruit concentrates sweetness and reduces water. Smoothies can be useful when carefully designed, but oversized blended drinks often turn several servings of fruit into a rapidly swallowed sugar load. Fruit-flavored products are the furthest distortion: sweetness without orchard, color without pigment complexity, and aroma without seasonal truth.

The hierarchy also protects the patient from the modern illusion that blending equals nourishment. A blender can be useful, but it can also erase the labor of eating. When a smoothie contains several bananas, dates, juice, sweetened powders, and no need for chewing, the experience is closer to a dessert beverage than a therapeutic fruit practice. A true Sim-Bo fruit serving should still feel like food. It should have texture, pace, fragrance, and a natural stopping point.

This hierarchy is not puritanical. It is practical. The digestive system responds to structure. The hand that peels an orange, the jaw that chews an apple, the tongue that tastes bitterness beneath sweetness - these are not irrelevant rituals. They are part of the metabolic event.

The Sim-Bo Fruit Practice

Fruit becomes therapeutic when it is practiced, not merely consumed.

- Eat fruit whole. Choose chewing over drinking.
- Use the morning as the primary window, especially for hydrating fruits and berries.
- Keep combinations simple: one or two fruits at a sitting.
- Favor seasonal, ripe, local fruit when possible. Freshness matters.
- Avoid commercial juice, syrup-packed fruit, sweetened dried fruit, and fruit-flavored products.
- Use berries, citrus, kiwi, pears, apples, cherries, plums, grapes, melon, and persimmon according to season, digestion, and clinical need.
- For weak or cold digestion, use stewed pear, baked apple, warm compote, or smaller portions rather than cold, raw abundance.
- For heat, dryness, constipation, and summer exertion, use watery fruits with discipline and attention.

With consistency, fruit becomes a morning meditation. The patient learns to taste fragrance before sweetness, texture before quantity, and completion before craving. The palate becomes quiet enough to enjoy what is real.

Fruit in the 3:2:1 Plate

In the 3:2:1 formula, fruit is the one part because light must be precise.

Too much grain can become heaviness. Too many vegetables can become coldness or digestive overwork in depleted patients. Too much fruit can become scattered sweetness, especially when appetite is unstable. The ratio protects each food from becoming excessive. It gives fruit a defined role: refresh, brighten, hydrate, and complete.

This is why fruit should not dominate the Sim-Bo plate. It is not the foundation. It is the final accent that keeps the meal alive. After the steady warmth of grain and the mineral movement of vegetables, fruit adds lift. The meal ends not with craving, but with clarity.

The one part also teaches restraint without deprivation. A small bowl of ripe berries, a sliced pear, or a seasonal citrus fruit can satisfy the desire for sweetness more elegantly than an elaborate dessert. The patient learns that pleasure does not require excess. It requires accuracy.

When this ratio is repeated, appetite becomes more intelligent. The palate stops demanding intensity and begins recognizing completion. That is the quiet genius of the Sim-Bo plate: it does not fight desire; it educates it.

Conclusion: Returning to Nature's Sweetness

Whole fruit proves that medicine does not need to be bitter to be serious.

It hydrates without heaviness, sweetens without corruption, colors the blood with plant intelligence, feeds the microbiome, supports elimination, refreshes the mind, and teaches the nervous system that pleasure can end in satisfaction rather than compulsion.

In a culture addicted to artificial stimulation, fruit restores gentleness. It reminds us that renewal can be bright, fragrant, and simple. It does not shout. It ripens. Its power comes from patience: the tree flowers, the fruit forms, the sugars mature, the acids soften, and the fragrance announces readiness. No factory can imitate that sequence.

Brown rice gave the Sim-Bo plate its ground. Fruit gives it light. That light must remain disciplined. Fruit used carelessly becomes another expression of appetite without order. Fruit used with season, timing, chewing, and proportion becomes one of the cleanest pleasures available to human nourishment.

Clinical Case Study 11: Clearing Oxidative Rust

Restoring Fascial Comfort Through Fruit, Sim-Bo Structure, Acupuncture, Cupping, and Blood-Moving Botanical Support

Patient: Laura C., 39-year-old female, graphic designer.

Chief concerns: widespread migrating myofascial pain, chronic trigger-point sensitivity, morning stiffness, poor sleep quality, processed-sugar cravings, and a long-standing pattern of fatigue after computer-intensive work.

Clinical Presentation

Laura's case illustrates the connection between stagnation, oxidative pressure, immobility, and the loss of clean nourishment. She spent long days seated at a computer, often twelve hours at a time, with shallow breathing, minimal sunlight, and high visual strain. Her meals were inconsistent and built around convenience foods: coffee, protein bars, sweet snacks, late dinners, and very little fresh fruit.

By the time she entered care, her pain pattern was not localized. It migrated through the neck, shoulders, upper back, ribs, hips, and calves. She described the sensation as internal rust: not sharp enough to be an injury, but constant enough to make ordinary life feel heavy.

Her history also revealed an emotional pattern that mattered clinically. She was not only sedentary; she was compressed. She held deadlines in her jaw, frustration in her shoulders, and fatigue behind constant productivity. Sweet foods were used at night as brief relief from a day without softness. This made fruit an important therapeutic bridge. It restored sweetness without returning her to the refined sugar cycle that intensified pain and sleep disruption.

The treatment was built around one central idea: replace dry stimulation with living moisture, color, and movement. Her plate had to become less frantic before her fascia could stop guarding.

Initial Findings

- hs-CRP: 4.2 mg/L, consistent with elevated inflammatory load.
- Pain scale: 8/10 on most days, with widespread myofascial

tenderness.

- Morning stiffness: two to three hours before she felt fully mobile.
- Tongue: pale and flabby with dark-purplish lateral edges and a thin sticky coating.
- Pulse: deep, choppy, and wiry, especially through the Liver position.

Her Traditional Asian Medicine presentation showed Liver Qi constraint with Blood Stasis, complicated by Spleen Qi weakness and Dampness. In clinical language, her system lacked movement, hydration, clean circulation, and nutritional brightness. The fascia felt undernourished and guarded; the blood picture suggested inflammation; the lifestyle pattern provided little opportunity for repair.

Treatment Principles

- Move Liver Qi and support Blood circulation to reduce fascial guarding and migratory pain.
- Use targeted whole fruit to deliver hydration, color-spectrum polyphenols, and antioxidant support in a simple form.
- Rebuild Spleen Qi through warm grains and cooked vegetables so fruit could be tolerated without cold digestive collapse.
- Reduce inflammatory dietary friction by removing refined sugar, industrial dairy, and seed oils.
- Use acupuncture, cupping, and botanical support to improve circulation, relax the myofascial field, and restore regulatory movement.

Plan and Intervention

Laura committed to a twelve-week Sim-Bo fascial rehabilitation plan.

The fruit prescription was precise, not casual. Morning fruit centered on dark berries, cherries, kiwi, and citrus in small, consistent portions. The goal was color density, hydration, and antioxidant support without creating glucose chaos or digestive coldness. Fruit was eaten alone in the morning or before warm grain meals.

In the first two weeks, portions remained modest so that the gut could adapt without bloating. By week three, she could tolerate a larger morning bowl of berries and kiwi, followed later by warm grain. By week six, she reported that the desire for packaged sweets had lost its urgency. The palate had begun to recognize real sweetness again.

The grain base was warm brown rice and Job's tears. This supplied grounding starch, digestive warmth, and steady energy. Vegetables focused on lightly steamed dark greens, dandelion, bok choy, and small amounts of sea vegetables to support mineral intake and Liver-Spleen movement.

Refined sweets, commercial fruit juice, sweetened dried fruit, industrial seed oils, and heavy dairy were removed. She was not deprived of sweetness. She was retrained toward sweetness that carried structure.

Acupuncture focused on moving Qi and Blood while calming sympathetic overactivation. LR3 and LI4 were used to open movement through the system; GB34 addressed tendon and fascial tension; SP6 and ST36 supported digestion and fluid transformation; BL17 and BL18 supported Blood and Liver regulation.

Emperor's Cupping Therapy® was applied across the upper back, shoulders, thoracic paraspinals, gluteal region, and iliotibial fascial lines to reduce myofascial restriction, support local circulation, and create a mechanical signal of release through guarded tissue.

Botanical support used a Blood-moving strategy based on Xue Fu Zhu Yu Tang principles, modified according to her presentation. The aim was to support circulation, reduce constraint, and help the fascia receive nourishment again.

Movement was kept simple. She walked for ten minutes after lunch and dinner, performed gentle thoracic opening stretches twice daily, and stood every hour during design work. The goal was not athletic performance. The goal was repeated circulation.

Sleep hygiene was also simplified. Screens were stopped earlier, late sweets were removed, and her evening meal was made warmer and less complex. As the night became less stimulating, morning stiffness began to loosen.

Follow-Up Changes

- Widespread pain decreased from 8/10 to 1-2/10, with occasional flares tied to prolonged computer work rather than constant baseline pain.
- Morning stiffness decreased from two to three hours to less than fifteen minutes on most days.
- hs-CRP improved from 4.2 mg/L to 1.1 mg/L during the follow-up period.
- Medication status was reviewed with the appropriate prescribing clinician as symptoms improved.

- Sugar cravings decreased markedly after the morning fruit cadence replaced refined sweets.
- Tongue presentation showed reduced purplish edging, less swelling, and a cleaner coating.
- Sleep became deeper, and she reported waking with less heaviness and better mental brightness.

Clinical Reflection

Laura's case demonstrates the teaching of this chapter: chronic pain often lives at the intersection of inflammation, stagnation, poor hydration, immobility, and emotional constraint. Fruit alone was not the treatment. Fruit was the light placed into a larger architecture of movement, warmth, proportion, acupuncture, cupping, and daily repetition.

The turning point came when sweetness stopped being stimulation and became nourishment. Her palate no longer reached for sugar to escape fatigue. It began to recognize color, moisture, and completion. The fascia softened as circulation improved. The nervous system became less guarded. The clinical picture moved from rust toward flow.

This is the quiet power of whole fruit in the Sim-Bo method. It does not fight the system. It refreshes the conditions under which the system can move again.

Transition: From Light to Flow

Fruit teaches renewal through brightness. It cools heat, moistens dryness, refreshes the mind, and restores the clean pleasure of natural sweetness. It also teaches timing. The ripe fruit must be gathered, eaten, and received before it collapses back into the soil. That lesson is part of its medicine: life is not meant to be hoarded. It is meant to circulate.

Healing cannot live on brightness alone. Renewal also requires movement: the sweeping current that clears residue, opens the gut, mineralizes the blood, and teaches the plate how to circulate.

Brown rice is earth. Fruit is light. Vegetables are the green current between them.

From the orchard, the Sim-Bo path moves into the field.

Chapter 12

Vegetables: The Cleansing Current

The Quiet Power of Green

If brown rice is the grounding grain and fruit is the light of renewal, vegetables are the current. They move what has become stagnant. They cool what has become irritated. They bring volume without heaviness, minerals without excess, texture without chaos, and a daily reminder that life depends on flow.

Vegetables do not need theatrical promises. Their power is quieter than that. Leaf, stem, root, bulb, sprout, and sea vegetable each carries a specific architecture: fiber, water, minerals, chlorophyll, polyphenols, bitter compounds, sulfur molecules, resistant starch, and texture. Together they create the two in the Sim-Bo 3:2:1 plate - the visible field of color and movement between the grounding grain and the renewing fruit.

The two is not a side dish. It is the cleansing current. Without vegetables, the Sim-Bo plate loses motion. Grains may ground the meal and fruit may refresh it, but vegetables keep the internal river moving: bile, stool, lymph, vascular tone, microbial fermentation, and emotional ease. The green portion of the plate is where stillness turns back into circulation.

The lesson is simple: a life that cannot eliminate cannot repair. Vegetables restore the ordinary pathways of release.

Chlorophyll and Liquid Sunlight

All plant life begins with light. Chlorophyll is the green architecture that allows a leaf to capture sunlight and convert it into living matter. When we eat dark greens, we are not eating magic. We are eating the memory of light organized into mineral, pigment, fiber, and water.

Chlorophyll shares a porphyrin-ring architecture with hemoglobin, though the two are not identical. Hemoglobin carries iron at its center and transports oxygen in human blood. Chlorophyll carries magnesium and allows plants to conduct photosynthesis. The comparison is still meaningful. Both structures reveal a deep continuity between light, mineral chemistry, oxygen movement, and life.

In the plate, chlorophyll-rich foods do not act by drama. They act by support. Dark greens provide magnesium, folate, vitamin K, carotenoids, nitrates, polyphenols, and fibers that assist vascular flexibility, redox balance, bowel regularity, microbial resilience, and normal hepatic work. They do not violently detoxify. They help the system remember how to move.

Spinach, lacinato kale, Swiss chard, parsley, cilantro, bok choy, watercress, and young leafy greens bring the green frequency into daily practice. The deeper the color, the more concentrated the plant's protective compounds tend to be. In Sim-Bo, greens are not decorative. They are daily instructions in cooling, circulation, and clarity.

The Language of Bitterness and Hepatic Flow

Modern taste has been trained away from bitterness. Industrial food prefers the addictive triad of refined sweetness, salt, and unstable fat. Bitterness asks more from the tongue. It slows the mouth. It sharpens attention. It signals that digestion is beginning.

Traditional Asian Medicine has long understood bitter flavor as descending and clearing. It drains excess, dries dampness, moves heat downward, and helps the system discharge what no longer belongs. Modern physiology describes part of the same wisdom through bitter taste receptors, vagal activation, bile flow, pancreatic secretion, gastric tone, and digestive readiness.

A small portion of bitter greens before or within a meal can awaken the digestive current. Dandelion greens, endive, mustard greens, arugula, radicchio, watercress, and bitter melon carry terpenes, flavonoids, alkaloids, glucosinolates, and other plant compounds that tell the liver-gallbladder axis to participate. Bile is not merely a fat emulsifier. It is one of the great streams of internal housekeeping.

When patients have lived for years on heavy, beige, low-fiber food, bitterness can feel medicinal at first. That is precisely its value. The palate becomes reeducated. Appetite becomes less ravenous. The digestive tract begins to move with more authority. When the current moves, the mind often lightens with it.

Root and Leaf: The Two Directions of Nourishment

Vegetables teach direction.

Leaves rise toward light. Roots descend into soil. The plate requires both movements. Leafy greens lift the meal with minerals, chlorophyll, nitrates, folate, and a cooling, spacious quality. Roots anchor the meal with sweetness, density, trace minerals, resistant starch, and the quiet satisfaction of earth.

Leafy vegetables - kale, spinach, collards, bok choy, napa cabbage, chard, lettuces, watercress - bring upward freshness. They lighten the meal, support vascular tone, and supply the green compounds that make the plate feel alive.

Root vegetables - carrots, beets, daikon radish, burdock, turnips, parsnips, sweet potato, taro, lotus root - bring downward steadiness. They ground the nervous system, add chewing, help stool formation, and give the digestive tract something substantial to organize.

A meal of only raw leaves can leave a depleted patient cold, anxious, or unsteady. A meal of only heavy roots can become too dense. The Sim-Bo plate pairs the two: leaf for lift, root for anchor; upward movement and downward settlement; cleansing without depletion.

Color as Chemistry: The Phytochemical Spectrum

Vegetable color is not decoration. It is chemistry made visible.

Deep green vegetables carry chlorophyll, magnesium, folate, vitamin K, carotenoids, nitrates, and polyphenols that support vascular tone, liver function, redox balance, and cellular protection.

Orange and yellow vegetables - carrots, squash, pumpkin, yellow peppers - carry carotenoids such as beta-carotene, lutein, and zeaxanthin. They nourish epithelial surfaces, visual function, mucosal barriers, and skin resilience.

Red vegetables - tomatoes, red peppers, beets, red cabbage, radicchio - bring lycopene, betalains, anthocyanins, nitrates, and vascular-supporting pigments that assist circulation and oxidative defense.

Purple and dark vegetables - eggplant skin, purple cabbage, purple carrots, purple sweet potatoes, black radish, sea vegetables, dark mushrooms - concentrate anthocyanins, mineral-rich polysaccharides, and deep-spectrum polyphenols that reinforce antioxidant defense and microbial diversity.

White and pungent vegetables - garlic, onion, leek, daikon, cauliflower, cabbage, radish - bring organosulfur compounds, quercetin, and glucosinolates that support immune surveillance, liver phase-II activity, respiratory resilience, and microbial balance.

A Sim-Bo plate should look like a garden in miniature. The colors do not exist for beauty alone. They are edible instructions. Diversity of color becomes diversity of defense.

THE INNER COSMOS

Correspondences of the Five Elements

Category	Wood	Fire	Earth	Metal	Water
Climate	Wind	Heat	Dampness	Dryness	Cold
Direction	East	South	Center	West	North
Season	Spring	Summer	Change of Seasons	Autumn	Winter
Color	Blue / Green	Red	Yellow	White	Black
Nature / State	Generation / Sprouting	Dispersion	Neutralization	Convergence	Condensation
Emotion	Anger	Joy	Worry / Thought	Sadness / Sorrow	Fear
Virtue	Benevolence	Propriety / Courtesy	Trust / Faith	Righteousness	Wisdom
Five Yin Organs	Liver	Heart	Spleen	Lungs	Kidneys
Five Yang Organs	Gallbladder	Small Intestine	Stomach	Large Intestine	Bladder
Body Tissues	Muscles / Sinews	Blood Vessels	Flesh / Muscle	Skin	Bones
Sense Organs	Eyes	Tongue	Lips	Nose	Ears
Taste	Sour	Bitter	Sweet	Spicy / Pungent	Salty
Five Fruits	Plum	Apricot	Jujube / Date	Peach	Chestnut

Figure 5. The inner cosmos: correspondences of the Five Elements.

The Mineral Current and Cruciferous Intelligence

Vegetables also carry mineral instruction. Potassium relaxes vascular tension and balances the sodium pressure that dominates processed food. Magnesium steadies nerve conduction, smooth muscle tone, and bowel motility. Nitrates in beets, arugula, celery, and leafy greens help support nitric-oxide pathways, widening the vascular river so blood can move with less resistance. Sulfur compounds in garlic, onions, leeks, cabbage, broccoli, radish, and mustard greens assist phase-two conjugation, glutathione activity, respiratory resilience, and the pungent movement of stagnant heaviness.

This is the hidden reason vegetables change how a patient feels. They do not merely add nutrients. They change fluid pressure, stool texture, vascular ease, microbial fermentation, bile movement, and the electrical weather of the nervous system. A plate without vegetables may still contain calories, but it lacks the mineral conversation that makes those calories behave.

Cruciferous vegetables deserve special respect. Broccoli, cabbage, bok choy, mustard greens, radish, watercress, turnip greens, cauliflower, kale, and Brussels sprouts carry glucosinolates that become active compounds through chewing, chopping, and microbial action. These compounds support the enzyme systems that help neutralize and package metabolic byproducts for elimination. They are not harsh detoxifiers. They are disciplined organizers of clearance.

Sea vegetables add another dimension. Kelp, wakame, nori, dulse, and hijiki carry iodine, trace minerals, alginates, and the mineral memory of the ocean. Used modestly and wisely, they bring salinity, depth, and thyroid-supporting mineral presence to the plate. They should not be consumed recklessly in large quantities; their strength is in precision. A strip of sea vegetable in soup or a small sheet of nori with rice can alter the mineral architecture of an entire meal.

The vegetable kingdom therefore teaches more than cleansing. It teaches conductivity. Minerals allow impulses to fire, vessels to relax, muscles to contract, bowels to move, and cells to hold water. Flow requires minerals. Vegetables bring them in a form the meal can understand.

The Gut's Green Ally: Prebiotic Mastery

Vegetables are among the great teachers of the microbiome.

Their fibers, resistant starches, pectins, mucilage, and polyphenols feed the native microbial community. When these fibers reach the colon, beneficial microbes ferment them into short-chain fatty acids such as butyrate, acetate, and propionate. Butyrate supports colon-cell energy needs, barrier integrity, immune tolerance, and a calmer mucosal environment.

This is why vegetables often succeed where probiotic pills alone disappoint. A probiotic attempts to introduce a few organisms. Fiber-rich plants feed the entire ecosystem. They do not merely add bacteria. They cultivate terrain.

Each bite of fibrous vegetable is an act of internal diplomacy. It gives beneficial microbes the food they require to remain dominant, encourages microbial diversity, and teaches the immune system the difference between nourishment and threat. When vegetables consistently occupy the center of the plate, the gut lining often becomes less reactive, stool becomes more regular, and the immune tone becomes less guarded.

A calm gut is not created by sterility. It is created by a thriving inner ecology that receives the same message every day: fiber is coming, minerals are coming, color is coming, there is no emergency.

Cooking with Compassion

How vegetables are prepared determines how they speak.

The Sim-Bo kitchen does not worship raw food or cooked food as ideology. It uses both with discernment. Raw vegetables are crisp, bright, cooling, and awakening. Cooked vegetables are warm, soft, grounding, and often easier for a depleted digestive tract to receive. A master plate understands texture, season, temperature, and constitution.

Gentle steaming, blanching, quick stir-frying, slow simmering, roasting, fermenting, and pickling each changes the vegetable's character. Heat may reduce some fragile compounds, but it can also soften fiber, improve digestibility, release carotenoids, reduce harshness, and make the meal kinder to a stressed stomach. The question is not raw versus cooked. The question is what the patient can assimilate.

Vegetables should never be rushed into violence. Scorched oil, deep frying, careless overheating, and repeated reheating can turn a healing food into a load the system must manage. The goal is to preserve color, texture, aroma, moisture, and vitality while making the plant easy to chew and digest.

Even the knife matters. To wash, trim, slice, steam, and plate vegetables with attention is not culinary decoration. It is part of digestion. The nervous system begins receiving the meal before the first bite. Preparation is the first medicine.

Seasonal Intelligence of Greens

Vegetables carry the intelligence of their season.

Spring brings tender greens, sprouts, peas, asparagus, young herbs, and bitter leaves. They move upward, quicken the liver-gallbladder current, and help clear the heaviness that accumulates through winter.

Summer brings cucumbers, zucchini, lettuces, celery, peppers, tomatoes, watercress, and cooling greens. They hydrate, refresh, and protect the system from heat, sweat, and excessive dryness.

Autumn brings squashes, roots, cabbages, mushrooms, onions, and dense vegetables that prepare the digestive tract for colder weather. Their sweetness and density help gather energy inward.

Winter favors cabbage, daikon, burdock, onions, leeks, sea vegetables, fermented greens, and hardy dark leaves. These foods warm, mineralize, and help the system endure a slower season.

Seasonal eating is not nostalgia. It is timing. A raw tomato in summer is refreshing; the same cold tomato in winter may be poorly suited for depleted, cold digestion. Sim-Bo honors the local cadence of climate and appetite. When the plate follows the land, physiology receives fewer mixed instructions.

Vegetables as Emotional Medicine

Green food changes mood because digestion and emotion are not separate systems.

Bitter greens often sharpen and clear the emotional field. Sweet roots settle worry. Pungent vegetables such as onion, garlic, scallion, radish, and mustard move breath and release pressure through the chest. Mineral-rich greens create a steadier nervous system because minerals participate in electrical balance, muscle tone, vascular relaxation, and neurotransmitter rhythm.

Patients often describe feeling lighter after several days of vegetable-centered meals. The effect is not mystical. It emerges from multiple converging mechanisms: improved bowel regularity, steadier glucose, less post-meal heaviness, higher fiber intake, microbial fermentation, vagal tone, and the psychological relief that comes when meals stop creating internal friction.

A vegetable-dominant plate is emotional hygiene. It reduces the heaviness that comes from stagnation. It gives the gut something useful to do. It gives the mind fewer chemical storms to interpret. It teaches the nervous system that nourishment can be clean, steady, and sufficient.

The Sim-Bo Green Bowl

A cleansing meal does not need complexity.

A simple bowl of warm grain, lightly cooked greens, raw accents, root vegetables, sprouts, a small amount of fermented food, and a modest drizzle of stable oil can contain the entire lesson of Chapter 12. It moves. It grounds. It hydrates. It feeds microbes. It teaches the palate that cleansing does not require punishment.

The Sim-Bo Green Bowl can be built as follows:

The ground: warm brown rice, barley, millet, or another simple grain.
The sweep: lightly steamed greens such as bok choy, kale, spinach, chard, napa cabbage, or watercress.
The anchor: roasted or simmered roots such as carrot, daikon, burdock, beet, turnip, lotus root, or squash.
The bright accent: shredded raw radish, sprouts, cucumber, herbs, or a few leaves of arugula.
The microbial note: fermented vegetables, miso broth, or a small portion of traditionally fermented tofu where appropriate.
The catalyst: lemon, vinegar, sesame, olive oil, sea salt, ginger, garlic, or scallion used with restraint.

This bowl is not a cleanse in the commercial sense. It is a daily lesson in flow. It asks for chewing. It gives bulk to the stool, minerals to the blood, work to the microbes, and steadiness to the meal. It is ordinary enough to repeat, and repetition is where Sim-Bo becomes medicine.

Vegetables and Longevity: The Flow of Vitality

Long-lived food cultures differ in many details, but they repeatedly return to a common pattern: plants are abundant, vegetables are ordinary, and the plate is not built around excess density.

Vegetables contribute to longevity not because they perform miracles, but because they lighten the daily load. They supply fiber, water, minerals, potassium, magnesium, folate, vitamin K, carotenoids, sulfur compounds, nitrates, and polyphenols while usually bringing fewer calories than dense processed foods. They demand chewing, slow the meal, fill the stomach without heaviness, and feed the microbial community that shapes immune tone.

Over decades, that difference matters. A meal built on vegetables asks less from the liver, less from the pancreas, less from the vascular system, and more from the act of presence. It replaces caloric compression with volume, color, and movement.

Longevity is not the absence of disease alone. It is the presence of continued flow: bowel flow, bile flow, lymphatic flow, blood flow, breath flow, and emotional flow. Vegetables are that principle placed directly on the plate.

The Daily Cadence of Vegetables

Vegetables work by repetition. A single green meal can refresh digestion, but daily vegetable rhythm rebuilds terrain. The Sim-Bo method therefore treats vegetables not as occasional garnish, but as the daily current that must appear again and again until the digestive tract trusts the pattern.

At breakfast or the first meal, use warm greens and roots to wake the bowel without shocking the stomach. At the middle meal, use the greatest variety: leaves, roots, crucifers, herbs, sea vegetables, fermented vegetables, and bitter accents. At the evening meal, simplify. Use soft-cooked greens, brothy vegetables, cabbage, daikon, squash, or bok choy to provide movement without overstimulation.

The vegetable portion should be generous enough to change the physical experience of eating. It should require chewing. It should create bulk. It should make the plate visually alive. In a true Sim-Bo bowl, vegetables are not hidden under sauce or chopped into decorative fragments. They are visible, audible, aromatic, and textural. The patient hears the crunch, sees the color, smells the steam, and feels the meal slow down.

This cadence also retrains appetite. Processed food teaches the tongue to demand intensity without substance. Vegetables teach the tongue to recognize subtler intelligence: bitter, pungent, mineral, sweet, earthy, watery, fibrous, cooling, warming. As the palate recovers, cravings lose volume. The patient no longer needs every meal to entertain the nervous system. Food can nourish without shouting.

The Practice of Gratitude

Every leaf once reached toward light. Every root once entered darkness to draw minerals from soil. To eat vegetables is to participate in that upward and downward movement.

Before eating, pause. Notice the color, the scent, the steam, the texture, the cut surface, the trace of land and season. Gratitude is not sentimental excess. It changes posture, breath, chewing, and attention. It moves the meal from consumption into relationship.

The Sim-Bo path is a daily practice of relationship: with food, with land, with timing, with appetite, with the intelligence of ordinary life. Vegetables remind us that healing is not conquest. It is cooperation.

Conclusion: Flow Restored

The grain grounds. The fruit renews. The vegetables move.

Together, they form the living trinity of the Sim-Bo plate: earth, light, and current. Vegetables keep the meal from becoming static. They bring color to the blood, fiber to the gut, bitterness to the liver, roots to the nerves, minerals to the cells, and quiet movement to the mind.

When vegetables take their rightful place at the center of daily eating, external cleansing rituals lose much of their glamour. The work becomes simpler and more demanding: cook the greens, chew the roots, welcome bitterness, honor season, and let elimination become reliable again.

Flow is not forced. It is restored by daily conditions that allow it to resume.

Clinical Case Study 12: The Cleansing Current

Restoring Hepatic Flow, Migraine Pattern, and Digestive Regularity Through Vegetable-Centered Sim-Bo Practice

Patient: Elena V., 42-year-old female, corporate accountant.

Chief Concerns: Chronic right-sided migraines, sluggish digestion with bowel movements approximately every four days, hormonal cystic acne along the jawline, and a persistent heavy sensation in the limbs.

Clinical Presentation

Elena illustrates a common pattern in patients whose meals have lost color and movement. Her diet was dominated by refined carbohydrates, dairy, dense proteins, and low-fiber convenience foods. The plate was beige, heavy, and dry. It contained calories, but little sweep.

Over time, this pattern appeared to contribute to constipation, skin eruptions, right-sided migraine tendency, and a sense of internal heaviness. In Traditional Asian Medicine observation, the presentation suggested Liver-Gallbladder constraint with heat, intestinal dryness, and sluggish downward movement. In practical language, the current was blocked.

Her work pattern intensified the presentation. Long hours at a desk, constant numerical concentration, skipped lunches, and late dinners left little room for movement or regular elimination. She drank coffee to push through afternoon heaviness, then craved dense evening foods because the system had been underfed and overstimulated all day. The result was not a lack of discipline. It was a loss of current.

The therapeutic strategy was therefore not to add a complicated detox program. It was to restore the most ordinary river: green food, bitter taste, warm grains, sufficient water, regular bowel movement, lateral-channel release, and enough simplicity for the liver-gallbladder system to stop holding tension.

Initial Findings

Blood pressure: 132/86 mm Hg at intake.

Tongue: dusky-red presentation with a thick, dry, yellow coating concentrated toward the root.

Pulse: wiry and sluggish, especially in positions associated with Liver-Gallbladder tension and digestive stagnation.

Bowel pattern: infrequent elimination, approximately every four days.
Skin: cystic jawline acne with cyclical hormonal worsening.
Pain pattern: recurrent right-sided migraine tendency along the temporal and lateral head pathway.

Traditional Asian Medicine Assessment

Liver-Gallbladder heat with Qi constraint: consistent with unilateral migraine tendency, irritability, jawline eruptions, and wiry pulse quality.
Intestinal dryness and stagnation: consistent with infrequent bowel movements, thick root coating, heaviness, and reduced downward movement.
Vegetable deficiency pattern: a clinical absence of bitter greens, fiber, minerals, and color in the daily plate.

Treatment Principles

The clinical objective was to restore flow: support bile movement, increase fiber, hydrate the stool, cool the heat pattern, move constrained Liver Qi, and give the digestive tract a daily green current it could trust.

Plan and Intervention

The Sim-Bo Dietary Prescription: Elena adopted a vegetable-centered version of the 3:2:1 plate.

Two parts vegetables: dark bitter greens such as dandelion, arugula, watercress, bok choy, and lacinato kale formed the central current of the meal. These were paired with roots such as daikon, burdock, beet, carrot, and turnip to guide movement downward and restore stool formation.
Three parts grains: brown rice and pearl barley replaced refined flour products and provided warmth, hydration, and bulk.
One part fruit: whole seasonal fruit was used earlier in the day to support hydration and refreshment without evening blood-sugar stimulation.
Preparation: vegetables were lightly steamed, simmered, or briefly stir-fried, with raw bitter accents used in modest amounts. Lemon, ginger, scallion, sesame, and small amounts of fermented vegetables

were used to keep the plate vivid without adding complexity.

Targeted Acupuncture Protocol: LR3 and GB34 were used to move Liver-Gallbladder constraint; SJ6 was selected to support bowel movement and lateral-channel release; ST36 and SP6 supported digestive resilience and fluid transformation.

Emperor's Cupping Therapy®: Cupping was applied along the lateral aspect of the body and the mid-thoracic Back-Shu region to reduce myofascial restriction, support local circulation, and release tension along the Gallbladder and Liver-associated pathways.

Botanical Medicine: Long Dan Xie Gan Tang was used within the Traditional Asian Medicine pattern to clear Liver-Gallbladder heat and support downward drainage. The formula was applied in a clinically monitored context and adjusted according to digestive tolerance and symptom response.

Twelve-Week Response

Migraine Pattern: The right-sided migraine pattern markedly decreased in frequency and intensity during the follow-up period.
Bowel Regularity: Elimination shifted from approximately every four days toward a regular daily or near-daily pattern by patient report.
Skin Presentation: Jawline cystic acne substantially softened, with fewer inflammatory eruptions during the observed cycle.
Limb Heaviness: The heavy, dragging sensation in the limbs decreased as bowel rhythm and meal structure improved.
Tongue Presentation: The thick, dry coating at the root thinned, and the dusky-red presentation became less intense within the Traditional Asian Medicine lens.
Daily Energy: Elena reported steadier afternoon energy and less post-meal heaviness.

Clinical Lesson

Elena's case demonstrates Chapter 12's central lesson: the internal river must move. Her improvement did not come from adding complexity. It came from restoring the missing current - bitter greens, fibrous roots, warm grains, hydration, meal timing, and a daily pattern of elimination.

The case also shows why vegetables must be understood as architecture, not garnish. The greens did not work alone. They worked in relationship with rice, barley, roots, acupuncture, cupping, herbal support, mealtime consistency, and deliberate chewing. The current returned because the entire environment became more coherent.

The lesson is not that vegetables perform miracles. The lesson is that stagnation has consequences, and flow has intelligence. When the plate becomes green enough, bitter enough, fibrous enough, and predictable enough, the pathways of release begin to reopen.

Transition: From Flow to Foundation

Vegetables teach movement. They keep the meal from hardening into density and the internal terrain from settling into stagnation. But every river depends on the soil beneath it. Clear current means little if the riverbed is depleted.

Beneath appetite, mood, immunity, elimination, and inflammation lives the human gut: a dense, intelligent ecology of microbes, mucosal tissue, immune surveillance, nervous system communication, and chemical translation. Vegetables sweep and feed this terrain. The microbiome decides what is fermented, absorbed, tolerated, rejected, remembered.

Green food is the daily practice of cleansing. The gut is the living memory of that practice.

Flow leads downward, into foundation. The river now meets the soil.

Part IV

The Science of Natural Healing

Beneath conscious effort and visible muscle lies a quieter network of repair: the gut, the immune system, the microbial terrain, and the antioxidant defenses that protect every cell from the wear of living.

Part IV moves into that inner architecture. The Sim-Bo method is not only a way of eating; it is a way of restoring the conditions under which immunity can discern, metabolism can regulate, and repair can proceed without constant interference. The gut teaches tolerance. The antioxidant system contains chemical sparks. Targeted support has value only when it strengthens the foundation rather than replacing it.

Natural healing begins where the terrain becomes readable again.

Chapter 13

The Gut: Where Immunity, Metabolism, and Mood Converge

The Forgotten Foundation and the Invisible Organ

The gastrointestinal tract is not a passive tube. It is a living borderland.

At one surface, it meets the outside world: food, water, microbes, pollen, chemicals, medicines, stress chemistry, and the countless fragments of modern life. At another surface, it opens into the bloodstream, the immune system, the liver, the nervous system, and the brain. No other organ system is asked to be so welcoming and so selective at the same time.

The gut receives the world and decides what becomes us.

Inside that terrain lives the microbiome: trillions of organisms, including bacteria, archaea, fungi, viruses, and their genetic material. They digest fibers human enzymes cannot break down. They generate short-chain fatty acids. They influence bile metabolism, immune tone, neurotransmitter pathways, epithelial repair, and inflammatory balance. They are not passengers. They are participants in the daily regulation of health.

When this ecosystem is diverse, well-fed, and protected by an intact mucosal barrier, digestion becomes clearer, immune judgment becomes steadier, and mood has a more stable chemical ground. When the terrain loses order, the consequences travel outward: bloating, irregular stool, skin irritation, fatigue, joint discomfort, brain fog, immune reactivity, and emotional volatility.

The gut is not the single source of every disease. It is more powerful than that simplistic claim. It is the crossroads where nourishment, immunity, metabolism, microbial ecology, and mood continually meet. Disturb that crossing long enough, and the entire organism feels the traffic.

The Living Soil Within

The most useful image for the gut is soil.

Fertile soil does not become rich by accident. It requires organic matter, moisture, microbial diversity, seasonal rest, and freedom from repeated chemical assault. The intestine obeys the same law. It needs fiber, water, minerals, plant compounds, warmth, chewing, calm, and intervals of rest. It needs food that can be fermented rather than food that merely stimulates the tongue.

Every meal plants something. Whole grains plant stability. Vegetables plant mineral current and fiber. Fruit plants hydration, color, and natural sweetness. Fermented foods, when tolerated, introduce living culture. Bitter greens awaken direction. Warm soups soften resistance. Highly processed food plants confusion: speed without structure, intensity without depth, calories without coherent architecture.

In healthy soil, many species coexist and restrain one another. Diversity creates resilience. In depleted soil, a few opportunistic organisms dominate. The same pattern appears inside the intestine. A fiber-rich, plant-centered plate encourages a broad microbial community. A pattern built on refined sugar, alcohol, low fiber, repeated ultra-processed meals, and chronic stress narrows that community and creates conditions where opportunistic species thrive.

The Sim-Bo philosophy uses simplicity to restore this internal agriculture. It does not overwhelm the gut with constant novelty. It gives the terrain repeated, recognizable inputs until digestion, microbial fermentation, elimination, appetite, and energy can be observed with clarity. Clean food builds readable soil. Readable soil creates reliable physiology.

The Three Gifts of a Healthy Microbiome

A healthy microbiome gives three practical gifts: fuel, tolerance, and chemical intelligence.

The first gift is fuel. When microbes ferment resistant starch and fibers from grains, vegetables, legumes, roots, and fruit, they produce short-chain fatty acids such as butyrate, acetate, and propionate. These compounds nourish colon cells, support barrier integrity, influence appetite signaling, and help regulate inflammatory tone. The patient feels this not as a laboratory concept, but as steadier stool, clearer energy, and less abdominal volatility.

The second gift is tolerance. A well-fed microbial community helps the immune system recognize the difference between food and invasion. This is one reason a therapeutic diet must contain more than restriction. Removing irritants matters, but feeding tolerance matters just as much. The intestine cannot learn peace from emptiness alone; it needs the right substrate.

The third gift is chemical intelligence. Microbial metabolites influence bile acids, hormone clearance, mineral absorption, epithelial repair, and gut-brain communication. The microbiome turns the ordinary meal into a pharmacy of small messages. A bowl of rice and vegetables becomes more than starch and fiber. It becomes fuel for a living community that returns medicine to the host.

This is the quiet genius of Sim-Bo nutrition. It does not attempt to micromanage every bacterial species. It changes the conditions of the forest: more fiber, more warmth, more timing, fewer irritants, less noise. The forest then begins to reorganize itself.

Dysbiosis: When the Garden Loses Order

Dysbiosis is not merely the absence of good bacteria. It is a loss of ecological order.

Antibiotic exposure, chronic alcohol intake, refined sugar, emulsifiers, pesticide residues, insufficient fiber, stress chemistry, sleep loss, and constant snacking can all disturb the microbial terrain. Beneficial organisms lose substrate. Mucus thickness may decline. Fermentation patterns shift. Opportunistic organisms gain room. The intestinal lining becomes more reactive.

The chain is clinically familiar:

Microbial diversity narrows and fermentation becomes less stable.
The mucus layer and epithelial barrier become more vulnerable.
Tight-junction regulation weakens, increasing intestinal permeability.
Bacterial fragments such as lipopolysaccharide, along with incompletely digested food antigens, can provoke immune alarm.
The liver, immune system, brain, skin, joints, and vascular system begin receiving the consequences of a disturbed gut terrain.

The symptoms rarely arrive wearing one label. One patient calls it IBS. Another calls it brain fog. Another calls it eczema. Another calls it anxiety. Another calls it autoimmune flare. The names differ; the underlying terrain often tells the same story: the border has become irritated, the soil has lost diversity, and the immune system is no longer receiving clear instruction.

Medication may quiet a symptom. It may reduce acid, suppress diarrhea, calm pain, slow inflammation, or steady mood. When needed, it has value. But a gut ecosystem cannot be rebuilt by symptom suppression alone. Soil is restored by changing what repeatedly enters it, how often it is disturbed, and whether the environment allows life to return.

The Gut-Brain Conversation

Mood is not sealed inside the skull.

The gut and brain speak through the vagus nerve, immune mediators, microbial metabolites, endocrine hormones, bile acids, blood sugar, sleep chemistry, and inflammatory tone. The enteric nervous system does not merely obey the brain. It reports to it. It warns, calms, contracts, relaxes, secretes, and withholds. A person can think with the mind while the gut is quietly voting on safety.

The intestine produces large amounts of peripheral serotonin and participates in many neurotransmitter pathways. That does not mean gut serotonin simply becomes brain serotonin. The relationship is more sophisticated. Microbes, immune cells, enteroendocrine cells, vagal pathways, tryptophan metabolism, and inflammatory cytokines all influence how emotional stability is felt. Mood becomes a whole-system event.

This is why digestive irritation so often accompanies anxiety, depression, panic, fatigue, and cognitive dullness. The gut lining becomes inflamed; the immune system sends alarm; the vagus nerve carries distress; sleep weakens; glucose becomes unstable; the brain receives a chemistry of threat. The patient experiences this as sadness, fear, irritability, or mental fog, but the roots may run through the belly.

The same connection runs in the opposite direction. Fear tightens motility. Chronic pressure alters secretion. Grief changes appetite. Anger heats the digestive terrain. A hurried meal eaten under stress is metabolically different from the same meal eaten with breath and attention. The gut records the weather of the mind.

Sim-Bo practice treats digestive and emotional regulation as one clinical field. Simple meals, warm texture, steady timing, diaphragmatic breathing, walking, gratitude, and silence before eating do not merely improve digestion. They change the nervous-system atmosphere in which digestion occurs.

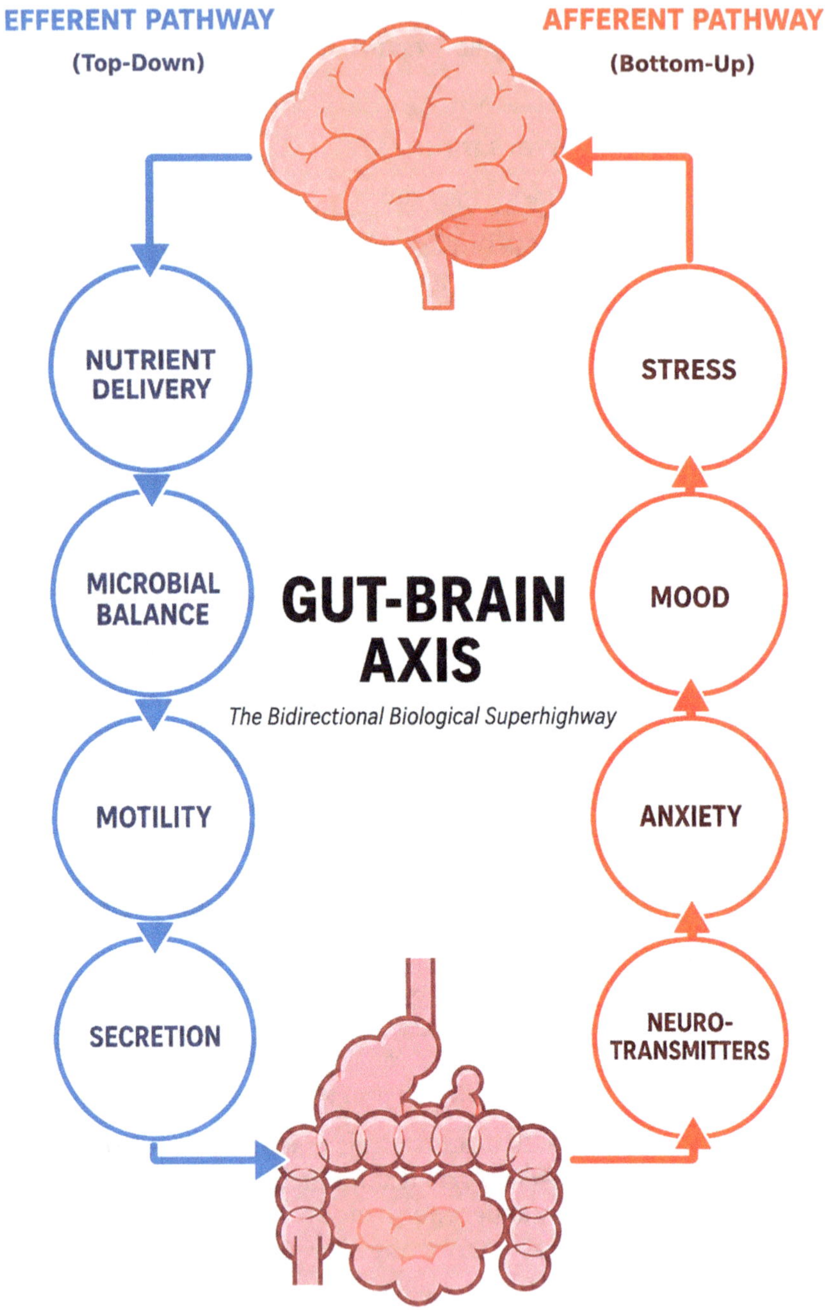

Figure 6. The gut-brain axis.

The Immune System's Classroom

The gut is the immune system's classroom.

A large portion of immune tissue is stationed along the gastrointestinal tract because the intestine is the place where the organism must constantly decide what to welcome and what to reject. Food proteins, microbes, airborne particles, environmental residues, and transient organisms pass through daily. The immune system must learn discernment, not constant aggression.

A stable microbiome helps teach that discernment. Beneficial microbes and their metabolites support regulatory T-cell activity, mucosal tolerance, epithelial repair, and calmer immune tone. When the terrain is diverse and well-fed, the immune response can become more intelligent: alert when necessary, tolerant when safe, restrained after the work is done.

When dysbiosis dominates, the lessons change. The immune system receives more alarm and less tolerance. Harmless foods may become suspicious. Pollen may provoke disproportionate response. Skin, joints, thyroid, or bowel tissue may become targets of misplaced defense. Allergic and autoimmune patterns rarely arise from one cause alone, but gut ecology often shapes the immune atmosphere in which those patterns intensify.

In this sense, the gut is not merely a digestive organ. It is an organ of discernment. It teaches the difference between nourishment and threat. Sim-Bo reduces confusion by reducing unnecessary variables: fewer processed ingredients, fewer chemical inputs, fewer erratic eating windows, fewer overstimulating meals, and more repeated contact with foods the system can recognize.

Intestinal Permeability: The Breach

The intestinal wall is delicate by design. It must allow nutrients to pass while keeping inappropriate material out of circulation. Its tight junctions are not cement walls; they are living gates, regulated by inflammation, microbes, stress, diet, toxins, medications, and the state of the mucosal barrier.

When that barrier is repeatedly irritated, intestinal permeability may increase. Bacterial fragments such as LPS, incompletely digested food proteins, and inflammatory signals can place the immune system on alert. The liver must process more inflammatory material. Cytokine activity rises. Symptoms appear at a distance: fatigue, skin eruptions, migraines, joint pain, mood instability, food sensitivity, and cognitive heaviness.

This is why the phrase "leaky gut" must be handled with precision. It is not a mystical explanation for every symptom, and it is not a standalone diagnosis that replaces clinical evaluation. It describes a real functional problem: a barrier meant to regulate exchange has become too permeable and too reactive. The result is not local discomfort alone. It is systemic communication changed at the border.

Repair begins when the daily injury decreases. The lining needs rest from irritants, substrate for renewal, adequate protein in proportion, minerals, butyrate-producing fiber, stable sleep, vagal tone, and meals that do not arrive as chemical chaos. The gut heals like soil: not through drama, but through repeated conditions that allow life to reestablish itself.

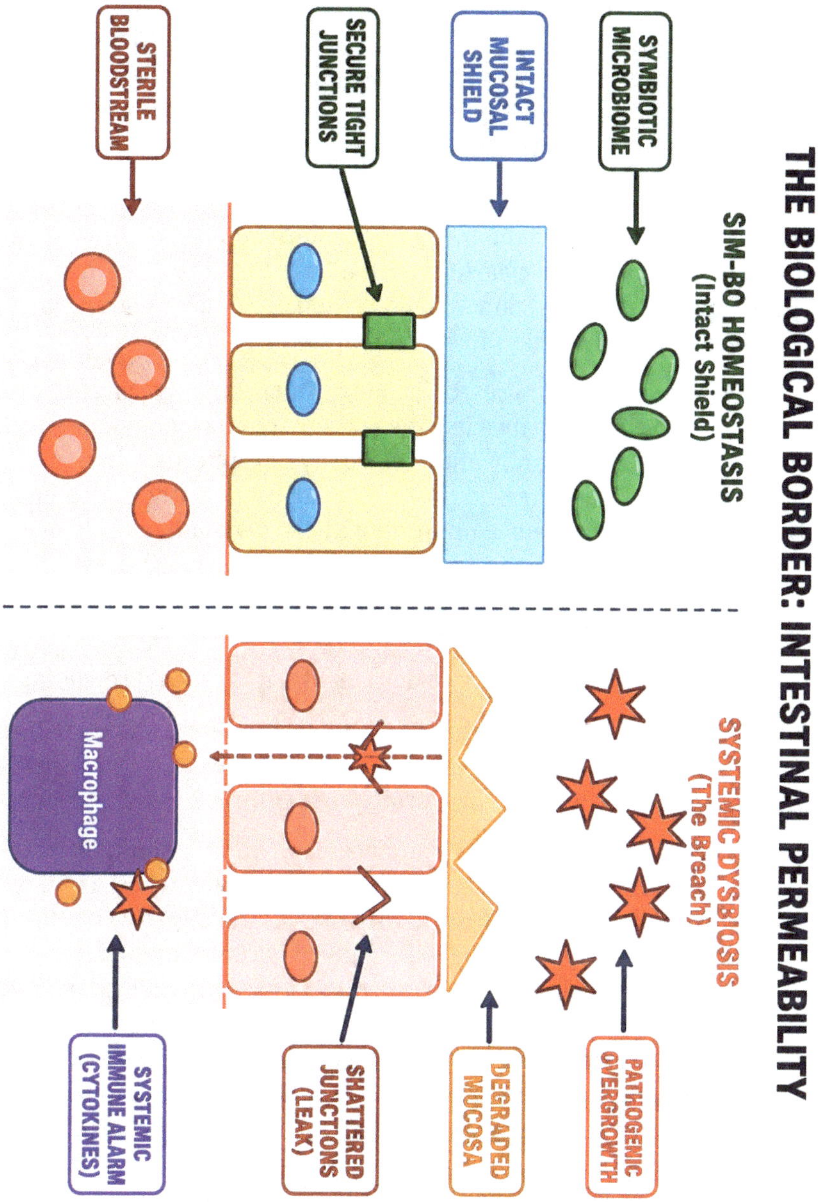

Figure 7. The biological border: intestinal permeability.

Mucus, Motility, and the Daily Sweep

The gut is protected not only by microbes, but by movement and mucus.

The mucus layer is a living shield. It keeps microbes at the proper distance from the intestinal wall, protects epithelial cells, and gives beneficial organisms a place to interact with the host without creating invasion. Fiber, polyphenols, adequate hydration, and microbial diversity help maintain that layer. Alcohol, chronic stress, poor sleep, low-fiber diets, and repeated irritants can thin the protection.

Motility is the other guardian. The intestine is meant to move in waves. Between meals, the migrating motor complex sweeps the upper gut like a housekeeper clearing residue from the floor. Constant grazing interrupts that sweep. Food arrives again before the previous signal has resolved. The system stays busy, but not clean.

This is why Sim-Bo uses both nourishment and spacing. The plate feeds the terrain; the pause lets the terrain organize. A patient who eats beautifully but constantly may still deny the intestine its rhythm of completion. A patient who fasts too intensely without feeding the microbiome may create emptiness without rebuilding resilience. The therapeutic answer is cadence: feed, digest, sweep, rest, repeat.

Restoring the Inner Garden: The Sim-Bo Protocol

Gut restoration is not a three-day cleanse. It is gradual rewilding.

The Sim-Bo approach rebuilds the terrain by making the daily environment simple enough for the intestine to repair and the microbiome to reorganize. The principles are direct:

Simplify the diet. Reduce unnecessary variety for a therapeutic period. Use unrefined grains, cooked vegetables, whole fruit, water, warmth, and clean protein in proportion. The digestive tract repairs more efficiently when the daily pattern becomes predictable.

Feed the microbiome. Prebiotic foods - cooked onions, leeks, garlic when tolerated, green banana, oats, barley, legumes, root vegetables, and cooled starches - provide substrate for beneficial fermentation. Fermented foods such as kimchi, sauerkraut, miso, and yogurt may be useful when appropriate, but they must match the patient's tolerance.

Remove repeated irritants. Alcohol, refined sugar, highly processed seed oils, artificial sweeteners, late-night eating, constant snacking, and unnecessary chemical exposure can all thin the terrain. The first medicine is often the removal of what keeps provoking the lining.

Restore digestive rest. Overnight fasting windows and clear spacing between meals allow the migrating motor complex to sweep the small intestine and help reduce the sense of constant digestive congestion. Rest is not deprivation. It is housekeeping.

Calm the vagus nerve. Breath before meals, slow chewing, upright

posture, gratitude, walking, and silence lower sympathetic tone. Blood flow returns to the gut. Secretion improves. Motility becomes more orderly.
Cook for reception. Many inflamed or depleted patients do better with warm, cooked, softened foods before they tolerate raw abundance. A softened vegetable can be more therapeutic than a heroic salad the intestine cannot receive.

Within weeks, many patients report less bloating, steadier elimination, calmer appetite, improved sleep depth, and more reliable energy. These changes are not stimulation. They are the visible signs of absorption returning.

The Gut-Brain-Immune Triangle

The gut, brain, and immune system form one living triangle.

The gut trains immunity. Immunity shapes mood. Mood alters digestion. Digestion changes microbial output. Microbial output modifies inflammatory tone. Each point of the triangle continually informs the others.

When the gut becomes irritated, immune vigilance rises and the brain may feel anxious or foggy.
When the brain lives under chronic stress, cortisol and sympathetic tone alter motility, secretion, permeability, and microbial ecology.
When immunity loses tolerance, inflammatory chemistry travels through skin, joints, blood vessels, nerves, and mood.

A single intervention rarely corrects all three points. Sim-Bo works because it acts through many simple inputs at once: food that is recognizable, timing that is stable, breath that settles the vagus nerve, movement that circulates lymph, sleep that restores barrier repair, and repetition that teaches safety.

The result is not artificial silence. It is a quieter internal conversation.

The Sim-Bo Gut Bowl

A therapeutic gut bowl should be simple enough for the intestine to recognize and complete enough for the microbiome to use.

Begin with a warm grain foundation: brown rice, barley, millet, oats, or Job's tears according to constitution and season. Add cooked vegetables in generous volume: leafy greens for mineral current, roots for anchoring, crucifers for sulfur pathways, and soft alliums for prebiotic depth. Add a small amount of clean protein when clinically appropriate. Finish with broth, warm water, ginger, miso, fermented vegetables, or bitter greens according to tolerance.

The goal is not culinary perfection. The goal is digestive legibility. The gut should know what is arriving, how much work is required, and when the work will end. This is why the same simple bowl repeated for several days can reveal more than a rotating menu of twenty "healthy" recipes. Repetition makes the response visible.

The patient watches: Does bloating decrease? Does stool become easier? Does appetite sharpen or soften? Does sleep deepen? Does the mind feel less fogged after lunch? The meal becomes a diagnostic instrument, not because it is complex, but because it is stable enough to observe.

Signs of a Healing Gut

When the gut begins to recover, the signs are usually practical before they are dramatic.

- Hunger becomes cleaner, appearing at appropriate times rather than as frantic craving.
- Bloating decreases and the abdomen feels less tense after meals.
- Stool rhythm becomes more consistent, with less urgency, straining, or incompletion.
- Sleep deepens because nighttime repair is no longer disrupted by digestive alarm.
- Brain fog begins to lift and mental focus becomes less effortful.
- Skin, allergy, and joint patterns may soften as inflammatory tone decreases.
- Energy becomes steadier because absorption is returning and the immune system is not consuming so much reserve.

These changes do not prove that every symptom came from the gut. They show that a restored digestive terrain gives every other healing effort better ground. When the soil becomes fertile, the rest of the system has something stable to grow from.

Ancient Observation, Modern Biology

Long before laboratories could sequence microbial DNA, healing traditions understood the centrality of digestion through observation. They saw that food altered mood, stool, skin, sleep, pain, and resilience. They recognized that a person could not be deeply well when digestion was chronically disturbed.

Modern biology has given this old observation new language: microbiome, intestinal permeability, GALT, short-chain fatty acids, vagal tone, enteroendocrine signaling, metabolic endotoxemia, and the gut-brain axis. The vocabulary changed. The central lesson did not.

Health is not built by fighting isolated symptoms forever. It is built by cultivating a habitat in which repair becomes easier than inflammation, tolerance becomes stronger than reactivity, and nourishment becomes more legible than noise.

The Sim-Bo method is practical microbiome medicine without theatrical complexity. It gives the inner soil what all soil requires: organic matter, rhythm, rest, water, warmth, and the absence of repeated assault.

Why Sim-Bo Begins Before Supplements

The modern gut market sells the fantasy of correction by capsule: probiotics, enzymes, powders, binders, cleanses, antimicrobials, and specialized formulas. Some of these tools can be useful when chosen with precision. None replaces terrain.

A probiotic placed into a hostile intestine is like seed thrown onto dry, chemical-soaked soil. A digestive enzyme swallowed before a chaotic meal may assist breakdown, but it cannot teach the nervous system to eat calmly. A fiber powder may change stool, but it cannot replace the broad architecture of vegetables, grains, fruit, water, chewing, and timing.

Sim-Bo begins before supplementation because the foundation determines whether the supplement becomes useful or merely another variable. First simplify. Then observe. Then add only what the case clearly requires. A master gardener does not begin by spraying the field. He studies the soil, water, season, and pattern of growth.

Conclusion: Healing Begins Below

The gut is where external nourishment becomes living tissue. It is where immunity learns tolerance, where appetite becomes honest, where microbial intelligence feeds metabolic order, and where emotion finds part of its chemical ground.

A damaged terrain makes every healing strategy work harder. A steadier terrain makes every intervention more effective: food, movement, rest, acupuncture, breath, botanical medicine, and disciplined simplicity. The foundation does not need to be glamorous. It needs to hold.

The gut teaches the first law of natural healing: cultivate the terrain before demanding the harvest.

Clinical Case Study 13: Clearing Cognitive Fog Through Gut Restoration

Patient: Michael P., 72-year-old male, retired financial analyst.

Chief concerns: anxiety, panic episodes, low mood, dense brain fog, erratic digestion with IBS-mixed pattern, and chronic fatigue. He reported that prior medication regimens reduced emotional intensity but left him apathetic and exhausted.

Clinical Presentation

Michael illustrates the gut-brain pattern at the center of this chapter.

For decades, his professional life was built around pressure: rushed meals, late nights, alcohol, processed carbohydrates, restaurant oils, and very little consistent fiber. His digestion became erratic long before his mood collapsed. He normalized bloating, irregular stool, poor appetite, and afternoon fatigue until anxiety and cognitive fog finally became impossible to ignore.

The clinical priority was not to treat his mind as separate from his intestine. His gut terrain, vagal tone, sleep, blood pressure, microbial substrate, and emotional chemistry had to be addressed as one field.

Initial Findings and Traditional Asian Medicine Assessment

Blood pressure: 148/92 mm Hg at baseline, in the setting of stress load and autonomic tension.

Tongue: swollen and dusky, with a thick greasy yellowish-white coating, consistent with Damp-Phlegm and Heat obstructing clarity within the Traditional Asian Medicine pattern.

Pulse: slippery and rapid, suggesting Phlegm-Heat with agitation of the Shen and digestive disturbance.

Primary pattern: Phlegm-Heat disturbing the Heart and misting the clear orifices, reflected in anxiety, panic, mental fog, and restlessness.

Secondary pattern: Spleen Qi deficiency with impaired transformation, reflected in erratic digestion, fatigue, and poor nutrient assimilation.

Treatment Principles

Reduce inflammatory and fermentative load from refined sugar, alcohol, seed oils, and ultra-processed foods.

Rebuild microbial substrate through cooked vegetables, whole grains, and measured fruit.

Support vagal tone before meals to improve motility, secretion, and the felt sense of safety.

Clear Phlegm-Heat and calm the Shen through acupuncture and botanical medicine.

Restore predictable meal timing and overnight digestive rest.

Plan and Intervention

Michael committed to a twelve-week Sim-Bo neuro-gut restoration plan.

The Sim-Bo dietary prescription: Alcohol, refined sugars, and fried seed-oil foods were removed. Slow-cooked brown rice and Job's tears served as the grain foundation. Lightly cooked, fiber-dense vegetables became the visible center of each meal. Whole fruit was used earlier in the day, away from heavy meals, to refresh hydration and reduce the need for refined sweetness.

Prebiotic rebuilding: Cooked onions, leeks, cabbage, root vegetables, oats, and barley were rotated to provide fermentable substrate while avoiding excessive raw load. Fermented foods were introduced cautiously and only as tolerated.

Autonomic reset: Diaphragmatic paced breathing was performed before meals to shift the nervous system toward parasympathetic readiness. Walking after meals was used to support glucose handling, motility, and mental settling.

Targeted acupuncture: PC5 and ST40 were selected to transform Phlegm and support clarity; Yin Tang and HT7 were used to calm the Shen; ST36 and SP6 supported digestion and recovery capacity.

Emperor's Cupping Therapy®: Sliding cupping was applied across the cervical-thoracic junction and upper back to reduce myofascial guarding, support local circulation, and ease the physical posture of chronic fear and mental strain.

Botanical medicine: Wen Dan Tang was used in a monitored clinical context for the observed Phlegm-Heat pattern, with the aim of supporting digestive regulation, reducing agitation, and clearing the sense of internal turbidity.

Medication coordination: Medication changes during the follow-up period were coordinated gradually with the prescribing psychiatrist and were not treated as a substitute for appropriate medical supervision.

Clinical Monitoring

Michael's progress was tracked through symptom rhythm rather than one isolated number: stool regularity, bloating, panic frequency, sleep continuity, morning energy, appetite, medication tolerance, tongue presentation, pulse quality, and ability to concentrate. The point was not to chase perfect data. The point was to watch whether the internal terrain became more coherent week by week.

The most important early sign was not dramatic euphoria. It was steadiness. He began waking with less dread. Meals produced less abdominal noise. His afternoon mind no longer collapsed into the same dense fog. The nervous system was not being forced into artificial calm; it was receiving fewer alarms from below.

Observed Outcomes After Twelve Weeks

Anxiety and panic: Panic episodes markedly decreased during the follow-up period, and Michael described a steadier internal state with fewer sudden surges of fear.

Cognitive clarity: Brain fog lifted significantly by patient report; he was able to read financial material again without repeatedly losing focus.

Digestion: IBS-mixed symptoms became more predictable, with less bloating, fewer urgency episodes, and steadier bowel rhythm.

Energy: Afternoon crashes decreased, and morning energy became more consistent.

Sleep: Sleep continuity improved, with fewer early-morning awakenings linked to anxiety.

Tongue and pulse: The greasy coating thinned, the dusky color softened, and the pulse became less rapid and less slippery as observed through Traditional Asian Medicine assessment.

Case Reflection

Michael's case illustrates the central law of Chapter 13: mental clarity requires clean terrain.

His improvement did not come from treating the brain as an isolated chemical container. It came from reducing inflammatory food patterns, rebuilding microbial substrate, restoring digestive rhythm, calming the vagus nerve, and addressing the Phlegm-Heat pattern that clouded both digestion and cognition. As the intestinal environment became less reactive, the nervous system received fewer danger messages. The mind had more room to settle.

The brain is not separate from the soil of the gut. When that soil becomes cleaner, steadier, and better fed, thought can return to order.

Transition: From Foundation to Firekeepers

The gut establishes the ground. It teaches tolerance, builds microbial order, and determines whether nourishment becomes clarity or alarm.

But even fertile ground faces the heat of living. Every breath, every meal, every step, and every immune response creates oxidative sparks. A healthy terrain can contain them. A depleted terrain lets them spread.

The gut reveals where healing takes root. The antioxidant network reveals how that root is protected when life inevitably burns.

Chapter 14

The Antioxidant Defense System

The Firekeepers Within

Every act of living creates a spark.

Every heartbeat, breath, movement, thought, and immune response depends on oxygen moving through the mitochondria to help produce ATP, the working currency of life. Oxygen gives us energy. It also leaves residue. A small portion of oxygen metabolism produces reactive oxygen species, often called free radicals: unstable molecules that seek electrons from nearby lipids, proteins, membranes, and DNA.

This is not a design flaw. Oxidation is part of living chemistry. A flame must release heat to warm a room; a mitochondrion must move electrons to generate energy. The danger begins when the sparks outnumber the firekeepers.

Oxidative stress is the internal rusting of physiology. It stiffens vessels, irritates nerves, weakens connective tissue, strains mitochondria, clouds cognition, and accelerates the visible signatures of aging. Skin loses elasticity. Joints lose ease. Vision becomes more vulnerable. Immune precision declines. Recovery takes longer.

Against this constant spark, the organism maintains an elegant defense network: the antioxidant system. It is not a single vitamin, not a celebrity supplement, and not a bottle on a shelf. It is a living grid of enzymes, minerals, plant compounds, breath, sleep, light, liver function, mitochondrial intelligence, and daily rhythm.

The great clinical mistake is to treat antioxidants as isolated rescue molecules while ignoring the terrain that generates oxidative strain. The Sim-Bo way begins elsewhere. It lowers the spark, feeds the firekeepers, restores cadence, and allows cellular repair to regain the advantage.

The Chemistry of Protection

A free radical is chemically restless. It lacks the stable electron arrangement it needs, so it takes from whatever is nearby. If it steals from a lipid membrane, the membrane becomes more fragile. If it steals from a protein, the protein may lose shape. If it strikes DNA, genetic integrity is challenged. One theft can trigger another, creating a chain reaction unless a protective molecule intervenes.

Antioxidants interrupt that chain. They donate an electron without becoming destructive themselves. Vitamin C, vitamin E, glutathione, carotenoids, flavonoids, polyphenols, and many plant pigments participate in this economy of protection. Their work is not theatrical. It is quiet maintenance at the level where aging begins.

There are two great classes of defenders.

Endogenous defenders are produced within physiology: glutathione, superoxide dismutase, catalase, peroxiredoxins, thioredoxin systems, and other enzymatic guardians.

Exogenous defenders arrive through food: colored plants, herbs, whole grains, legumes, seeds, fruits, vegetables, and their mineral co-factors.

The distinction matters. A supplement can donate a compound. A lifestyle builds the network. Glutathione requires amino acids. Superoxide dismutase depends on trace minerals such as zinc, copper, and manganese. Glutathione peroxidase requires selenium. Mitochondria require B-vitamins, magnesium, CoQ10, and a stable supply of energy.

Antioxidant defense is therefore not a pill-based event. It is a coordinated architecture. Food supplies the material. Breath regulates the chemistry. Sleep resets the repair window. Movement circulates the waste. Calm conserves the reserves. Rhythm keeps the system intelligible.

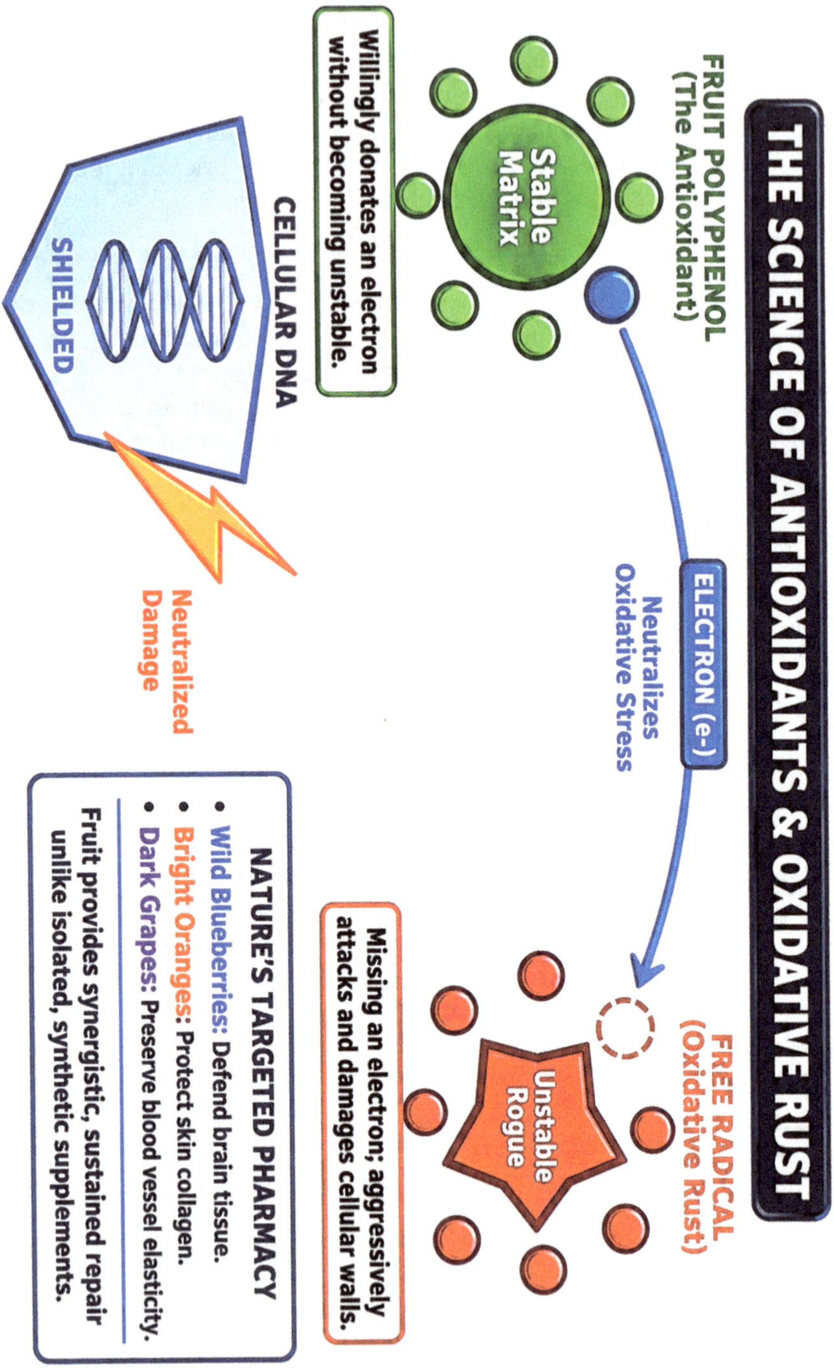

Figure 8. The science of antioxidants and oxidative rust.

Oxidation and Inflammation: The Closed Loop

Inflammation and oxidation are intimate partners.

During acute infection or injury, immune cells use reactive oxygen species as weapons. A controlled oxidative burst helps destroy pathogens and clear damaged tissue. In that moment, the spark is useful. It belongs to the repair sequence.

The damage begins when the repair sequence never resolves. Chronic inflammation keeps immune chemistry active. Active immune chemistry produces more reactive oxygen species. Oxidative injury then irritates tissue and calls for more immune activity. The loop tightens: inflammation creates oxidation; oxidation feeds inflammation.

This is why chronic stress, poor sleep, unstable blood sugar, air pollution, alcohol, industrial oils, emotional pressure, and sedentary living are not separate problems. They all increase the same internal cost: more sparks, fewer firekeepers, weaker resolution.

Breaking the loop requires more than suppressing a symptom. It requires restoring the conditions under which the antioxidant network can work: simple food, mineral sufficiency, cellular hydration, daily movement, darkness at night, natural light in the morning, and a nervous system no longer forced to live under continuous emergency.

Food as Antioxidant Architecture

The Sim-Bo plate is antioxidant architecture in edible form.

Brown rice, vegetables, and fruit do more than fill the stomach. They deliver minerals, fiber, slow carbohydrate, phytochemicals, water, color, and microbial fuel in a pattern physiology can read. The colors on the plate are not decoration. They are protective chemistry made visible.

Deep red foods — tomatoes, pomegranates, cherries, and berries — provide lycopene, anthocyanins, and polyphenols that support vascular resilience and endothelial protection.

Orange and yellow foods — carrots, winter squash, citrus, persimmon, and sweet roots — deliver carotenoids and vitamin C patterns that nourish mucosal barriers, skin structure, and visual tissues.

Dark green foods — leafy vegetables, herbs, bok choy, kale, chard, and parsley — provide magnesium, chlorophyll-associated compounds, lutein, folate, and a mineral current that supports liver work, bile flow, and ocular protection.

Blue and purple foods — blueberries, black grapes, plums, purple

cabbage, eggplant skin — concentrate anthocyanins and dark-spectrum polyphenols that support neurovascular and mitochondrial defense.
Earth-toned foods — intact grains, sesame, flax, sprouted seeds, legumes, and nuts — deliver vitamin E patterns, selenium, zinc, lignans, and trace mineral scaffolding for enzymatic defense.

The genius of whole food is not one compound. It is the matrix. A berry is not only anthocyanin. A carrot is not only beta-carotene. A green leaf is not only magnesium. Each arrives with water, fiber, mineral co-factors, organic acids, aroma, texture, and digestive pacing.

This matrix is why the Sim-Bo method favors food before capsules. A capsule can isolate. A plate can orchestrate.

Many plant compounds also speak through Nrf2, the transcriptional pathway that helps regulate endogenous antioxidant enzymes. Colorful plants do not merely donate protection; they instruct cellular defense to organize itself. This is the higher intelligence of food: it does not simply fight the spark. It teaches the firekeepers to stand ready.

Color as Clinical Intelligence

Color is one of the simplest clinical languages available at the table.

A pale plate usually tells a pale metabolic story. Beige meals built from white flour, white sugar, fried starch, and processed oils may satisfy hunger quickly, but they provide little instruction for antioxidant defense. They ask the mitochondria to burn fuel without providing enough pigment, mineral, and fiber intelligence to manage the residue.

A living plate looks different. It carries red, orange, yellow, green, purple, brown, and black. Each shade carries its own chemistry, but the deeper lesson is synergy. Lycopene needs fat and a digestive system ready for absorption. Carotenoids are better received when the meal contains warmth and a small amount of stable lipid. Polyphenols interact with the microbiome, becoming smaller metabolites that communicate with the gut lining, liver, vessels, and immune system.

This is why Sim-Bo does not chase one famous antioxidant. It builds a field. A single compound may be impressive in a laboratory. A daily plate must survive digestion, fermentation, bile flow, absorption, circulation, and cellular use. The clinical power is not in spectacle. It is in repetition.

Color must also be timed. Heavy raw salads in a cold, depleted digestive state can burden assimilation. Overcooked vegetables stripped of texture and vitality lose part of their message. The master meal respects temperature, season, constitution, and preparation. A carrot steamed with care can become easier medicine than a raw vegetable swallowed in haste.

Breath and Light: Environmental Regulators

The antioxidant system does not live inside the diet alone. It responds to air, light, darkness, and respiratory cadence.

Oxygen is both fuel and challenge. Shallow, rapid breathing keeps the chest tense, limits diaphragmatic movement, and reinforces sympathetic tone. Slow diaphragmatic breathing changes the internal atmosphere. It improves respiratory efficiency, supports vagal regulation, assists carbon dioxide balance, and tells the nervous system that the emergency has passed.

A long exhalation is one of the simplest forms of metabolic hygiene. It does not perform detoxification as a trend. It restores the chemistry of calm. When the breath slows, cortisol pressure decreases, heart rhythm becomes more coherent, and inflammatory tension has fewer reasons to persist.

Light is another antioxidant regulator. Morning sunlight helps anchor circadian timing, which organizes cortisol, melatonin, mitochondrial repair, temperature, appetite, and sleep depth. Melatonin is more than a sleep molecule; it participates in antioxidant defense, mitochondrial protection, and nighttime repair.

Moderate natural sunlight also supports nitric-oxide signaling and vascular tone. The lesson is not reckless exposure. It is intelligent contact with the natural day: light in the morning, darkness at night, and less blue artificial stimulation after sunset.

Breath and light teach the same law as food: the dose, timing, and rhythm determine whether a life-giving element restores or strains.

The Internal Antioxidant Pharmacy

The most important antioxidant pharmacy is already built into the cells.

It does not advertise. It does not require a label. It works continuously, provided the terrain supplies the minerals, amino acids, rest, and metabolic clarity required to keep it active.

Glutathione is the central intracellular defender. Built from glutamine, glycine, and cysteine, it helps neutralize reactive species, supports phase-two liver conjugation, and regenerates other antioxidants so they can return to work.

Superoxide dismutase converts superoxide radicals into less reactive compounds that can be further processed. It relies on mineral co-factors and functions as an early responder in oxidative defense.

Catalase helps convert hydrogen peroxide into water and oxygen, preventing accumulation of a compound that can become highly damaging in the wrong chemical setting.

Coenzyme Q10 sits in the mitochondrial electron-transport chain, helping shuttle electrons for ATP production while limiting leakage that would otherwise increase oxidative strain.

Melatonin participates in nighttime antioxidant regulation and mitochondrial repair, linking sleep depth directly to cellular resilience.

These defenders do not work as isolated celebrities. They function as a relay. One molecule donates. Another regenerates. One enzyme converts a radical. Another completes the neutralization. The network is the medicine.

This is why mineral-poor dieting, chronic sleep loss, alcohol, emotional strain, and processed food weaken antioxidant defense even when a person swallows expensive supplements. The internal pharmacy cannot run on slogans. It requires raw material, rest, timing, and simplicity.

The Mineral Keys

Antioxidant enzymes are mineral-dependent instruments.

Without minerals, the orchestra cannot play. Zinc and copper help superoxide dismutase function. Selenium supports glutathione peroxidase. Manganese participates in mitochondrial antioxidant defense. Magnesium steadies the electrical and enzymatic environment in which repair occurs. B-vitamins help move energy through the pathways that keep cells from drowning in unfinished combustion.

This is where restrictive, fashionable dieting quietly weakens resilience. A person may remove calories and still lose the trace elements required for defense. A person may drink expensive green powders and still lack the warm, mineral-rich, fiber-bound meal that digestion can receive. Depletion often hides behind discipline.

Whole grains, legumes, seeds, vegetables, sea vegetables, herbs, and fruits supply these mineral keys in a pattern the digestive system understands. The Sim-Bo plate therefore does not merely offer antioxidants. It provides the metal co-factors that allow endogenous antioxidant enzymes to exist.

The goal is not nutritional decoration. It is enzymatic competence.

When Antioxidants Become Noise

More is not automatically wiser.

Oxidation is not purely evil. In small amounts, reactive oxygen species act as adaptation signals. Exercise uses them. Immune defense uses them. Mitochondria use them to communicate demand. A life with no oxidative challenge would be a life with no growth.

The clinical problem is excess without recovery. The solution is not to smother every spark with random megadoses of isolated antioxidants. In the wrong person, at the wrong dose, and at the wrong time, excessive supplementation can create confusion, blunt adaptive signals, or compete with the internal network that should have been strengthened by food, sleep, and movement.

This is why Sim-Bo respects hierarchy. Food builds the terrain. Breath lowers the pressure. Sleep restores the night chemistry. Movement creates useful stress and then resolution. Only after that foundation is restored does an isolated nutrient deserve a role.

A capsule should never become a substitute for a life that has stopped generating balance.

The Sim-Bo Detox: Cleansing Without Depletion

A detox that depletes is not detoxification.

Modern commercial cleansing often misunderstands the liver. Punishing fasts, sugar-heavy juice programs, stimulant laxatives, and oversized supplement stacks may make a patient feel dramatic sensations, but drama is not proof of repair. True detoxification requires binding, transformation, conjugation, bile flow, bowel movement, kidney filtration, lymphatic circulation, sweating, breath, and sleep.

The Sim-Bo detox does not bypass this system. It strengthens it. The goal is fewer variables, cleaner inputs, slower eating, predictable elimination, and enough minerals to finish what the liver begins.

> Simplify variety, not nourishment. For a short clinical window, meals are narrowed to plain brown rice, lightly cooked vegetables, whole fruit, clean water, and gentle herbal teas. This lowers dietary noise and gives digestion a clear pattern.

Hydrate deliberately. Water supports kidney filtration, bowel movement, bile flow, and the movement of water-soluble waste. It is taken steadily, not forced in punishing volumes.
Move lightly and consistently. Walking, stretching, and diaphragmatic breathing support lymphatic movement and circulation without creating another stress burden.
Protect deep sleep. Nighttime repair is when antioxidant systems, brain clearance, hormonal rhythm, and mitochondrial restoration converge.
Exhale fully. Carbon dioxide is a metabolic by-product. Slow complete exhalation helps regulate acid-base balance and supports parasympathetic tone.

The Sim-Bo detox is not a harsh purge. It is a restoration of flow. When the intake becomes simple, the exits become clearer. When digestion rests from novelty, repair becomes audible again.

The Antioxidant Lifestyle

A true antioxidant lifestyle is recognizable by its calm.

It does not chase extremes. It does not confuse punishment with discipline. It does not try to buy protection one capsule at a time. It lowers avoidable sparks and strengthens the network that handles the necessary ones.

The rusting pattern is easy to identify: chronic psychological pressure, suppressed anger, late-night light, alcohol, smoking, fried food, refined sugar, repeatedly heated oils, sleep debt, sedentary days, shallow breathing, and emotional speed. Each adds oxidative pressure.

The renewal pattern is equally clear: dawn light, clean hydration, whole grains, green vegetables, colorful fruit, slow breathing, daily walking, adequate minerals, meaningful work, emotional honesty, and darkness at night. Each restores the firekeepers.

Emotional regulation belongs in antioxidant medicine. Anger, fear, grief, and resentment are not abstractions; they alter breath, blood pressure, cortisol, glucose, gut motility, and immune tone. A calm mind does not merely feel better. It changes chemistry.

Peace preserves physiology. Not sentimental peace, but trained peace: the daily practice of choosing a slower breath, a simpler plate, a darker room, a steadier schedule, and fewer unnecessary conflicts with nature.

The Clinical Rules of Antioxidant Medicine

Antioxidant medicine follows a strict hierarchy.

First, reduce the obvious oxidizers: fried food, smoke, alcohol excess, late screens, sleep debt, emotional speed, chronic overwork, and meals eaten under pressure. Removing these inputs is not glamorous, but it immediately lowers the number of sparks the system must manage.

Second, restore the daily carriers of repair: mineral-rich grains, green vegetables, colored fruit, steady hydration, bowel regularity, morning light, darkness at night, and breath that reaches the diaphragm. These are not accessories. They are the infrastructure of cellular defense.

Third, use concentrated tools only with a defined purpose. Vitamin C, CoQ10, selenium, NAC, glutathione support, carotenoids, or botanical formulas may have value when the terrain calls for them, but they must enter a working system. A bridge helps only when there is a road on both sides.

This hierarchy protects the patient from the common error of modern wellness: adding more while changing nothing. The Sim-Bo path is different. It removes what increases the spark, restores what feeds the firekeepers, and reserves targeted tools for seasons of genuine demand.

The Sim-Bo Antioxidant Plate

Every Sim-Bo meal can be built as edible defense.

The base: brown rice, oats, millet, or quinoa, prepared warm and soft, providing steady glucose and trace minerals for enzyme function.
The greens: bok choy, spinach, chard, kale, herbs, or cruciferous vegetables, providing magnesium, folate, chlorophyll-associated compounds, fiber, and bitter intelligence for liver and bile flow.
The color: carrot, beet, red cabbage, winter squash, purple vegetables, or peppers, adding carotenoids, anthocyanins, and polyphenol architecture.
The accent: sesame, flax, walnuts, pumpkin seeds, or sprouted legumes, adding vitamin E patterns, zinc, selenium, and mineral support for antioxidant enzymes.
The fruit: berries, citrus, pomegranate, apple, pear, or seasonal fruit, providing vitamin C patterns, soluble fiber, organic acids, hydration, and color-based protection.

The meal must be eaten slowly. Chewing is not mechanical delay; it is the first antioxidant act of digestion. It reduces stress, initiates salivary chemistry, signals safety, and prevents the gut from receiving nourishment as an emergency.

A plate eaten in panic cannot become the same medicine as a plate eaten with presence. The chemistry of the food and the chemistry of the eater meet at the table.

Oxidative Stress and Mitochondrial Economy

The mitochondria are where energy and oxidation meet most intimately.

When fuel arrives in a steady rhythm and the cell has oxygen, minerals, and rest, electron flow remains orderly. ATP is produced, heat is managed, and only a manageable number of radicals escape. When fuel arrives in excess, especially after a large sedentary meal, the system backs up. Electrons leak. Reactive species rise. The engine smokes.

This is why the same meal can behave differently under different conditions. A bowl of warm grain and vegetables eaten after a walk and followed by rest enters one metabolic environment. The same calories eaten late at night, in stress, under blue light, after alcohol, enter another. Oxidative chemistry is shaped by context.

Post-meal movement is therefore antioxidant medicine. Ten quiet minutes of walking after eating increases glucose disposal, supports circulation, and reduces the metabolic pressure inside the mitochondria. The meal burns cleaner because the muscles are open for fuel.

This is one of the simplest laws of energy: a system designed to move cannot process abundance well while motionless.

The Organs That Reveal Oxidative Strain

Oxidative stress is systemic, but it often announces itself through the most delicate tissues first.

The eyes are early witnesses. Retinal and macular tissue carry high metabolic demand, constant light exposure, and lipid-rich membranes. When antioxidant reserve thins, glare becomes more irritating, visual stamina decreases, and recovery after long screen or flight exposure slows. Food cannot replace eye care, but ocular tissue still depends on the same terrain as every other tissue: circulation, sleep, color, minerals, hydration, and mitochondrial steadiness.

The vessels speak next. The endothelial lining is injured by blood-sugar swings, oxidized lipids, smoking, hypertension, stress chemistry, and inflammatory load. Oxidative pressure changes the behavior of cholesterol and proteins inside the vessel wall. The issue is not a single number on a lab panel; it is the condition of the river those numbers move through.

Skin records the same process visibly. Collagen, elastin, hydration, pigment, wound repair, and texture all depend on the balance between oxidative exposure and repair capacity. Sunlight used with wisdom supports circadian timing; sunlight used without respect adds wear. The same law governs food, work, stress, travel, and exercise: dose determines whether a stimulus trains or damages.

Joints also reveal the redox state. Cartilage, fascia, synovial tissue, and tendons are sensitive to oxidative pressure because repair is slower and circulation is more limited. When sparks accumulate, movement becomes stiff. When the inner terrain clears, movement often feels easier before any dramatic external change is visible.

This is why antioxidant medicine cannot be reduced to a capsule. It is ocular medicine, vascular medicine, skin medicine, connective-tissue medicine, immune medicine, and mitochondrial medicine at once. The network protects the entire terrain.

Clean Aging

Every breath creates a spark. Every meal, step, and thought alters how that spark is handled.

The antioxidant defense system proves that physiology is not passive. It has firekeepers: enzymes, minerals, pigments, sleep, breath, and rhythm.

Sim-Bo protects those firekeepers through clean food, plant color, mineral sufficiency, slow breath, darkness, movement, and daily repetition.

The daily economics are simple. If the sparks generated by work, food, thought, and environment exceed the repair available through sleep, minerals, color, movement, and calm, the system spends more than it earns. Wrinkles, fatigue, pain, vascular stiffness, visual strain, and immune fragility are not random penalties; they are unpaid invoices.

Sim-Bo changes that economy by reducing unnecessary expense and increasing quiet repair. The method does not promise escape from aging. It teaches a cleaner way to age: fewer oxidized inputs, more plant color, steadier digestion, better breath, reliable darkness, and enough repetition for repair to compound.

Conclusion: The Calm Between Sparks

Every breath creates a spark. Every meal, step, thought, conflict, and recovery period alters the way that spark is handled.

The antioxidant defense system proves that physiology is not passive against the wear of life. It is equipped with firekeepers. It knows how to convert strain into repair when the terrain is not overwhelmed.

To live with vitality is not to hide from oxidation. It is to master the conditions around it: clean food, slow breath, mineral sufficiency, deep sleep, steady light, daily movement, and a life quiet enough for repair to complete its work.

The Sim-Bo law remains intact: food first, rhythm always, targeted tools only when the terrain asks for them.

Clinical Case Study 14

Restoring Antioxidant Capacity Under Oxidative Strain

Patient: Thomas G., 59-year-old male, commercial airline pilot.

Chief concerns: progressive visual blurring associated with early macular-degeneration monitoring, frequent prolonged respiratory infections, accelerated skin aging, and persistent fatigue.

Clinical Presentation

Thomas lived inside an oxidative profession. Long flights, high-altitude exposure, circadian disruption, airport food, irregular sleep, dehydration, and repeated time-zone shifts created a constant internal demand. He was not collapsing from one dramatic disease event. He was being worn down by sparks that never fully cleared.

His work pattern narrowed sleep, reduced melatonin rhythm, disturbed digestion, and kept him dependent on dry processed food during travel. His visual decline, respiratory vulnerability, skin changes, and fatigue formed one clinical picture: oxidative strain outpacing antioxidant renewal.

Initial Findings

hs-CRP: 4.6 mg/L, consistent with elevated inflammatory burden.

Tongue: red and dry, with a peeled center and dark prickles at the tip.

Pulse: rapid, floating, and empty at the deeper level.

Traditional Asian Medicine assessment: Liver and Kidney Yin depletion with heat signs affecting the eyes; Lung Qi deficiency with reduced respiratory resilience.

Treatment Principles

Build a colorful Sim-Bo plate rich in phytochemicals, minerals, fiber, and hydration.

Support endogenous antioxidant pathways with food-based trace minerals and regular sleep timing.

Nourish Liver and Kidney Yin within the Traditional Asian Medicine framework.

Reduce processed airport-food exposure and industrial oils during

travel.
Restore circadian anchors: morning light, darker evenings, travel hydration, and scheduled sleep recovery.
Use acupuncture, cupping, and botanical medicine to support visual pathways, respiratory resilience, fascia, and recovery.

Clinical Strategy

The protocol was not built around a single antioxidant. It was built around three clinical corrections: remove the strongest sources of oxidative pressure, restore circadian repair, and feed the endogenous defense network with color and minerals.

For a pilot, perfection was not realistic. Airports, night flights, recycled cabin air, dehydration, and irregular time zones could not be eliminated. The intervention had to be portable, repeatable, and simple enough to survive travel.

Plan and Intervention

Thomas committed to a twelve-week Sim-Bo antioxidant restoration plan.

The antioxidant shield: processed carbohydrates, fried airport foods, and industrial seed-oil snacks were removed from his travel pattern and replaced with packed Sim-Bo meals.
Macular defenders: orange and yellow vegetables, leafy greens, carrots, winter squash, bok choy, parsley, and dark greens were used daily to supply carotenoid and mineral patterns supportive of ocular tissue.
Neurovascular color: blueberries, black grapes, pomegranate, and dark seasonal fruit were used as the one-part fruit component, providing anthocyanin-rich color and soluble fiber.
Grounding grains: oats, quinoa, brown rice, and millet supplied steady carbohydrate and trace minerals required for enzymatic defense.
Acupuncture: GB37, LR3, KI3, ST36, and selected eye-supportive points were used to support Liver-channel circulation, foundational Yin, digestive resilience, and fatigue recovery.
Emperor's Cupping Therapy®: sliding cupping was applied along the posterior chain and upper back to reduce myofascial restriction, support local circulation, and assist respiratory ease.
Botanical medicine: Qi Ju Di Huang Wan was used within the Traditional Asian Medicine framework to nourish Liver and Kidney Yin and support visual comfort.

Clinical Markers and Patient Report

Inflammatory marker: hs-CRP improved from 4.6 mg/L to 0.8 mg/L.
Vision: visual blurring stabilized by patient report; ophthalmologic monitoring continued with the appropriate eye-care clinician.
Immune resilience: recurrent respiratory infections decreased during the follow-up period.
Energy: fatigue improved, with steadier stamina during travel days.
Skin and tissue quality: dryness and visible photo-aging appeared less pronounced by clinical observation and patient report.
Tongue and pulse: the tongue became less dry, the coating improved, and pulse quality became steadier within the Traditional Asian Medicine pattern assessment.

Clinical Meaning

Thomas's case illustrates the central law of Chapter 14: aging pressure accelerates when oxidative strain outpaces antioxidant repair. His improvement did not come from a single miracle compound. It came from restoring the network.

Color returned to the plate. Darkness returned to the night. Breath returned to the diaphragm. Travel food became planned rather than desperate. Acupuncture and botanical medicine supported the terrain, but the daily architecture did the deeper work.

The lesson is exact: the cell does not need theatrical detox. It needs fewer sparks, stronger firekeepers, and enough daily order to complete repair.

Thomas also demonstrates why antioxidant medicine must be practical. A beautiful plan that fails at the airport is not medicine. His success came from preparing travel meals, carrying dark fruit instead of packaged snacks, drinking water before coffee, using light deliberately, and protecting recovery sleep after flights. The prescription became portable.

Transition: From Firekeepers to Targeted Tools

When the antioxidant network is nourished, the ordinary sparks of living burn cleaner. Plants provide color. Minerals steady enzymes. Breath regulates the inner atmosphere. Sleep restores the night crew. Movement clears the channels.

Still, seasons of high demand arrive: illness, antibiotics, travel, winter darkness, emotional pressure, heavy training, poor soil, depleted food quality, or clinical deficiency. In those moments, targeted nutrients can serve a precise role.

A supplement is not a substitute for the forest. It is a temporary tool carried into difficult terrain. It works best when the foundation is already alive: food first, cadence always, capsules only with purpose.

The shelf of targeted tools now comes into view. The question is not how many bottles a person can take. The question is which support is necessary, clean, temporary, and worthy of entering the Sim-Bo order.

Chapter 15

Targeted Supplements: Strategic Support, Not Substitution

The Supplement Paradox

The modern supplement shelf is crowded because modern life is depleted.

Capsules, powders, tinctures, extracts, probiotics, peptides, greens blends, mineral drops, and isolated tonics now occupy the space once held by whole meals, sunlight, rest, soil, and seasonal eating. The promise is seductive: swallow the missing molecule and repair the damage created by industrial food, indoor living, chronic stress, sleep loss, pollution, and relentless pace.

The Sim-Bo view is simpler and stricter. A supplement is a tool. It is not a lifestyle. It is not a replacement for food. It is not a license to keep violating the conditions that created the deficiency.

The word supplement already contains its proper role. It adds support to a foundation that must already exist. When the foundation is weak, supplementation becomes cosmetic scaffolding around a house whose frame is still rotting. When the foundation is strong, a targeted nutrient can be elegant: a precise bridge across a temporary gap, a short-term reinforcement during repair, a focused clinical instrument used with timing and restraint.

This is the paradox. The more people chase bottles, the more they often drift from the original medicine: food in its matrix, breath in its depth, sunlight in its timing, sleep in its darkness, movement in its daily repetition, and emotional chemistry quiet enough for repair to occur.

Supplements are most powerful when they are treated with humility.

Why Functional Gaps Appear

Even disciplined patients can develop functional nutrient gaps in the modern world.

Soil quality has changed. Agricultural speed, depleted mineral cycles, long-distance shipping, chemical exposure, and storage time can reduce the density and vitality of food before it reaches the plate. Indoor living reduces sunlight exposure. Chronic stress increases demand for B-vitamins, magnesium, vitamin C, and antioxidant reserves. Alcohol, sleep disruption, medications, digestive inflammation, low bile flow, dysbiosis, and poor stomach acid can alter absorption and utilization. Pollution and emotional strain increase oxidative demand. Aging changes digestive efficiency and metabolic reserve.

This is not the old picture of deficiency. Scurvy, rickets, and beriberi are extreme end-stage absences. Modern patients more often present with functional insufficiency: enough nutrient to avoid collapse, not always enough to support resilience under load. A blood test may look acceptable while the patient's clinical pattern tells a different story: fatigue, poor stress tolerance, muscle tightness, low mood, fragile immunity, slow wound healing, brittle sleep, hair shedding, restless legs, poor digestion, or loss of reserve.

This is the narrow doorway where supplementation has value. It does not replace Sim-Bo. It helps the patient cross a demanding season while food, timing, digestion, sleep, breath, and bowel flow rebuild the ground beneath the symptom.

The order matters: remove the interference, rebuild the foundation, target the gap, then withdraw what is no longer needed.

When a Supplement Earns Its Place

A supplement earns its place only when three conditions are present: a credible need, a clean form, and a defined exit strategy.

Credible need may appear through laboratory data, clinical signs, medication history, dietary gaps, travel stress, chronic illness, digestive limitation, or a season of unusual demand. Clean form means the product contains what it says, avoids unnecessary additives, protects fragile compounds from oxidation, and respects dose. Exit strategy means the tool is not allowed to become identity. It is used, observed, adjusted, and eventually retired when the foundation can carry the work.

This hierarchy protects the patient from the most common supplement error: confusing intensity with intelligence. A large stack creates the feeling of control. It also creates too many variables. When twenty compounds are swallowed every morning, the practitioner can no longer read the terrain. If sleep improves, which ingredient helped? If anxiety rises, which dose provoked it? If digestion worsens, which capsule created irritation? Complexity makes observation impossible.

Sim-Bo restores a clean clinical experiment. Simplify the diet. Stabilize meal timing. Remove processed noise. Introduce one tool at a time.

Observe energy, sleep, bowels, mood, skin, pain, cravings, pulse, tongue, and laboratory markers. This is not slow medicine. It is accurate medicine.

Correct the terrain first: food, sleep, breath, movement, hydration, digestive rhythm, and elimination.
Introduce only what has a defined purpose.
Use one new tool at a time whenever possible.
Track the response through signs the patient can feel and markers the clinician can measure.
Pause periodically to confirm that the foundation, not the bottle, is carrying the recovery.

The Three Laws of Sim-Bo Supplementation

1. Matrix First

The original delivery system for nutrients is whole food.

A berry does not deliver vitamin C alone. It delivers water, fiber, polyphenols, minerals, acids, aroma, texture, color, and digestive pacing. A seed does not deliver oil alone. It delivers minerals, lignans, protein, fiber, and a structure that slows absorption. A leaf does not deliver magnesium alone. It arrives with chlorophyll, folate, potassium, bitterness, nitrate, and the intelligence of sunlight converted into edible architecture.

The matrix governs meaning. Isolated nutrients can be useful, but they are fragments. The intact food pattern remains the mother language of metabolism.

2. Minimum Effective Dose

Dose determines direction.

A nutrient can correct a gap, irritate a system, or distort a pathway depending on amount, form, timing, and the person receiving it. Zinc can support immunity; excess zinc can disturb copper balance. Iron can restore oxygen-carrying capacity when truly needed; unnecessary iron can feed oxidative stress. Vitamin D can restore light deficiency; reckless dosing can disturb calcium regulation. High-dose antioxidants can be useful in selected circumstances; they can also blunt adaptive signals when used without purpose.

Sim-Bo supplementation uses the minimum effective dose for a defined reason. The question is never, How much can I take? The question is, What precise support does this terrain require now?

3. Cycle, Observe, Withdraw

A supplement should earn its place repeatedly.

The disciplined method is simple: use it for a defined period, observe the clinical response, remove it when the terrain stabilizes, and watch whether the baseline holds. If vitality remains steady after withdrawal, the system has recovered a measure of self-regulation. If the same pattern returns, the deeper cause still remains: poor sleep, unresolved stress chemistry, weak digestion, low fiber, alcohol, inadequate light, chronic inflammation, medication interaction, or a food pattern that continues to create need.

The goal is not a larger supplement protocol. The goal is fewer bottles and a stronger patient.

When Support Becomes Clinically Useful

The clean clinical question is not whether a patient should take supplements. The cleaner question is what the system is attempting to do, and what it lacks in order to complete that work.

A mineral may be useful when the nervous system cannot downshift. Vitamin D may be useful when light exposure, immune resilience, and mineral metabolism require restoration. Probiotic support may be useful after antibiotics, travel, infection, or a long period of digestive disruption. Omega-3 support may be useful when the lipid terrain is dry, inflamed, or dominated by processed oils. Vitamin C may be useful when connective tissue, immune response, or oxidative strain requires more support than food alone is currently providing.

In each case, the tool serves the terrain. It does not become the terrain. The supplement is not the hero of the story; the physiology is. The supplement provides one missing brick while the house is being rebuilt through food, sleep, movement, breath, and daily order.

This principle protects the patient from the most common error in modern wellness: using advanced tools to avoid simple discipline. A person who sleeps four hours, eats late, avoids vegetables, breathes shallowly, lives under resentment, and swallows twenty capsules is not practicing sophisticated medicine. That person is decorating disorder.

Clinical usefulness appears when the tool serves a clear purpose: replenish, protect, regulate, or bridge. Replenish means intake is insufficient or absorption is impaired. Protect means a temporary season of oxidative, infectious, travel, toxic, or emotional strain has increased demand. Regulate means a pathway needs assistance while the broader pattern is corrected. Bridge means the patient is not yet strong enough to rely on food and rhythm alone.

Once the bridge has done its work, it should become less important. This is the sign of good supplementation: the patient gradually becomes less impressed by the bottle and more faithful to the structure of the day.

The Minimalist Clinical Shelf

A healthy supplement shelf should look like a quiet clinic, not a marketplace.

The Sim-Bo shelf is small, purposeful, and easy to explain. Every product has a reason. Every reason has a time frame. Every time frame has an observation point. If a patient cannot say why a product is present, what it is meant to support, and when it will be reassessed, the product is probably serving anxiety rather than healing.

The minimalist shelf protects digestion. Each capsule carries excipients, binders, coatings, oils, sweeteners, flavors, or botanical compounds that must be processed. A patient with bloating, reflux, constipation, loose stools, nausea, or food sensitivity can become overwhelmed by the supplement stack itself. In those cases, stopping the stack is often the first medicine.

This is why the Sim-Bo method often begins with subtraction. Remove the nonessential. Keep only what is targeted. Let the digestive tract become quiet enough to reveal the true pattern. Then support that pattern with precision.

A disciplined supplement plan should be able to fit on one page: product, purpose, dose, timing, duration, food pairing, caution, and reassessment. Anything more chaotic than that belongs to commercial wellness, not clinical restoration.

Reading the Response

A supplement plan is only as intelligent as the observation that follows it.

The patient must learn to read response through energy, bowel rhythm, sleep continuity, mood steadiness, appetite, skin, pain, cravings, temperature, and tolerance. A helpful tool produces a cleaner pattern. An unsuitable tool produces noise: agitation, insomnia, loose stool, constipation, headache, nausea, skin eruptions, racing thoughts, or a heaviness that the patient cannot explain.

This is not failure. It is communication. The system is showing whether the tool fits the terrain.

The most important response is not the first burst of energy. Many patients mistake stimulation for healing. Caffeine feels impressive. High-dose B vitamins can feel impressive. Strong adaptogens can feel impressive. But the deeper test is stability: sleep continuity, digestive ease, emotional steadiness, fewer crashes, calmer focus, and less reliance on rescue.

Sim-Bo clinical observation prefers the quiet improvement. The nervous system becomes less dramatic. The bowel becomes predictable. The patient needs fewer rescue tools. The day becomes easier to repeat. This is how the terrain speaks.

The Core Sim-Bo Support Tools

Certain nutrients deserve recurring clinical attention because modern life repeatedly drains them. They are not universal prescriptions. They are common tools: useful when the pattern calls for them, unnecessary when the foundation already supplies them.

Vitamin C: The Electron Donor

Vitamin C is a water-soluble antioxidant, collagen cofactor, immune support nutrient, and recycling partner for other antioxidants. Because humans do not synthesize it internally, intake must come from food or targeted support.

The Sim-Bo foundation favors citrus, kiwi, bell pepper, berries, parsley, cabbage, leafy greens, and other whole-food sources. When stress, travel, infection exposure, poor wound healing, smoking history, high oxidative load, or low intake increases demand, supplemental vitamin C can be used strategically. Smaller, divided amounts often serve better than heroic dosing that irritates the stomach and bowel.

Vitamin C belongs to repair, not performance theater.

Vitamin D3 and K2: Light and Calcium Direction

Vitamin D is more than a vitamin. It is a hormone-like signal shaped by sunlight, skin, liver, kidney, immune tone, fat tissue, and circadian pattern. Indoor living has made low vitamin D status common, especially in patients with limited sun exposure, darker skin, higher body fat, chronic inflammation, or long winters.

When supplementation is needed, vitamin D3 works best inside a larger mineral and fat-soluble context: magnesium sufficiency, vitamin K2, adequate dietary fat, and sensible light exposure. D3 helps increase calcium absorption; K2 participates in routing calcium into the tissues where structure is needed. The point is not to flood the bloodstream with calcium. The point is coordinated direction.

Sunlight remains the original teacher. Supplementation is the backup lantern.

Omega-3 Fatty Acids: Lipid Resolution

Omega-3 fatty acids are lipid messengers. They influence membrane fluidity, inflammatory resolution, vascular tone, brain structure, and cellular communication. Their value lies not in trendy anti-inflammatory language, but in the quiet chemistry of resolution: helping the system complete a response rather than remain trapped inside it.

Flax, chia, hemp, walnuts, and leafy greens supply alpha-linolenic acid, or ALA. Marine algae oil supplies direct EPA and DHA without relying on fish as the intermediary. Quality matters. Oxidized oil is no medicine. The best omega-3 strategy combines fresh plant fats, algae-based support when needed, low intake of repeatedly heated industrial oils, and a plate rich in vegetables and whole grains.

A clean lipid signal requires both the right oil and the absence of the wrong smoke.

Magnesium: The Mineral of Release

Magnesium participates in ATP handling, nerve conduction, muscular relaxation, vascular tone, glucose regulation, bowel motility, and stress physiology. It is the mineral of release: the unclenching of muscle, vessel, nerve, and mind.

Leafy greens, seeds, legumes, cacao, nuts, and whole grains provide the natural foundation. Stress, sweat, alcohol, poor intake, low stomach acid, medications, and depleted food patterns can increase need. Glycinate is often used for nervous system calm; malate for muscular energy; citrate for bowel motility in selected patients. Oxide is common, inexpensive, and poorly tolerated by many patients.

The right form matters because the mineral must arrive where the pattern needs it.

Probiotics: Transient Gardeners

Probiotics are not lasting rulers of the gut. They are transient gardeners.

After antibiotics, travel, stress, infection, processed food exposure, or digestive disruption, targeted strains can help reintroduce microbial diversity and restore ecological communication. Their work depends on terrain. Without fiber, polyphenols, hydration, bowel movement, sleep, and lower stress chemistry, even excellent strains pass through a hostile landscape with little lasting effect.

The Sim-Bo method pairs probiotics with prebiotics: brown rice, vegetables, fruit, legumes when tolerated, seeds, roots, greens, and resistant starch. The garden does not thrive because seeds are thrown on concrete. It thrives when soil is prepared.

The Conditional Tools

Some supplements require more caution because the difference between correction and excess is narrow.

Iron belongs only where iron status, symptoms, menstrual pattern, absorption, ferritin, inflammation, and clinician judgment support its use. Unneeded iron can intensify oxidative pressure.

Zinc can support epithelial integrity, immune resilience, taste, wound repair, and reproductive function. Chronic excess can disturb copper balance and weaken the very system it was meant to support.

Iodine and selenium influence thyroid function. Their value depends on terrain, autoimmunity pattern, dietary intake, medication status, and clinical assessment.

Methylated B-vitamins can be useful in selected patients with methylation strain, low intake, medication effects, anemia patterns, neuropathy, or homocysteine concerns. They can also overstimulate sensitive patients when used without discrimination.

NAC, glutathione, digestive enzymes, bile support, berberine, curcumin, and botanical formulas are not casual wellness accessories. They are clinical tools for defined patterns.

The more powerful the tool, the more precise the hand must be.

Methylation Without Mania

Methylation is one of the most misunderstood territories in modern nutrition.

The methylation cycle helps regulate DNA maintenance, neurotransmitter metabolism, detoxification, histamine handling, homocysteine conversion, cell division, and nervous system stability. It depends on folate, B12, B6, riboflavin, choline, betaine, magnesium, zinc, protein status, liver function, gut absorption, and genetic variation.

The supplement industry often reduces this elegant network to a single obsession: take methylated vitamins. Sim-Bo rejects that shortcut. A pathway is not repaired by throwing one methyl donor at it indefinitely. Overmethylated patients may become anxious, wired, insomniac, irritable, or headache-prone. Undermethylated patients may remain flat, fatigued, histamine-reactive, or slow to recover. The answer is not ideology. The answer is observation.

Folic acid, folinic acid, and 5-MTHF behave differently. B12 forms behave differently. Choline and glycine shape the cycle differently. The clinician must read the person, not worship the pathway.

Methylation is not a supplement category. It is a regulatory conversation.

Whole-Food Synergy: The Matrix of Intelligence

No capsule replicates the full intelligence of intact food.

A laboratory can isolate ascorbic acid. It cannot recreate the full architecture of a mandarin orange: water, fiber, flavonoids, fragrance, acidity, mineral pattern, sweetness, texture, peel chemistry, and the pace of chewing. A capsule can provide magnesium. It cannot reproduce the green matrix of chard, the bitterness that awakens bile, the fiber that feeds microbes, or the ritual of a warm meal that tells the vagus nerve the environment is safe.

This is why whole-food synergy is central to Sim-Bo. Nutrients behave differently inside a living matrix. The same molecule can carry a different metabolic meaning depending on its companions, timing, dose, and terrain. Food is architecture. Supplements are extracted tools.

The wise clinician uses both in proper order.

The Four-Step Supplement Sequence

Sim-Bo supplementation follows a sequence.

1. Remove

Remove the inputs that create need: ultra-processed food, alcohol excess, late screens, sleep fragmentation, unstable oils, refined sugar, overtraining, emotional suppression, chronic snacking, and supplement clutter.

2. Rebuild

Rebuild with the 3:2:1 plate, warm hydration, bowel regularity, morning light, chewing, movement, and consistent sleep. Food rhythm repairs more pathways than scattered capsules ever can.

3. Target

Target the remaining gap with the cleanest, simplest, lowest effective tool. Choose form, dose, timing, and duration with a clinical purpose.

4. Withdraw

Withdraw what is no longer needed. A patient who cannot stop a supplement without collapsing has not yet restored the root. The bottle is still carrying the work that daily life must eventually resume.

The Future of Precision Supplementation

The future of supplementation will be smaller, cleaner, and more intelligent.

The old model sells long-term stacks: dozens of pills taken daily by habit, fear, and marketing. The next model will measure more carefully, dose more lightly, and withdraw more often. Wearable physiology, metabolomics, microbiome mapping, continuous glucose data, dried blood spot testing, salivary hormone patterns, and at-home biomarker tools will gradually expose what the clinician has always known: need changes by season, stress, sleep, digestion, illness, and recovery phase.

A tired patient after surgery, a depleted mother postpartum, a traveler after antibiotics, a patient recovering from viral illness, an older adult with low appetite, and a high-stress executive with poor sleep do not require the same bottle. They require different support, different duration, and a different exit plan.

The future belongs to precision, not accumulation.

The Supplement of Simplicity

The strongest supplement is the one that reduces the need for supplementation.

A steady meal schedule lowers stress chemistry. Brown rice and vegetables feed the microbiome. Fruit supplies water, color, and gentle sweetness. Morning light sets the clock. Walking moves glucose into muscle. Breath lowers sympathetic tone. Sleep restores immune intelligence. Emotional completion removes the chemical background noise that no pill can outshout.

These are not lifestyle decorations surrounding the real intervention. They are the intervention.

When this foundation becomes stable, supplements become smaller. The protocol simplifies. The shelf quiets. The patient stops collecting external rescue and begins trusting internal regulation again.

The ultimate supplement is cadence: the quiet repetition of food, sleep, breath, movement, light, and peace in an order the organism can believe.

Conclusion: Strategic Support, Not Substitution

Supplements occupy a narrow and important place in natural healing.

They can correct a gap, assist a repair phase, support a depleted pathway, restore a missing nutrient, or carry the patient through a demanding season. They can also become another form of noise: more inputs, more fear, more expense, more complexity, more distance from the original medicine of simple living.

The Sim-Bo standard is clear. Food first. Rhythm first. Digestion first. Sleep first. Breath first. Then targeted support.

A bottle should never become the center of the healing story. It should stand quietly at the edge, useful when called, removed when the foundation can hold.

Reading the Response

A supplement protocol must produce clearer signals, not more confusion.

When a targeted nutrient is well matched, the response is usually orderly. Sleep becomes deeper without morning heaviness. Bowels become more predictable without dependence. Energy becomes steadier without stimulation. Pain softens without dullness. Mood becomes less reactive without emotional flattening. Laboratory markers may improve, but the patient often feels the change first as coherence.

When a supplement is poorly matched, the system speaks quickly. Magnesium may loosen the bowel too much. Methylated B vitamins may create agitation in sensitive patients. Ashwagandha may feel grounding to one constitution and heavy to another. Probiotics may improve bloating in one patient and increase pressure in another when the microbial terrain is not ready. Iron may restore vitality when truly needed and create oxidative heaviness when taken without cause.

The practitioner listens to these responses the way an experienced musician listens to tuning. The goal is not to force the note. The goal is to restore harmony.

Nature never asks the patient to swallow complexity forever. It asks for the daily discipline that makes complexity unnecessary.

Clinical Case Study 15: Restoring Endocrine Stability with Targeted Support

Patient: Arthur M., 58-year-old male, civil engineer.

Chief concerns: twelve-year history of type 2 diabetes, erratic glucose control despite metformin and exogenous insulin, severe fatigue, central weight gain, and burning numbness in the lower legs consistent with peripheral neuropathy symptoms.

Clinical Presentation

Arthur arrived with the familiar pattern of advanced metabolic exhaustion: excess glucose, reduced insulin sensitivity, inflammatory weight gain, neuropathic discomfort, and fear of progressive vascular damage. His case belonged in a chapter on supplements because the first temptation was to add more: more nutrients, more capsules, more glucose-lowering agents, more external control.

The deeper clinical need was order. Supplements could support the process, but the primary therapy had to remove the daily inputs that kept glucose, inflammation, and vascular strain active.

Initial Findings

HbA1c: 8.7% at baseline.
Fasting blood glucose: 184 mg/dL at baseline.
Neuropathy pattern: daily burning and numbness in the lower legs and feet by patient report.
Tongue presentation: dusky red with central cracks and a dry, sticky yellow coating.

Pulse: rapid, thready, and slippery in the right middle position.

Traditional Asian Medicine Assessment

Arthur's presentation was consistent with Wasting and Thirsting pattern, or Xiao Ke, complicated by Yin depletion, Phlegm-Heat, Spleen-Stomach weakness, and Blood Stasis in the collaterals. The burning and numbness in the lower extremities reflected impaired distal circulation and a long-standing failure of nourishment to reach the periphery.

Treatment Principles

Restore glycemic cadence by removing refined sugar, processed flour, and late eating.
Support insulin sensitivity through predictable meals, movement

after food, and high-fiber Sim-Bo structure.
Nourish Yin and fluids while reducing Phlegm-Heat and digestive stagnation.
Support distal circulation through acupuncture, movement, breath, and myofascial release.
Use targeted support only where it served the endocrine terrain, never as a substitute for the dietary foundation.

Plan and Intervention

Arthur committed to a twelve-week Sim-Bo endocrine-restoration plan. Medication changes were coordinated with his prescribing endocrinologist and were never treated as a substitute for appropriate medical supervision.

The Sim-Bo dietary prescription was built around a glycemic lock: no refined sugars, no processed flours, no liquid calories, and no late-night eating.

Three parts grain: buckwheat, Job's tears, brown rice, and other intact grains supplied steady fuel with fiber and minerals.
Two parts vegetables: bitter melon, dandelion greens, bok choy, daikon, and leafy greens were emphasized to support bile flow, fiber intake, mineral restoration, and glucose regulation.
One part fruit: tart green apple and berries were used in measured portions, placed away from heavy meals and paired with movement when appropriate.
Targeted support: magnesium, algae-based omega-3, vitamin D/K2 when clinically indicated, and gut-supportive prebiotic fiber were used as tools, not as the center of care.
Acupuncture: EX-B3, ST36, SP6, and Bafeng were used to support endocrine regulation, digestive strength, and distal circulation.
Emperor's Cupping Therapy®: stationary decompression across the mid-thoracic and paraspinal regions supported circulation and softened protective tissue restriction.
Botanical medicine: Yu Quan Wan was used within the TAM framework to nourish Yin, generate fluids, clear Stomach Heat, and support the Wasting and Thirsting pattern.

Follow-Up Pattern

HbA1c improved from 8.7% to 5.8%.
Fasting blood glucose improved from 184 mg/dL to 92 mg/dL.
Neuropathic burning and numbness markedly decreased; Arthur reported restoration of sensation in the feet during the follow-up

period.
Insulin was discontinued under endocrinologist supervision, and metformin was reduced by 50% by the prescribing clinician.
Energy, morning clarity, and post-meal stability improved by patient report.
Tongue coating, color, and pulse qualities improved through Traditional Asian Medicine observation.

Interpretive Note

Arthur's case demonstrates the central law of targeted support: the tool works best after the daily terrain stops generating the same demand. His improvement did not come from supplement accumulation. It came from sequence: remove refined inputs, restore meal cadence, rebuild the plate, support the gut and circulation, use selected nutrients and botanicals with purpose, and let the prescribing physician guide medication adjustments as objective markers changed.

The endocrine system responds to order. Supplements can assist that order. They cannot replace it.

Arthur also demonstrates the discipline of sequence. The intervention did not begin by adding more products to an already stressed system. It began by removing the strongest metabolic provocations. Only after the daily pattern became simpler could targeted support be read clearly.

His case also shows why supplementation belongs inside a broader clinical ecology. Magnesium without movement would have been incomplete. Algae-derived omega-3 support without removal of industrial oils would have been diluted. Botanical medicine without meal timing would have been forced to work against the patient's own habits. The tools became useful because the terrain stopped arguing with them.

Transition: From Bottles to Breath

When the supplement shelf becomes quiet, attention turns inward.

A capsule can fill a physical gap. Breath changes the chemistry that decides whether repair is allowed to begin. Food supplies materials. Sleep restores the command center. Movement spends glucose and circulates lymph. But the mind determines whether the nervous system lives in safety or alarm.

From targeted tools, the path now turns toward the medicine that no bottle can contain: thought, feeling, forgiveness, gratitude, grief, restraint, and the trained calm that changes physiology from the inside out.

The mind is the next terrain of nourishment. It can inflame or settle digestion before the first bite is swallowed. It can keep cortisol alive after danger has passed. It can turn memory into chemistry, fear into gastric tension, resentment into vascular strain, and gratitude into a measurable softening of the system.

The supplement chapter closes the science of targeted tools. The deeper work now moves into the interior climate: emotion, attention, forgiveness, purpose, and the practiced state of safety. When those forces become orderly, even the most precise nutrient works better because physiology is no longer defending itself against the person who lives inside it.

This is why the supplement shelf must remain subordinate to the lived day. A bottle can deliver magnesium, but it cannot teach a patient to stop living in emergency. A capsule can deliver vitamin D, but it cannot replace the morning act of stepping into light. A probiotic can influence the intestinal garden, but it cannot create the humility of eating plants every day.

Targeted support ends at the edge of behavior. Beyond that edge begins the medicine of attention: the repeated choice to breathe before reacting, to eat before exhaustion, to sleep before collapse, to forgive before bitterness hardens into chemistry. The next form of healing is not another product. It is the trained interior life becoming safe enough for physiology to repair.

Part V

Living Without Medication

The first four parts of this book rebuilt the foundation: modern disease, inflammatory chemistry, food as instruction, and the Sim-Bo architecture of grains, vegetables, fruit, gut ecology, antioxidant defense, and targeted supplementation. But no meal plan can complete healing while the nervous system remains at war.

Part V moves from nourishment into execution. Here, the work becomes daily and embodied: emotional steadiness, physical movement, sleep timing, sunlight, and the six-month transformation plan. Food creates the terrain. Mind, motion, and circadian order determine whether that terrain can finally repair.

Chapter 16

Mind and Emotion: The Missing Medicine

Emotion as Chemistry

Every emotion is a chemical event.

Love, fear, anger, grief, gratitude, shame, trust, and relief do not remain sealed inside the private theater of the mind. They move through the nervous system, endocrine system, immune network, digestive tract, breath pattern, vascular tone, and muscular fascia. Emotion is not an invisible mood floating above physiology. It is physiology speaking in a different accent.

The brain and the rest of the human system are not separate kingdoms. They are one continuous conversation. A thought changes breath. Breath changes heart rhythm. Heart rhythm changes vagal tone. Vagal tone changes digestion. Digestion changes microbial chemistry. Microbial chemistry changes immune behavior. Immune behavior changes mood.

This is why a pristine meal eaten in panic does not land the same way as the same meal eaten in calm. The food may be identical. The receiving system is not. Stress makes nourishment harder to interpret. Safety makes the same nutrients easier to receive.

In the Sim-Bo philosophy, emotional hygiene is not a luxury. It is part of the prescription. Food gives the cells material. Emotional steadiness gives them permission.

The Meal as an Emotional Event

A meal is never only a nutrient event. It is an emotional event received by the gut, the liver, the pancreas, the microbiome, and the nervous system. Two patients can eat the same bowl of brown rice and vegetables and receive it differently. One eats while arguing, scrolling, and breathing from the throat. The other eats seated, quiet, grateful, and unhurried. The ingredients match. The internal atmosphere does not.

This is why the Sim-Bo table is deliberately plain. Its simplicity removes sensory chaos, but its deeper purpose is to restore the emotional posture of eating. The patient learns to sit, breathe, chew, receive, and stop. That sequence repairs a forgotten relationship: food is no longer swallowed as anesthesia, reward, punishment, distraction, or escape. It becomes nourishment again.

Emotional eating is often misnamed as weakness. More precisely, it is an attempt at nervous system regulation through taste. Sweetness, salt, fat, crunch, and heat can temporarily change chemistry. The problem is not the desire for comfort; the problem is using processed stimulation as the only language of comfort. Sim-Bo gives the patient another vocabulary: warmth, regularity, breath, chewing, gratitude, and enough.

The Biology of Stress: Survival Chemistry

The human stress response was built for survival. The hypothalamic-pituitary-adrenal axis, or HPA axis, coordinates the release of cortisol and adrenaline when danger requires immediate adaptation. In a short emergency, this chemistry is brilliant. Cortisol mobilizes glucose. Adrenaline sharpens attention. Blood flow shifts toward action. Pain sensitivity changes. Digestion slows so the organism can run, fight, lift, escape, or endure.

The injury begins when survival chemistry becomes the atmosphere of daily life.

Modern stress rarely arrives as a single visible predator. It arrives as financial pressure, family tension, unfinished tasks, comparison, screens, fear of failure, resentment, overresponsibility, and the subtle humiliation of never feeling caught up. The danger is not always physical, but the chemistry is real.

Chronic stress reshapes regulation in predictable ways:

- Glucose rises as cortisol asks the liver for quick fuel, making blood sugar and insulin coordination more difficult.
- Digestion weakens as blood flow and attention are redirected away from the gut.
- The microbiome becomes less stable because motility, acid secretion, bile flow, and immune tolerance are altered by sympathetic tone.
- Immune discernment becomes less precise: some defenses weaken while inflammatory vigilance remains high.
- Sleep becomes lighter, and the repair cycles that depend on darkness and parasympathetic dominance lose their depth.

A system that never feels safe cannot allocate its full resources to repair. This is not psychology dressed in poetic language. It is stress physiology. Every slow diaphragmatic breath is a mechanical message to the autonomic nervous system: the danger has passed; regulation may resume.

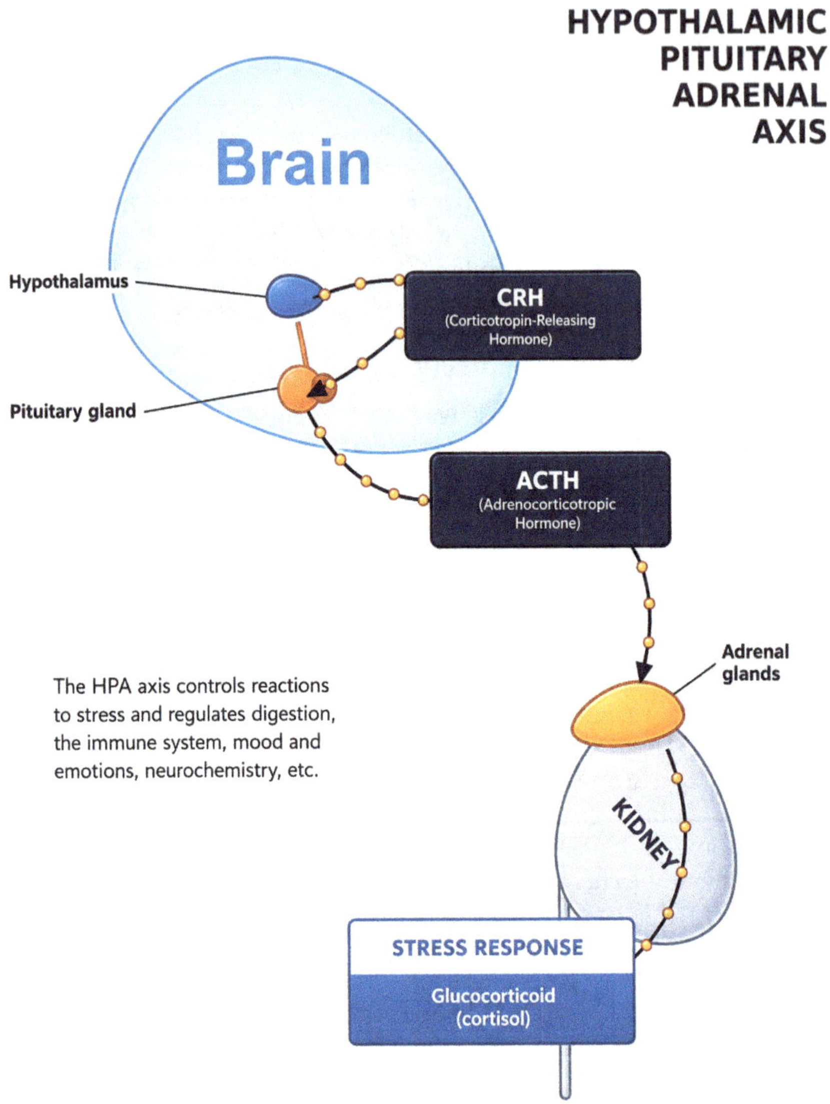

Figure 9. Hypothalamic-pituitary-adrenal axis.

The Vagal Highway

The vagus nerve is the great bridge between emotional life and organ function. It travels from the brainstem into the throat, heart, lungs, stomach, liver, pancreas, intestines, and beyond, carrying messages in both directions. It tells the gut what the mind feels, and it tells the mind what the gut is enduring.

When psychological pressure rises, the stomach tightens, digestive secretion changes, motility becomes irregular, and microbial ecology shifts. The gut then returns its own weather report through immune molecules, microbial metabolites, vagal afferents, and blood sugar fluctuation. Anxiety can disturb digestion; disturbed digestion can intensify anxiety. The loop is not imaginary. It is the architecture of the gut-brain-emotion circuit.

Simple practices restore this circuit because they speak the language of the vagus nerve: slow breathing, longer exhalation, prayer, gratitude before meals, warm touch, walking after emotional strain, and eating without screens. These are not decorative wellness rituals. They are mechanical interventions in autonomic tone.

In Sim-Bo living, emotional hygiene begins before digestion. A meal should not enter a battlefield. It should enter a system that has been invited back into order.

The Hidden Cost of Suppressed Emotion

Suppressed emotion becomes physiological posture.

Unspoken anger tightens the jaw, neck, diaphragm, chest wall, and gut. Unresolved grief changes breath. Chronic fear narrows movement. Shame collapses the shoulders. Long-held resentment keeps the nervous system rehearsing danger after the event has ended. The conscious mind may try to forget, but the tissues continue to hold the pattern.

Emotion must move. Not explosively. Not theatrically. But honestly. Crying, laughing, sighing, writing, speaking truthfully, walking, stretching, singing, praying, and breathing from the diaphragm all give emotion a physical path. Without a path, emotional charge becomes tension, tension becomes altered chemistry, and altered chemistry becomes another source of inflammatory strain.

Emotional fluency is the goal: the ability to feel without drowning, express without harming, and release without pretending nothing happened. Sim-Bo healing does not ask the patient to become emotionally numb. It asks the patient to become clean in emotional metabolism.

The Physiology of Forgiveness

Forgiveness is not moral approval. It is release from internal captivity.

When resentment remains active, the nervous system continues to replay the threat. The event may be gone, but the chemistry is rehearsed daily: cortisol, adrenaline, shallow breath, tightened vessels, guarded sleep, and inflammatory readiness. Forgiveness interrupts that rehearsal. It tells the organism that the old threat no longer deserves the present moment.

This is why forgiveness is medical in the deepest sense. It lowers the demand placed on the stress system. It frees attention from repetition. It reduces the need for defensive posture. It returns energy to digestion, sleep, immunity, creativity, and service.

The Sim-Bo evening practice is simple: before sleep, exhale what does not belong in the night. Name one resentment, one unfinished tension, or one fear that the day activated. Breathe out slowly. Let the ribcage soften. Sleep should not begin with the nervous system still arguing with ghosts.

The Medicine of Gratitude

Gratitude is not politeness. It is orientation.

Fear trains attention to search for threat. Gratitude trains attention to recognize sufficiency. A warm meal, a quiet room, a stable breath, a patient friend, a functioning hand, a moment of sunlight - each recognition shifts the nervous system toward safety. The chemistry of safety changes digestion, vascular tone, heart rhythm, breath depth, and immune behavior.

A brief moment of thanks before eating is therefore more than a spiritual gesture. It changes how the meal is received. The jaw softens. The breath drops. The stomach prepares. The vagus nerve hears the message. The meal becomes less like an interruption and more like a conversation.

In Sim-Bo practice, gratitude is the invisible cofactor of nourishment. The plate provides material. Gratitude prepares the internal terrain to accept it.

Mindfulness and Simplicity

Mindfulness is the mental form of Sim-Bo.

To live simply is to give one act the dignity of full attention: one bite, one breath, one step, one conversation, one moment of washing rice, one cup held with both hands. The modern mind is trained to divide itself across screens, tasks, anxieties, and imagined futures. Divided attention consumes energy without producing completion.

Attention is metabolic. Fragmentation has a cost. When awareness scatters, breath shortens, posture collapses, and digestion loses its rhythm. When attention gathers, the system steadies.

Begin with three small disciplines:

Take one slow breath before answering a message.
Feel the temperature of water when washing your hands.
Chew the first three bites of every meal with undivided attention.

These acts are small only to the ego. To the nervous system, they are proof that life has returned to the present tense.

Neuroplasticity: Practicing Peace

The brain becomes skilled at what it repeats.

A patient who rehearses worry daily develops efficient pathways for fear. A patient who practices resentment develops speed in anger. A patient who practices calm, breath, forgiveness, and attention creates a different neural architecture. The mind does not change because it is commanded once. It changes because a new pattern is repeated until it becomes familiar.

Peace is not passive. It must be practiced with the same seriousness that an athlete gives to strength or a musician gives to scales. Morning, mid-afternoon, and evening, pause for one minute. Inhale quietly. Exhale longer than you inhale. Let the shoulders drop. Let the tongue rest. Let the abdomen move. The practice is simple because the nervous system learns through repetition, not spectacle.

Consistency turns fleeting chemistry into character.

The Emotional Microbiome

The gut contains a microbial ecosystem. The mind contains an emotional one.

Both require diversity, movement, and balance. A healthy inner life does not mean constant happiness. It means thoughts and feelings can arrive, be recognized, metabolized, and released. Anxiety, grief, anger, joy, desire, tenderness, frustration, awe - all have a place when they move. The problem is stagnation: one emotional species taking over the entire landscape.

Journaling, honest conversation, silent time in nature, prayer, creative work, and unhurried breath act like psychological fiber. They keep the inner ecosystem moving. They prevent emotional constipation.

Forced positivity is not health. Emotional sterility is not peace. True calm is not the absence of weather; it is the capacity to remain coherent as weather passes through.

Boundaries as Nervous System Medicine

Many patients misunderstand emotional healing as endless accommodation. They believe peace means absorbing every demand without complaint. That is not peace. That is collapse disguised as kindness.

A boundary is the shape of emotional metabolism. It tells the nervous system where the self ends and the world begins. Without boundaries, every request feels like an invasion, every silence feels like abandonment, and every conflict becomes a threat to survival. The stress response remains active because the inner gate has no clear threshold.

The calmest patients are not those who never experience conflict. They are those whose internal architecture is clear. They know when to say yes. They know when to pause. They know when to leave a conversation, close the screen, end the meal, protect sleep, or refuse the familiar emotional bargain that steals vitality.

In Traditional Asian Medicine, emotional constraint often appears as tight ribs, sighing, throat pressure, digestive irregularity, menstrual tension, headaches, and a wiry pulse. In biomedical language, the same pattern may appear as sympathetic overactivation, altered breathing mechanics, elevated vascular tone, and digestive dysregulation. The languages differ. The clinical reality is the same: unexpressed pressure must find tissue.

A clean boundary is therefore not selfish. It is circulatory. It keeps emotional force moving instead of letting it pool inside the chest, jaw, abdomen, and blood vessels.

The Sim-Bo Emotional Hygiene Practice

Emotional hygiene must be as ordinary as brushing the teeth. A patient should not wait for a crisis before clearing the mind. The daily practice is simple because the nervous system learns from repetition.

Morning begins with orientation. Before the phone, before messages, before news, one hand rests over the lower abdomen and one hand over the chest. Three slow breaths establish ownership of the day. The patient names one priority, one boundary, and one act of gratitude. This prevents the mind from being immediately colonized by external demand.

Before meals, the practice is reception. The fork does not move until the breath has dropped. The shoulders soften. The jaw relaxes. The patient gives the digestive tract a clear message: this is not danger; this is nourishment. Even one minute can change the entire chemistry of the meal.

At night, the practice is release. The patient writes one sentence: "Today I am finished carrying..." and completes it honestly. The page receives what the nervous system no longer needs to rehearse in sleep. Then the exhalation lengthens. The system enters darkness without dragging the day into the bed.

This is not sentimental self-care. It is regulatory discipline. Sim-Bo emotional hygiene removes psychological debris before it hardens into sleep disruption, digestive tension, vascular strain, and inflammatory readiness.

Peace as Immune Intelligence

Calm is strength.

A regulated person is not weak, detached, or passive. Regulation is advanced physiology: adaptable heart rhythm, proportionate immune responsc, stable breath, flexible digestion, clear attention, and the ability to recover after stress without remaining captured by it.

Emotions train immunity. Chronic fear teaches hypervigilance. Chronic anger teaches defense. Gratitude teaches sufficiency. Love teaches tolerance. Purpose teaches endurance. The goal is not emotional perfection; it is immune discernment. The system must learn when to defend and when to stand down.

Emotional intelligence becomes immune intelligence when the nervous system no longer mistakes every internal sensation for danger.

Conclusion: The Peaceful System

No medication can replace the chemistry of safety.

Medicine can stabilize risk, relieve suffering, and save life when danger is acute. But a life that remains emotionally inflamed continues to send the system into defense. Food can be pristine, supplements can be targeted, sleep can be planned, but unresolved emotional alarm will continue to shape digestion, blood sugar, vascular tone, immune behavior, and repair.

Peace is not escape from life. It is the internal order that allows life to be processed without constant injury.

Each act of forgiveness, each breath before a meal, each moment of gratitude, each honest word, each quiet pause tells the human system: the emergency is over. The work of repair may continue.

Stillness gathers the chemistry. Movement will carry it.

This chapter is not an invitation to sentimental living. It is a demand for emotional precision. The patient who wants to live without unnecessary medication must learn the chemistry of resentment, the posture of fear, the digestion of grief, the vascular tone of anxiety, and the immune instruction of peace. What is not felt clearly will often be acted out physically.

The missing medicine is not a pill, a mantra, or a mood. It is the disciplined return of emotional truth to daily physiology. A clear mind softens the breath. A soft breath steadies the heart. A steady heart changes the meal, the sleep, the gut, and the immune response. This is how inner life becomes treatment terrain.

Clinical Case Study 16: Restoring Vascular Calm Through Emotional Safety

Endothelial Strain, Angina Pattern, and Heart Blood Stasis

Patient: Victoria H., 61-year-old female, homemaker.

Chief concerns: activity-limiting chest pressure with exertion, systemic fatigue, shortness of breath, elevated blood pressure, and established coronary artery disease under cardiology care.

Clinical Presentation

Victoria arrived carrying the visible exhaustion of a life spent in service to everyone except herself. Her meals were quick, convenient, and often built around processed family foods. Her sleep was light. Her breathing was shallow. Her household responsibilities were constant. She described decades of swallowed frustration, private worry, and the feeling that her chest had become "tight from holding everything in."

Conventional care had appropriately focused on risk control: blood pressure, lipids, beta-blockade, antiplatelet strategy, and the prevention of acute cardiac events. Those tools mattered. The Sim-Bo question was different: what daily pattern kept her vascular system guarded, inflamed, and unable to recover?

Within Traditional Asian Medicine observation, her presentation was consistent with Heart Blood Stasis complicated by Phlegm-Turbidity and constraint. The biomedical picture pointed toward endothelial strain, elevated inflammatory load, oxidative lipid stress, poor nitric-oxide tone, and chronic sympathetic activation.

Initial Findings and Assessment

Blood pressure: 148/92 mm Hg at baseline, despite medication support.
hs-CRP: 6.4 mg/L, consistent with elevated inflammatory risk.
Tongue and pulse: dusky-purple tongue, engorged sublingual veins, and a deep, choppy pulse quality within Traditional Asian Medicine assessment.

Functional pattern: exertional chest pressure, breath limitation, fatigue, emotional suppression, processed-food exposure, and shallow breathing converging into vascular guardedness.

Treatment Principles

The clinical objective was not to replace cardiology care. It was to reduce the daily inputs that kept her vascular terrain under pressure: inflammatory oils, refined sugars, emotional compression, shallow breath, sedentary stagnation, and poor endothelial nourishment.

Medication decisions remained under cardiology supervision. The Sim-Bo intervention focused on food architecture, breathing, emotional release, movement tolerance, acupuncture, cupping, and botanical support.

Plan and Intervention

Victoria committed to a twelve-week Sim-Bo cardiovascular restoration plan.

3 parts grains: red quinoa, whole oats, and brown rice provided soluble fiber and steady energy, supporting bile clearance and metabolic steadiness.
2 parts vegetables: beetroot, arugula, bok choy, celery, parsley, and leafy greens supported nitrate availability, fiber intake, mineral density, bowel flow, and vascular relaxation.
1 part fruit: pomegranate, berries, and hawthorn-containing preparations supplied color-dense polyphenols and cardiovascular antioxidant support.
Emotional hygiene: a nightly forgiveness breath, morning gratitude, and five minutes of expressive writing gave long-held tension a daily exit path.
Breath practice: slow exhalation before meals and before sleep was used to shift autonomic tone and reduce chest guarding.
Movement: short, supervised walks were introduced below the threshold of chest pressure and gradually expanded as tolerance improved.
Targeted acupuncture: PC6 and HT7 were used to regulate chest tension and emotional steadiness; BL15 and SP10 were used within the TAM framework to support Heart Blood movement and circulation.
Emperor's Cupping Therapy®: gentle sliding decompression was applied across the upper thoracic region and pectoral fascia to reduce myofascial restriction, improve breathing mechanics, and support local circulation.
Botanical medicine: Dan Shen Yin with hawthorn was used within a monitored clinical context to support circulation and cardiovascular resilience. This was coordinated carefully with medication status

because cardiovascular herbs require professional oversight when blood-thinning or cardiac medications are involved.

Clinical Reasoning

Her cardiovascular plan was built around one principle: lower the inflammatory pressure on the endothelium while increasing the signals that invite vascular relaxation. Food reduced the oxidative load. Beets, arugula, leafy greens, berries, pomegranate, and oats supported nitric-oxide availability, fiber intake, bile clearance, and antioxidant capacity. Breath practice reduced sympathetic tone. Emotional release reduced chest guarding. Walking restored a safe mechanical demand that the heart could answer gradually.

The treatment did not frame her arteries as clogged pipes waiting for a single chemical solution. It treated the vascular system as living tissue: reactive, emotional, muscular, endothelial, inflammatory, and responsive to repeated daily conditions.

Twelve-Week Treatment Response

Chest symptoms: exertional chest pressure markedly decreased during the follow-up period; walking tolerance improved from approximately one block to longer neighborhood walks by patient report.
Inflammatory marker: hs-CRP improved from 6.4 mg/L to 0.9 mg/L.
Blood pressure: resting blood pressure improved from 148/92 mm Hg to 118/76 mm Hg, with medication status reviewed by her cardiologist.
Breath and fatigue: shortness of breath and daily fatigue decreased, and morning energy became more stable.
Emotional state: Victoria reported less chest tightness during family stress and greater ability to pause before reacting.
Tongue and pulse: sublingual vein congestion softened and pulse quality became less choppy within TAM observation.

Clinical Takeaway

Victoria's case illustrates the central teaching of Chapter 16: emotional life is not separate from vascular life. A guarded heart is not only a metaphor. Long-term stress changes breath, fascia, blood pressure, endothelial tone, sleep, digestion, and inflammatory chemistry.

Her improvement did not come from one heroic intervention. It came from coherence: food that cooled the vascular terrain, breathing that lowered sympathetic tone, emotional release that reduced internal compression, movement that restored circulation, and cardiology-supervised risk management that remained in place where needed.

The heart is not a pump floating outside the story of a life. It listens to every breath, every meal, every fear, every resentment, every act of relief. When the inner atmosphere becomes safer, circulation can begin to soften.

Transition: From Stillness to Motion

Inner peace prepares the chemistry. Movement circulates it.

Emotion settles into posture, fascia, breath, gait, and muscular tone. Worry rounds the shoulders. Grief narrows the ribs. Anger clenches the jaw. Fear shortens the step. The next medicine is therefore not another idea; it is motion.

Deep feeling becomes biological flow when it is given a physical path: walking, stretching, lifting, breathing, carrying, reaching, opening the chest, and letting the limbs complete what the nervous system has been holding.

The Sim-Bo order continues: simple thoughts, simple breath, simple motion. Stillness makes the system safe. Movement teaches it to flow.

Chapter 17

Movement as Medicine

The Healing Power of Motion

Life is motion before it is thought. The embryonic heart begins to pulse before language, before ambition, before identity. Cerebrospinal fluid moves in quiet waves. Lungs expand and release. Blood circulates, lymph drifts, fascia glides, joints hinge, and muscles speak to the nervous system with every contraction. Stillness has its place, but stagnation is never neutral.

Modern fitness culture reduced movement to a punishment for eating, a transaction of calories burned against calories consumed. That reduction stripped motion of its dignity. Movement is not a penalty. It is participation. It is one of the primary ways physiology confirms that the environment is safe, resources are available, and repair can proceed.

In the Sim-Bo philosophy, movement serves three governing purposes: circulation, coordination, and clearance. It moves blood through vessels, lymph through channels, glucose into working muscle, breath through the diaphragm, emotion through posture, and attention through space. Every joint is a pump. Every muscle fiber is a messenger. Every deliberate step is a vote for order.

We do not build physical capacity merely to achieve an aesthetic ideal. We build it to carry a demanding life without collapse: to work with clarity, serve with endurance, lead without exhaustion, and remain useful when difficulty arrives. Movement is not separate from healing. It is healing made visible.

The Circulatory Symphony and Endothelial Shear

The cardiovascular system is the tireless courier of human life. With each heartbeat, oxygen, nutrients, immune cells, hormones, and heat are delivered through an immense vascular network. Waste returns for processing through the liver, kidneys, lungs, and skin. Yet the heart was never meant to carry the entire circulatory task alone. Skeletal muscle is the second pump.

When muscles contract, they compress veins and help return blood toward the chest. This simple mechanical action assists venous flow, reduces pooling, and improves delivery of oxygenated blood to working tissue. Movement also changes the inner surface of arteries. As blood moves across the endothelium, shear stress stimulates nitric oxide production, relaxing vascular tone and supporting healthier circulation.

A ten-minute walk after a meal may look ordinary, but its physiology is precise. Working muscle increases glucose uptake, improves insulin sensitivity, supports triglyceride handling, and calms the nervous system through rhythmic motion. The meal is no longer simply sitting in the bloodstream; it is being escorted into use.

Circulation is not only a matter of the heart beating. It is the entire human frame cooperating with the heart. Walking, climbing stairs, stretching the calves, rising from a chair, carrying groceries, and sweeping the floor all keep the vascular river moving. The smallest daily motions, repeated with consistency, become cardiovascular medicine.

The Lymphatic River

The lymphatic system is the quiet river of immunity and fluid balance. Unlike the cardiovascular system, it has no central heart-like pump. It depends on motion: skeletal muscle contraction, joint movement, diaphragmatic breathing, posture, and the one-way valves that guide lymph forward.

Lymph carries immune cells, excess fluid, proteins, inflammatory byproducts, and cellular debris through a slow-moving drainage network. When life becomes sedentary, that river loses momentum. Fluid pools. Joints feel stiff. Tissue feels heavy. Morning swelling, sluggish recovery, and low-grade fatigue often reflect more than age; they reflect a system that has not been moved enough to clear itself.

Gentle daily movement reawakens this current. Walking, tai chi, mobility work, fascial stretching, and slow strength practice create repeated compression and release. The diaphragm adds an internal pump, drawing lymph upward from the abdomen and lower limbs with every deep breath.

Sweating also has its place. The liver and kidneys remain the primary organs of detoxification, yet the skin participates in heat regulation, mineral exchange, and physical release. A light, honest sweat from walking, gardening, mobility practice, or slow repetitive work signals that circulation has reached the surface and internal heat is moving outward. This is not exhaustion. It is flow.

Movement and the Brain: Neuroplasticity in Motion

Motion feeds the mind. Rhythmic walking, coordinated movement, and sustained physical practice influence the hippocampus, frontal networks, motor planning, memory consolidation, and emotional regulation. The brain was not designed to solve life from a chair alone. It thinks more clearly when the frame moves through space.

Physical activity supports the release of Brain-Derived Neurotrophic Factor, or BDNF, a neurotrophic molecule involved in synaptic plasticity, learning, and resilience. Movement does not merely strengthen muscle; it changes the conditions under which the nervous system learns, adapts, and recovers.

This is why a brisk walk can soften anger, why stretching can loosen grief held in the chest, and why slow hiking can untangle thoughts that refused to move at a desk. Catecholamines and cortisol are not meant to remain trapped in abstract mental loops. They are meant to be spent through breath, stride, reach, contraction, and release.

The mind often needs motion before it can find stillness. A patient may speak about stress for months and remain stuck; then, after weeks of daily walking, the same emotional knot begins to loosen without force. Movement gives psychology a physical exit.

Thc Myth of Intensity

Modern commercial fitness sells intensity because intensity is easy to market: heavier weight, louder music, harder classes, higher heart rates, more sweat, more exhaustion. But healing movement is not measured by punishment. It is measured by restoration.

Relentless overtraining can resemble chronic stress. Excessive volume without recovery may elevate stress chemistry, irritate joints, disturb sleep, suppress immune resilience, and convert exercise into another burden. A depleted patient does not need to be broken down. A depleted patient needs skillful motion that rebuilds trust.

The longest-lived communities did not build health around punishing workouts. They walked, gardened, climbed, carried, knelt, squatted, cooked, cleaned, danced, and moved through the day because life required it. Movement was woven into existence, not bolted onto it as a corrective ritual.

The Sim-Bo question is not, "How much pain did I endure to burn calories?" The better question is, "How well did I move today?" Smoothly, rhythmically, without panic, without performance, without injury. Healing favors consistency over spectacle.

The Future of Physical Longevity

The future of movement medicine will not belong to the loudest gym or the most punishing protocol. It will belong to practices that restore coordination, joint integrity, fascial glide, muscle memory, breath control, balance, and everyday strength. Technology may help map movement patterns, but the highest goal will remain ancient: a human being able to walk, rise, squat, carry, breathe, bend, reach, and recover without fear.

Longevity training will increasingly move away from isolated vanity metrics and toward functional fluency. The question will shift from how much a person can lift once to how well they can inhabit daily life for decades. Fluid movement, strong feet, mobile hips, stable shoulders, responsive breath, and resilient connective tissue will become the true markers of physical intelligence.

The elite future is not a life with less motion. It is a life where motion returns everywhere: into work, transportation, worship, cooking, conversation, aging, and rest.

Breath as the Primary Movement

Even in apparent stillness, the diaphragm moves thousands of times each day. It is the original internal engine. With every descent, it massages the liver, stomach, intestines, and abdominal fascia; changes pressure gradients; supports venous and lymphatic return; and helps regulate autonomic tone.

Breath is therefore not merely oxygen intake. It is mechanical therapy. Slow diaphragmatic breathing lengthens the exhale, supports vagal activity, steadies heart-rate variability, and teaches the nervous system that danger has passed. The lungs move, the ribs widen, the pelvic floor responds, the abdomen softens, and the entire internal architecture receives a signal of safety.

A shallow chest breath belongs to urgency. A slow abdominal breath belongs to repair. When breath becomes steady, digestion receives permission, posture softens, and attention settles. This is the smallest unit of movement medicine: available anywhere, requiring no equipment, no gym, no performance, and no injury risk.

In Sim-Bo healing, breath is the bridge between stillness and motion. It is the hidden exercise that prepares every visible exercise to become therapeutic.

Gentle Strength and Myokines

Strength is not brutality. True strength is organized engagement.

Skeletal muscle is more than mechanical tissue. It is an endocrine organ. When muscle contracts, it releases myokines—chemical messengers involved in immune modulation, glucose handling, fat metabolism, and communication with distant organs. In this sense, contracting muscle speaks to the liver, fat tissue, vascular system, brain, and immune network.

Gentle resistance training two or three times a week can preserve bone density, improve joint stability, support glucose regulation, and maintain the muscle reserve required for aging with independence. The work does not need to be theatrical. Slow bodyweight squats, wall push-ups, bands, carries, step-ups, controlled lunges, and floor-to-stand practice can create profound change when performed with attention and breath.

The purpose is not ego-driven hypertrophy. The purpose is to maintain a strong, responsive frame capable of serving life. A muscle that can contract smoothly, relax fully, and coordinate with breath is more valuable than a muscle trained only for appearance.

The Muscle as Metabolic Organ

Muscle is often judged by appearance, but its deeper value is metabolic. Active skeletal muscle is one of the largest sites of glucose disposal. After a meal, contracting muscle creates a place for circulating fuel to go. It lowers pressure on the pancreas, improves the usefulness of insulin, and turns nourishment into work instead of storage. This is why the Sim-Bo plate is completed by walking. Food provides the structure; muscle opens the gate.

The lower leg deserves special respect. The calf and soleus complex functions like a peripheral pump, especially in a culture of long sitting. Standing, walking, heel raises, and slow ankle movement restore one of the simplest engines available to a sedentary patient. No machine is required. No specialized identity is required. The lower leg simply has to remember its duty.

Post-meal motion is one of the most underused clinical tools in modern life. The ten or twenty minutes after eating decide whether fuel becomes clarity or heaviness. A person who walks gently after the main meal teaches glucose, triglycerides, bile, lymph, breath, and thought to move in the same direction. The effect is humble, but the physiology is elegant.

A sedentary day asks the pancreas to solve what the legs should have helped solve. A moving day distributes the task. This is one reason patients often notice that cravings soften when daily walking becomes consistent. The meal no longer leaves energy stranded in circulation. It is carried into use.

Joint Oil and Fascial Fluency

A joint is nourished by motion. Synovial fluid does not circulate through a powerful central pump. It depends on loading, unloading, compression, rotation, and glide. A joint that never bends loses confidence. A spine that never rotates forgets its length. Hips that never open begin to imprison the pelvis. Shoulders that never reach upward teach the breath to stay shallow.

Fascia follows the same law. It is not dead wrapping around muscle; it is living connective tissue shaped by hydration, pressure, emotion, habit, and daily position. Long sitting tells fascia to shorten. Guarded emotion tells it to grip. Repetitive stress tells it to thicken. Gentle variation tells it to glide again.

This is why Sim-Bo movement values circles, spirals, reaching, squatting, standing, crawling, lengthening, and slow strength. The purpose is not to shock the tissues into obedience. The purpose is to reintroduce forgotten directions. When the tissues regain directions, pain loses much of its authority.

The patient who cannot squat, twist, reach, or rise from the floor does not merely lack flexibility. The patient has lost vocabulary. Movement restores the alphabet of daily living one letter at a time.

The Sim-Bo Movement Prescription

The most effective movement plan is the one simple enough to repeat under stress. A patient does not need a heroic transformation. A patient needs daily architecture that the nervous system can trust: brief morning activation, post-meal circulation, subtle movement throughout the workday, and evening release. Each element carries a different task.

Morning activation: five to fifteen minutes of sunlight walking, joint circles, spinal extension, calf raises, or dynamic stretching. The purpose is to wake the endocrine day and place attention back inside the physical frame.

Post-meal circulation: ten to twenty minutes of easy walking after the largest meal. The purpose is glucose handling, gastric comfort, lymphatic flow, and mental clarity.

Workday interruption: three minutes of standing, breathing, shoulder circles, hip opening, stair climbing, or calf activation every thirty to sixty minutes. The purpose is to break the spell of chair physiology.

Evening release: slow stretching, floor breathing, hip mobility, tai chi, or a quiet walk. The purpose is descent from output into repair.

This prescription is built on reliability. A patient who moves gently every day often outperforms the patient who trains punishingly twice a week and then collapses into immobility. Consistency is the medicine. The day is the clinic.

Micro-Movements and the Fascial Web

The healthiest systems rarely stop moving. Not frantic motion, not restless agitation, but subtle continuity. The human frame was designed for shifting: turning the spine, widening the ribs, squatting, reaching, twisting, bending, standing, kneeling, and rising.

Fascia responds to hydration, pressure, glide, and varied direction. When movement narrows to sitting, typing, driving, and scrolling, the fascial web loses range. Tissues feel sticky. Joints feel compressed. Posture collapses into predictability. Pain then appears in areas that were never moved through their full vocabulary.

Native biomechanical fluency returns through small acts repeated often:

Stand, walk, or change position for several minutes every half hour.

Circle the shoulders, wrists, neck, and ankles during transitions.

Stretch the calves and engage the lower legs while seated to support the muscle pump.

Squat or hinge daily within a safe range.

Breathe deeply when moving from sitting to standing.

Carry ordinary objects with awareness instead of outsourcing every load.

These micro-movements turn ordinary life into physical practice. Sweeping a floor, pulling weeds, washing vegetables, folding laundry, and preparing brown rice become more than chores. They become repetitions of useful motion. Daily life becomes the training ground.

Walking: The Original Clinical Instrument

Walking is the most underestimated therapy in modern medicine. It requires no membership, no machine, no costume, and no complicated calculation. Yet it recruits the feet, ankles, knees, hips, spine, arms, eyes, lungs, heart, vestibular system, and attention in one integrated act. It is rhythmic enough to calm the nervous system and demanding enough to change metabolism. It is ordinary enough to repeat and complex enough to train the whole frame.

A post-meal walk deserves special respect. After food enters circulation, skeletal muscle becomes the most generous sink for glucose. The step tells the meal where to go. Instead of leaving glucose and triglycerides crowded in the bloodstream, walking invites them into tissue for use and storage in a more orderly form. Ten or fifteen quiet minutes after lunch may be more clinically useful than an ambitious workout performed later in a state of exhaustion.

Walking also restores orientation. The eyes look outward. The breath expands. The feet receive texture from the ground. The mind stops circling itself and begins moving through space. For patients locked in worry, grief, anger, or decision fatigue, walking is often the first emotional medicine that requires no explanation.

The Sim-Bo standard is direct: walk every day, especially after the largest meal. Walk without performance. Walk until the system remembers that energy is meant to circulate.

Joint Nourishment and Synovial Intelligence

Joints are nourished by motion. Cartilage has limited direct blood supply. It depends heavily on compression and decompression to move fluid, distribute nutrients, and clear waste from the joint space. When a joint never moves through its available range, the internal environment becomes dry, stiff, and poorly signaled. Pain creates guarding, guarding creates immobility, and immobility deepens the pattern.

The answer is not reckless stretching or harsh manipulation. The answer is frequent, respectful articulation: circles, bends, rotations, controlled squats, gentle spinal waves, ankle mobility, shoulder opening, and breath-led range. The joint should be reminded that it is safe to move before it is asked to perform.

Morning mobility matters for this reason. Before the mind enters the demands of the day, the joints should receive a quiet tour of their capacity. Neck, shoulders, wrists, spine, hips, knees, ankles, and toes all deserve attention. These small motions are not trivial. They are the first renewal of circulation after the long stillness of sleep.

A joint that moves daily remains in conversation with the nervous system. A joint that is ignored eventually speaks through stiffness.

Movement as Emotional Release

Every emotion has posture. Fear tightens the belly and hip flexors. Anger narrows the chest and jaw. Grief rounds the spine and restricts breath. Joy widens the ribs and opens the face. The nervous system writes its history into muscle tone.

Movement gives trapped emotion a path. A long walk can spend the chemistry of anger. Slow stretching can open the chest after grief. Rhythmic breathing can soften anxiety. Dance can return pleasure to a frame that has been living only in survival.

This is why patients who begin consistent gentle movement often report more than improved sleep or digestion. They report emotional clarity. They do not simply feel fitter; they feel less trapped. Lymph moves, breath deepens, posture changes, and the mind receives new evidence: the emergency has passed.

The abstract work of "letting go" often becomes possible only when the physical system practices release. Every deliberate step forward is a rehearsal in forgiveness.

The Healing Cadence: Circadian Motion

Movement becomes more medicinal when it respects time. The same activity carries different meaning depending on when it is performed.

Morning — Awaken the Current: Gentle mobility, fascial stretching, or a brisk walk in early light helps shift the system from nocturnal repair into daytime engagement. Morning motion pairs well with sunlight because both tell the endocrine clocks that the day has begun.

Midday — Circulate the Meal: A moderate walk after the main meal supports digestion, glucose handling, lymphatic movement, and afternoon clarity. This is one of the simplest ways to convert nourishment into usable energy.

Evening — Release and Restore: Slow stretching, tai chi, soft walking, or diaphragmatic breathing helps the nervous system step down from performance into repair. The goal is not intensity. The goal is transition.

This cycle—awaken, circulate, release—mirrors the daily movement of light, temperature, appetite, and sleep pressure. The wisdom is simple: move with the day, not against it.

The Minimum Effective Movement Dose

The modern patient often fails because the prescribed plan is too dramatic to repeat. Sim-Bo movement begins with the minimum effective dose: small enough to perform on a difficult day, meaningful enough to change physiology when practiced consistently.

A healing dose may be ten minutes of walking after the main meal, five minutes of joint mobility before breakfast, three sets of controlled chair squats, or one breath-led stretching sequence before sleep. The power is not in the novelty of the exercise. The power is in the repeated instruction. Tissues adapt to what they receive every day.

This is why consistency is superior to intensity for many chronically inflamed patients. A single exhausting class cannot replace a week of distributed motion. The vessels need frequent flow. The joints need regular lubrication. The lymph needs repeated compression. The nervous system needs many small experiences of safety, not occasional episodes of punishment.

The minimum dose grows naturally. Ten minutes becomes twenty. A short walk becomes a hill. A chair squat becomes a full squat. A light carry becomes real strength. The patient does not leap into resilience; resilience accumulates through repeated, well-timed acts of participation.

The Joy of Play

The word exercise often carries the weight of duty. Play carries the chemistry of freedom.

Children do not run to burn calories. They run to explore. They climb to test the world. They dance because rhythm has entered them before self-consciousness has. Somewhere in adulthood, motion became moralized, quantified, and judged. The healing task is to recover pleasure without losing discipline.

Hike a trail. Garden deeply. Dance badly. Play catch. Walk while talking with someone you love. Stretch on the floor. Practice balance while waiting for tea to steep. The immune system rewards repeated participation, not theatrical suffering.

When laughter joins oxygenated breath and moving muscle, the nervous system receives one of the oldest signals of safety: life is still worth entering fully.

Conclusion: Motion as Medicine

Movement is medicine because life is motion. Blood must circulate. Lymph must drain. Breath must expand. Joints must glide. Muscles must contract. Fascia must receive pressure and release. The mind must move through space to complete many of its emotional loops.

To move is to join the ancient dialogue between gravity, ground, breath, and time. The feet speak to the earth. The lungs speak to the atmosphere. The heart speaks to the rhythm of effort and rest. Motion returns abstract health advice to physical reality.

Healing begins when movement stops being punishment and becomes cadence: walking as naturally as breathing, breathing as naturally as gratitude, strength as service, and motion as a quiet daily vow to remain alive in the world.

Clinical Case Study 17

Restoring Pelvic Flow in Fibroids and Hormonal Strain

Patient: Rachel T., a 44-year-old corporate director.

Chief concerns: Heavy menstrual bleeding lasting up to ten days, pelvic pain, cyclical breast tenderness, mood volatility before menstruation, and three diagnosed uterine fibroids.

Clinical Presentation

Rachel's case illustrates the endocrine consequences of stagnation. Her professional life was highly sedentary and psychologically demanding. Long hours in a chair, shallow breathing, late meals, minimal daily motion, frequent exposure to plastics and synthetic cosmetics, and low fiber intake created a pattern in which estrogen clearance, bowel elimination, pelvic circulation, and stress chemistry were moving in the wrong direction.

Conventional care viewed the fibroids primarily as a uterine problem. Clinically, the pattern was broader. The uterus was the visible site of distress, but the deeper terrain involved liver clearance, bowel rhythm, pelvic blood flow, inflammatory tone, and autonomic pressure.

Within Traditional Asian Medicine observation, her presentation was consistent with Liver Qi Stagnation transforming into Blood Stasis, complicated by Spleen Qi deficiency and Damp-Phlegm. The language is old, but the pattern was unmistakable: poor movement, poor clearance, poor flow.

Initial Findings

Pelvic ultrasound confirmed three submucosal uterine fibroids; the largest measured 5.2 cm.

Menstrual bleeding lasted up to ten days with clotting by patient report.

Pelvic pain reached 9/10 at peak intensity and required frequent medication use.

Tongue presentation was dusky with purplish petechiae along the lateral margins and swollen sublingual veins.

Pulse quality was deep, wiry, and choppy in positions traditionally associated with Liver and reproductive patterns.

Treatment Principles

Support hepatic estrogen clearance through whole-food structure and cruciferous vegetables.
Increase bowel regularity so metabolized hormones could leave efficiently through bile and stool.
Restore pelvic circulation through movement, breath, acupuncture, and myofascial decompression.
Reduce xenoestrogen exposure from plastics, industrial cosmetics, alcohol, and highly processed foods.
Move Blood, soften constraint, and support menstrual rhythm within the Traditional Asian Medicine framework.

Plan and Intervention

Sim-Bo dietary prescription: Rachel adopted a 3:2:1 endocrine-support pattern anchored in brown rice, quinoa, steamed cruciferous vegetables, leafy greens, berries, citrus, and adequate hydration. Industrial dairy, alcohol, plastic food storage, and highly processed foods were removed from the daily pattern.
Grains as binders: Fiber-dense brown rice and quinoa supported bowel regularity and bile-associated elimination. The goal was not starvation or restriction; it was steady clearance through predictable structure.
Vegetables as hepatic allies: Broccoli sprouts, cabbage, bok choy, and leafy greens supplied fiber and sulfur-containing compounds associated with hepatic detoxification pathways. These foods became daily architecture rather than occasional side dishes.
Movement protocol: Rachel began two ten-minute walks daily, a slow post-meal walk after lunch, pelvic mobility work, diaphragmatic breathing, and gentle hip-opening stretches. The purpose was to restore flow without provoking exhaustion.
Acupuncture: SP8, LR3, SP6, and Zi Gong were used to regulate menstrual discomfort, soften Liver constraint, support Spleen function, and encourage pelvic circulation.
Emperor's Cupping Therapy®: Cupping was applied along the sacral and gluteal fascia to reduce myofascial restriction, support local circulation, and ease pelvic tension.
Botanical medicine: Gui Zhi Fu Ling Wan was used within the Traditional Asian Medicine framework to address Blood Stasis patterns, support pelvic circulation, and assist menstrual regulation. Formula use was individualized and monitored clinically.

Clinical Changes During Follow-Up

Menstrual bleeding decreased from up to ten days with heavy clotting to approximately four days of moderate flow with markedly fewer clots by patient report.
Pelvic and premenstrual pain decreased from 9/10 at peak intensity to approximately 1-2/10 during the follow-up period.
Medication use for menstrual pain decreased by patient report, with ongoing care decisions kept within appropriate medical oversight.
Follow-up ultrasound documented reduction of the largest fibroid from 5.2 cm to 2.8 cm; interpretation and surgical planning remained under gynecologic supervision.
The planned hysterectomy was reassessed and deferred by her gynecologist during the follow-up period.
Breast tenderness, mood volatility, bowel irregularity, and pelvic heaviness improved substantially.
Tongue color, sublingual vein congestion, and pulse quality improved within the Traditional Asian Medicine clinical lens.

Case Meaning

Rachel's case does not reduce fibroids to one cause or one intervention. It shows how a pelvic condition can exist inside a larger architecture of stress, stagnation, estrogen exposure, poor clearance, low movement, and disrupted timing. The therapeutic aim was not to attack the uterus. The aim was to restore flow: food flow, bowel flow, lymphatic flow, blood flow, breath flow, and daily cadence.

When movement returned, the pelvis was no longer an isolated site of congestion. It became part of a living circulation again. That is the deeper lesson of Chapter 17: motion is not decoration. It is the physical language of renewal.

Transition: From Motion to Timing

Motion opens the channels; timing teaches them when to repair. Muscles move blood and lymph, breath steadies the nervous system, and walking turns nourishment into usable energy. But movement alone does not complete the healing rhythm. The day itself must become ordered.

Light must arrive at the right hour. Darkness must return with authority. Sleep must be protected as the night's deepest medicine. The pumps of the muscles prepare the terrain, but circadian timing conducts the repair.

The same walk that improves glucose handling in daylight can disturb sleep when performed with too much intensity at night. The same breath that steadies digestion before a meal can deepen restoration when practiced before bed. The same nervous system that needs effort during the day needs permission to withdraw when darkness comes. Motion is never separate from time.

This is the next discipline of living medicine: not simply moving more, but moving in season with the day. Morning asks for orientation. Midday asks for circulation. Evening asks for release. Night asks for surrender. When these phases are honored, physical practice stops being an isolated habit and becomes part of a larger solar architecture.

A life can be active and still remain dysregulated if its timing is broken. A patient can walk every day and still feel depleted if sleep is shallow, meals arrive unpredictably, and artificial light erases the boundary between evening and morning. Movement opens the door, but the clock decides whether repair enters.

From motion, we enter the medicine of light, sleep, and the ancient clockwork of the sun.

Chapter 18

Sleep, Sunlight, and Circadian Healing

The Medicine of Night and Day

Every living system keeps time with light.

Plants open and close their leaves by the sun. Birds migrate through seasonal cues. Hormones rise and fall according to daylight, darkness, temperature, feeding, fasting, and rest. Human physiology is no exception. We are not separate from the rotation of the earth; we are organized by it.

At the center of this order sits the suprachiasmatic nucleus, the master clock located above the optic chiasm. It receives light information from the eyes and translates that information into timing for the entire human system: cortisol release, melatonin production, body temperature, digestive readiness, insulin sensitivity, immune activity, mitochondrial efficiency, and emotional steadiness.

When this master clock is aligned with natural light and darkness, energy arrives with greater clarity. Hunger appears at sensible times. Sleep descends more easily. Digestion anticipates its work. The mind wakes with less resistance and settles with less force. When the clock is ignored, downstream systems lose their cadence. The stomach works at the wrong hour. The brain remains alert in the dark. The immune system receives confused instructions. Metabolism begins to drift.

Modern life placed artificial suns inside every room and every hand. Screens glow after dusk. Overhead lights flatten evening into a second afternoon. Mental work continues long after the nervous system should have begun its descent. Heavy meals arrive late. Caffeine delays the signal to rest. The result is not merely poor sleep. It is a collapse of timing.

In the Sim-Bo philosophy, circadian order stands beside food, movement, and emotional hygiene as a pillar of recovery. Nutrients provide material. Timing determines whether that material is used for repair or held in confusion.

The Master Clock and the Peripheral Clocks

The brain contains the central clock, but every major organ keeps its own local time.

The liver times detoxification, glucose storage, bile flow, and cholesterol metabolism. The pancreas times insulin secretion. The gut times enzyme release, motility, microbial fermentation, and barrier repair. The muscles time glucose uptake and protein synthesis. Immune cells time surveillance and renewal. These clocks do not operate as isolated devices. They are musicians in one orchestra.

Light is the conductor. Food is the percussion. Movement is the pulse. Sleep is the rest between notes. When these signals agree, physiology becomes coherent. When light says morning, food says midnight, stress says emergency, and darkness never arrives, the entire system loses its score.

This is why a person can eat a clean diet and still remain exhausted if they live outside the clock. A perfect meal eaten at the wrong hour does not carry the same meaning. A brilliant supplement cannot replace the nightly fall of melatonin. A workout cannot fully compensate for a nervous system kept under artificial noon until midnight.

Circadian medicine begins with a simple law: timing is not decorative. Timing is part of the treatment.

Sleep as Nighttime Repair

Sleep is not passive unconsciousness. It is the most organized repair state in human life.

During deep non-REM sleep, growth hormone rises, tissue repair accelerates, immune memory consolidates, glucose regulation improves, and the nervous system processes the emotional load of the day. During REM sleep, memory, creativity, mood regulation, and adaptive learning are reorganized. The night is not empty. It is occupied by maintenance work that waking consciousness cannot perform.

One of the most remarkable processes of sleep is glymphatic clearance. As sleep deepens, fluid exchange through the brain improves. Cerebrospinal and interstitial fluids move more efficiently through neural tissue, supporting the clearance of metabolic waste, including proteins associated with neurodegenerative vulnerability. The older phrase of a brain 'washing itself' is not a poetic exaggeration. It is a useful image for a real physiology of nighttime clearance.

This nightly cleaning does not belong to the brain alone. Sleep also changes vascular tone, temperature regulation, hormonal rhythm, appetite control, mitochondrial recovery, and immune balance. A night of fragmented sleep can disturb glucose handling, increase blood pressure tendency, raise inflammatory tone, and sharpen cravings the following day. Chronic sleep loss does not create one problem. It weakens the entire regulatory field.

The deepest damage from poor sleep is not always visible the next morning. It appears as a lower threshold for life: sharper cravings, shorter patience, stronger pain, poorer temperature control, weaker concentration, and greater reactivity to ordinary stress. The patient calls it fatigue, but fatigue is only the surface of a timing injury.

Many people try to solve this chemistry with stimulation. They add caffeine, harsher exercise, stronger willpower, brighter screens, louder entertainment, or another supplement. Each solution drives the same exhausted system harder. The night is not asking to be conquered. It is asking to be completed.

Sim-Bo treats sleep as nighttime digestion. The day is swallowed by experience. The night breaks it down, sorts it, stores what is useful, and clears what should not remain. Without that nocturnal processing, the person wakes still carrying yesterday.

The Sun's Daily Script

Sunlight writes a daily script through the eyes, skin, nervous system, and endocrine network.

- Morning light acts as ignition. Bright outdoor light shortly after waking tells the master clock that the day has begun. Cortisol rises in its proper morning pulse, body temperature climbs, alertness sharpens, and digestive readiness begins to return.
- Midday light acts as reinforcement. Strong daytime brightness anchors wakefulness, supports mood chemistry, and strengthens the contrast between day and night. The brighter the day, the more convincing darkness becomes later.
- Evening darkness acts as the seal. As light fades, melatonin rises, core temperature begins to fall, blood pressure trends downward, and the nervous system prepares for repair.

Melatonin is often reduced to a sleep hormone, but it is more than that. It is a timekeeper, antioxidant, immune modulator, mitochondrial signal, and messenger of darkness. When screens and bright indoor light suppress melatonin at night, the loss is not simply an hour of sleepiness. It is the loss of a repair instruction.

Natural light restores order by reestablishing contrast. Bright morning. Honest day. Dim evening. True darkness. The master clock does not require exotic technology. It requires unmistakable signals.

Duration matters, but placement gives duration its meaning. Seven hours of sleep from 3:00 AM to 10:00 AM does not always carry the same regulatory value as seven hours held closer to darkness. The clock reads more than quantity. It reads position in the solar day.

This is why circadian healing can feel strangely powerful. It does not add a new chemical. It gives the existing chemistry a schedule. The system stops receiving contradictory instructions and begins to organize itself around a stable day.

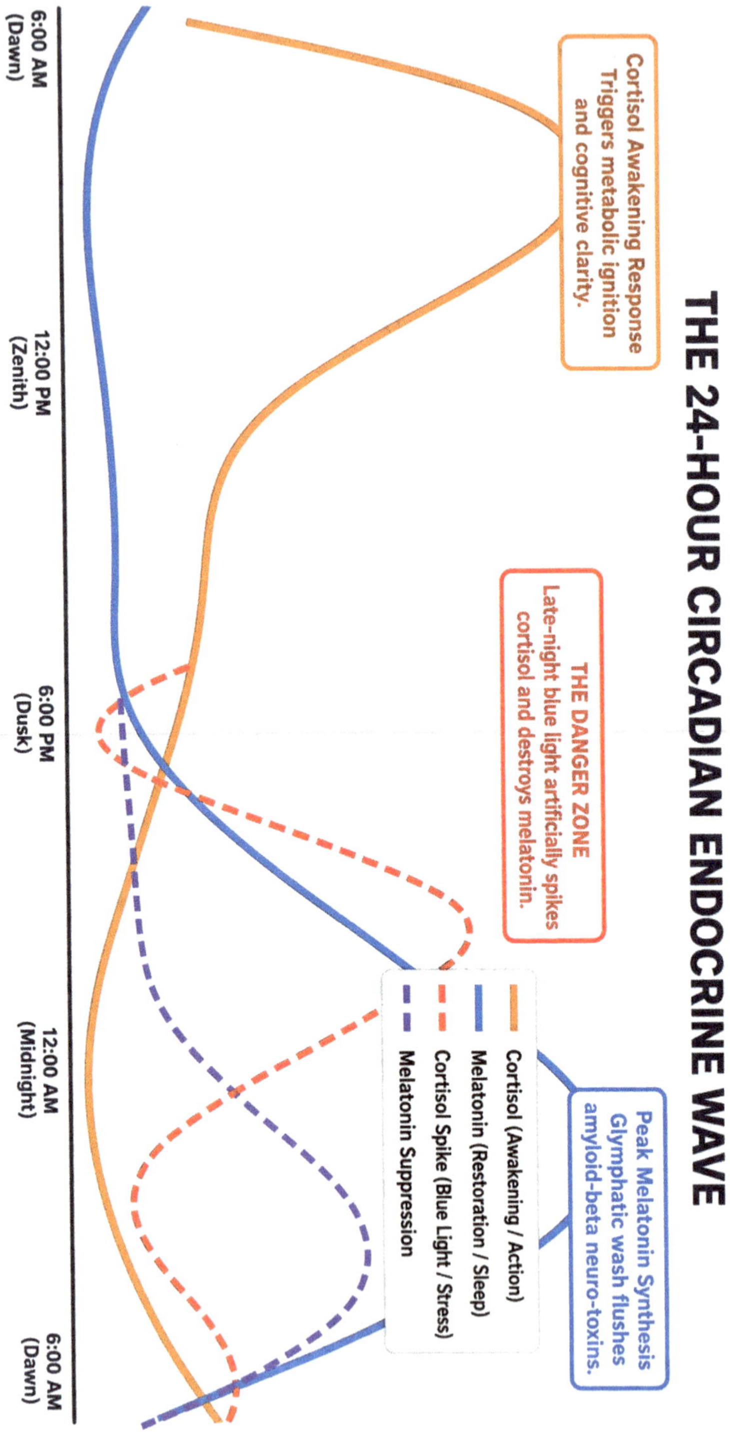

Figure 10. The 24-hour circadian endocrine wave.

The Language of Light and Darkness

Day and night are not enemies. They are partners.

Daylight stimulates, mobilizes, warms, and clarifies. Darkness integrates, cools, repairs, and protects. The alternation between them shapes enzyme release, hormone rhythm, appetite, sleep pressure, immune timing, and mood. A life without real darkness becomes a life without full repair.

The modern evening is biologically confusing. Brilliant LEDs, late meals, digital conflict, inbox checking, and entertainment streams keep the nervous system in daylight mode long after the sun has disappeared. The person lies down, but physiology remains standing. The room is dark enough for the eyes to close, but the internal day has not ended.

The Sim-Bo cadence is deliberately simple: work, move, and eat with the sun; dim, fast, reflect, and restore with the night. This is not romantic nostalgia. It is the oldest timing system physiology understands.

Modern Insomnia and Hyperarousal

Many patients who say they cannot sleep are not suffering from a broken sleep switch. They are trapped in an overactive wake state.

The nervous system remains guarded because the day never fully closes. Caffeine lingers. Screens stimulate. Financial pressure follows the person into bed. Social conflict remains unresolved. Late meals keep blood flow, heat, and digestive work active. The mind tries to sleep while the internal environment continues to negotiate unfinished business.

Sleep cannot be forced by willpower. The harder a person tries to sleep, the more alert the system becomes. Sleep must be invited through predictability. Darkness, temperature, timing, breath, and ritual all deliver the same message: the day is complete; the environment is safe; repair may begin.

This is why the Sim-Bo sleep method begins long before the pillow. It begins with the evening.

The Sim-Bo Sleep Ritual

Healing sleep begins before bedtime because the nervous system requires twilight.

> Dim the home one hour before bed. Turn off overhead lights. Use warm, low light. Let the visual field receive the message that day is ending.

Close the digital gate. Screens, news, messages, and work tasks should end before the sleep window. A nervous system cannot enter repair while still negotiating demands.

Eat early and light. Late, heavy meals raise core heat, increase digestive demand, and keep the metabolic engine active when temperature should be falling.

Unwind through breath and length. Gentle stretching, slow exhalation, quiet journaling, prayer, or stillness helps move the system from sympathetic readiness into parasympathetic descent.

Release one grievance and keep one lesson. Forgiveness lowers the emotional volume of the day. Gratitude gives the mind a safe final orientation.

Sleep in cool darkness. The room should be dark, quiet, and slightly cool. Darkness feeds melatonin. Coolness supports the natural thermal descent required for deep rest.

The ritual works because it replaces negotiation with sequence. The same sequence, practiced nightly, becomes an instruction the nervous system begins to trust.

Chrononutrition: Eating With the Clock

Food has a clock.

The same meal eaten at noon and at midnight does not create the same metabolic effect. Earlier in the day, insulin sensitivity is usually stronger, digestive readiness is higher, and the system is better prepared to handle fuel. Late at night, physiology is moving toward repair, cooling, fasting, and cellular maintenance. A heavy meal at that hour asks the wrong system to do the wrong work.

Sim-Bo meal timing follows the sun. Breakfast or the first meal should arrive after morning light and after the person has truly awakened. The main meal should occur while the day is bright and digestive fire is strongest. Evening food should be simple, warm, and modest, leaving enough space for sleep to begin without gastric conflict.

This pattern is not deprivation. It is respect for sequence. The liver should not be asked to process a large meal at the same time the brain is preparing glymphatic clearance and melatonin is rising. The stomach should not be forced into labor when the nervous system is trying to descend.

A disciplined eating window gives the peripheral clocks a stable anchor. The gut learns when to open. The pancreas learns when to answer. The liver learns when to store, when to release, and when to repair.

Sunlight as a Metabolic Nutrient

Sunlight is not merely illumination. It is environmental nutrition.

Morning light anchors the master clock. Sensible sunlight on skin supports vitamin D synthesis when season, latitude, skin tone, and exposure permit it. Light exposure influences mood, nitric oxide biology, immune timing, and the distinction between wakefulness and sleep. A life lived entirely indoors asks the endocrine system to keep time without the primary signal it was built to read.

The Sim-Bo approach does not worship reckless sun exposure. It honors appropriate contact with natural light: morning outdoor light, midday brightness when safe, and the deliberate reduction of artificial brightness after sunset. The goal is not burning. The goal is orientation.

A patient who has not seen morning light for years often does not need another stimulant first. They need dawn. They need the sky to enter the eyes and tell the brain what hour it is.

Temperature, Breath, and the Descent

Sleep requires a descent: light descends, temperature descends, effort descends, and thought descends.

A cooler room, warm feet, gentle stretching, and slow breathing all help shift the system toward rest. The diaphragm is especially important. Slow exhalation tells the vagus nerve that danger has passed. The heart rate becomes steadier. The jaw softens. The abdomen loosens. The gut receives permission to repair instead of guard.

Modern sleep advice often focuses on supplements, trackers, mattresses, or devices. These may have a place, but the core physiology is older: darkness, coolness, safety, timing, breath, and repetition. The human system sleeps best when the environment stops arguing with the night.

Sleep and Immunity

The immune system does not rest during sleep. It reorganizes.

At night, immune cells refine memory, surveillance, and tolerance. Inflammation that was necessary during the day should resolve. Tissue repair accelerates. The nervous system shifts from defensive scanning toward internal maintenance. When sleep is shortened or fragmented, immune behavior becomes less precise: more reactive in some places, weaker in others, less tolerant, less disciplined.

This is why chronic insomnia and chronic inflammatory disease travel together so often. Sleep loss raises the volume of immune alarm. Immune activation disturbs sleep. The loop continues until timing is restored.

Rest is not laziness. Rest is immune intelligence.

This is especially clear in patients with autoimmune tendency, recurring viral flares, inflammatory skin patterns, or chronic allergy. The immune system becomes more disciplined when night is protected. It learns when to defend, when to tolerate, and when to stand down.

The Art of Waking

The morning matters as much as the night.

A jarring alarm can throw the nervous system into emergency before the day has begun. A calmer awakening changes the entire hormonal tone. Rise at a consistent time. Let natural light touch the eyes. Stretch before speaking. Drink warm water. Take several slow breaths. Allow the first minutes of the day to belong to orientation rather than reaction.

The first ten minutes after waking are not trivial. They establish posture, breath, thought, light exposure, and autonomic tone. A person who begins the day by checking crisis signals on a phone has already invited disorder before breakfast. A person who begins with light, breath, water, and gratitude has already practiced medicine.

Circadian Disruption and Metabolism

Circadian disruption is not only a sleep problem. It is a metabolic problem.

The liver, pancreas, gut, muscle, and adipose tissue all read time. When wake time changes daily, meals drift late, light exposure is weak in the morning, and screens extend the evening, metabolic organs lose coordination. Glucose that would be handled with relative efficiency during daylight can become more difficult to manage at night. The same meal can produce a different response depending on the hour, the light environment, the previous night of sleep, and the state of the nervous system.

This explains a common clinical pattern: a patient eats reasonably well, yet remains fatigued, hungry at night, inflamed in the morning, and foggy after meals. The problem is not always the ingredient list. Sometimes the deeper disorder is timing. Food arrives when the digestive clock is unprepared. Work continues when the repair clock should be active. Stress peaks when the temperature rhythm should fall. Metabolism receives good material in a disordered schedule.

Sim-Bo corrects this through repeatable architecture. Morning light anchors the central clock. Daylight meals anchor the peripheral clocks. Movement during the day improves glucose disposal. Evening dimness protects melatonin. Overnight fasting gives the gut, liver, and brain a quiet window. These are not separate lifestyle tips. They are one timing system.

Night Eating and the Loss of Repair

Night eating is one of the quietest ways to interrupt repair.

A late meal asks digestion to dominate the same hours assigned to cooling, glymphatic exchange, hormonal recalibration, and immune resolution. Heart rate may remain elevated. Core temperature may stay warmer. Reflux may worsen. Blood sugar may remain more variable. The person may technically be asleep, but the internal labor of digestion competes with the deeper work of restoration.

The Sim-Bo evening meal is therefore intentionally simple and early. It is not a moral rule. It is a mechanical courtesy to the night. When the stomach is quiet, the heart can slow. When the heart slows, the brain can descend. When the brain descends, sleep becomes a repair state rather than a sedated struggle.

The Evening Boundary

The evening boundary is the missing medicine in many modern lives.

Without a boundary, the day leaks into the night. Work follows the patient into bed. Family conflict remains unresolved. The phone becomes the final object seen before sleep and the first object touched upon waking. The nervous system receives no ceremony of completion.

A boundary does not require luxury. It requires repetition. Close the kitchen. Close the laptop. Lower the lights. Put the phone outside the bedroom. Write down the unfinished task so the mind does not have to hold it all night. Wash the face. Stretch the spine. Breathe slowly. Let the same acts appear in the same order until the nervous system no longer debates rest.

The strongest sleep ritual is not complicated. It is believable. The system trusts what repeats.

When the Clock Breaks: The Clinical Pattern

A broken clock produces recognizable symptoms.

The patient wakes tired, becomes alert too late in the day, craves stimulation in the afternoon, eats heavily at night, falls asleep with difficulty, wakes between 2:00 and 4:00 AM, and begins the next morning already behind. Caffeine becomes the morning replacement for sunlight. Sugar becomes the afternoon replacement for rest. Screens become the evening replacement for closure.

Over time, the pattern touches every system: appetite becomes less trustworthy, digestion becomes less predictable, pain sensitivity rises, mood becomes less stable, and the immune system becomes easier to provoke. This is why circadian repair is not cosmetic. It is one of the most direct ways to reduce the daily noise surrounding the immune and endocrine systems.

The first correction is almost embarrassingly simple: wake at a consistent time, step into morning light, eat in daylight, move before evening, dim the home, and protect the night. Simplicity works here because the master clock does not need novelty. It needs a clear signal repeated until order returns.

Conclusion: The Rhythm of Light

Every cell carries memory of dawn and dusk.

To live against that memory is to fight the most ancient clock in physiology. To live with it is to let the day organize energy and the night organize repair. Sleep, sunlight, darkness, meal timing, breath, and waking ritual are not separate habits. They are one circadian architecture.

The Sim-Bo way turns that architecture into daily practice: wake with light, eat with clarity, move in daylight, dim the evening, release the day, and sleep in darkness. The result is not forced discipline. It is relief. The system stops guessing what time it is.

Healing depends not only on what we consume, but on when we live.

Clinical Case Study 18

Restoring the Circadian Master Clock

Patient: Julian L., 37-year-old male, active job seeker.

Chief concerns: systemic inflammatory symptoms, chronically swollen lymph nodes, sudden hives, severe fatigue, and diagnosed Hashimoto's thyroiditis. He had been prescribed corticosteroids and antihistamines, which reduced symptoms temporarily but did not restore stability.

Clinical Presentation

Julian's pattern reflected severe circadian drift. Under the pressure of unemployment and financial anxiety, he spent most nights under blue light until nearly 4:00 AM, submitting applications, searching job boards, and scanning messages. He slept until late morning or noon and rarely received direct morning light. His meals shifted later. His mind never left the arena of threat.

The clinical picture was not simply insomnia. His entire timing system had lost its anchor. Without morning light, consistent sleep onset, stable meals, and evening darkness, his immune and endocrine rhythms had no reliable reference. The skin, lymphatic system, thyroid terrain, and nervous system all reflected the same disorder: the day had invaded the night, and the night no longer repaired the day.

Initial Findings

hs-CRP: 8.5 mg/L, consistent with elevated systemic inflammatory load.

Skin and lymphatic status: recurrent hives with persistent lymph-node swelling by patient report and clinical observation.

Energy: severe fatigue with anxious dread on waking.

Tongue: red and dry, with swollen lateral margins, red petechiae, and a sticky yellow root coating.

Pulse: rapid and wiry across several positions.

Traditional Asian Medicine Assessment

Julian's presentation was consistent with Liver Fire and Heat in the Blood complicated by Kidney Yin depletion and lymphatic congestion. The timing disorder was central. Late-night wakefulness consumed cooling reserves, aggravated heat signs, and left the immune terrain reactive rather than regulated.

The clinical principle was to anchor the clock, restore darkness, clear heat, support Yin, improve lymphatic movement, and reduce the inflammatory load without treating symptom suppression as the only strategy.

Plan and Intervention

Circadian anchor: morning outdoor light within the first part of the day, paired with a consistent wake time. The goal was to teach the master clock when morning had arrived.

Digital sunset: all job searching, screens, and work-related communication ended in the evening. The night was protected as repair territory.

Sim-Bo nutrition: simple warm meals built around cooling grains, vegetables, and fruit, with careful attention to timing. Evening meals were kept modest and early to lower digestive heat before sleep.

Mineral and sea elements: mineral-rich vegetables and small culinary amounts of sea vegetables were used when clinically appropriate, avoiding high-dose iodine exposure.

Acupuncture: LI11 and SP10 were used to clear heat; LR3 and KI3 supported regulation of Liver constraint and Yin depletion; additional points were selected according to sleep, pulse, and skin presentation.

Emperor's Cupping Therapy®: gentle sliding decompression was applied along the cervical and thoracic regions and upper back to reduce myofascial restriction, support local circulation, and assist lymphatic movement.

Botanical medicine: a heat-clearing and blood-level strategy was used, including principles associated with Shi Wei Bai Du San and Long Dan Xie Gan Tang, adjusted to presentation and monitored clinically.

Medication context: corticosteroid and antihistamine decisions remained under the supervision of the appropriate prescribing clinician.

The first two weeks were corrective rather than dramatic. Julian felt the discomfort of losing nocturnal stimulation. The phone had become both anxiety outlet and false companion. Removing it from the night revealed how restless his mind had become.

By the third week, morning light began to create a recognizable start to the day. By the sixth week, the evening cutoff no longer felt like punishment; it felt like relief. The clinical lesson was clear: circadian healing often begins with resistance because the nervous system has become loyal to the pattern injuring it. Once the pattern is repeated long enough, the system begins to prefer order.

Observed Changes Over Twelve Weeks

Inflammatory tracking: follow-up testing showed a marked downward trend from the elevated baseline inflammatory pattern.
Skin and lymphatic symptoms: hives markedly decreased during follow-up, and lymph-node swelling softened by patient report and clinical observation.
Sleep timing: bedtime shifted earlier and became more consistent; waking moved closer to morning light.
Energy: crushing fatigue decreased, and morning dread was replaced by steadier daytime function.
Medication reliance: steroid and antihistamine use was reviewed and adjusted only with the appropriate prescribing clinician.
Tongue and pulse: heat signs reduced within the Traditional Asian Medicine lens.

Clinical Pattern

Julian's case illustrates the central law of Chapter 18: immune stability is inseparable from circadian order. The inflammatory pattern was not merely a skin problem, a thyroid problem, or a lymphatic problem. It was a timing disorder expressed through multiple tissues.

By restoring morning light, protecting darkness, simplifying meals, lowering evening stimulation, supporting lymphatic movement, and addressing heat through acupuncture and botanical medicine, the system received a coherent temporal message again. The repair did not begin with force. It began with time restored.

Food can provide clean material. Movement can circulate it. Emotional hygiene can quiet the alarm. But sleep and light decide the hour in which those efforts are integrated. Without timing, even the right tools arrive in disorder.

Transition: From Timing to Routine

Light sets the score. Routine plays the music.

Sleep, sunlight, meals, movement, emotional steadiness, and simplicity become medicine only when repeated long enough to become climate. A good day matters. A repeated day changes the terrain.

Circadian order gives the final dimension of the Sim-Bo method:

when. The work now becomes sequence, duration, repetition, and embodiment. Food, movement, sleep, breath, sunlight, and emotional hygiene must be arranged into a living calendar the nervous system can trust.

A circadian life is built through small repetitions that appear ordinary from the outside: the same waking hour, the same morning light, the same quiet evening, the same protected dark, the same respectful meal timing. These repetitions are not small to the nervous system. They are the architecture of trust.

The patient who can repeat a wise day has already crossed the threshold from information into embodiment. The calendar becomes the treatment room. The meal becomes the cue. The bedroom becomes the sanctuary. The morning becomes the reset.

From timing, routine begins: the disciplined transformation of knowledge into six months of daily practice.

Chapter 19

The Six-Month Sim-Bo Transformation Plan

From Knowledge to Practice: The Architecture of Execution

Knowledge becomes medicine only when it becomes practice.

A philosophy may calm the mind, but only repeated action teaches physiology a new order. The Sim-Bo method was never designed to remain an idea. It is a daily architecture: food prepared simply, meals timed consistently, movement performed steadily, breath used deliberately, sleep protected with reverence, and emotional noise reduced before it becomes chemistry.

This plan converts simplicity into a sequence that can be lived without confusion. It does not punish. It does not shock the system into submission. It removes noise in stages, then replaces chaos with cadence.

The progression follows six movements: Detox, Adapt, Strengthen, Balance, Maintain, and Thrive. Each has a distinct purpose. The early weeks remove the loudest irritants. The middle months rebuild metabolic confidence. The final weeks transform effort into identity. By the end, Sim-Bo is no longer a diet being followed from the outside; it becomes a pattern the nervous system recognizes as safe.

Detox -> Adapt -> Strengthen -> Balance -> Maintain -> Thrive

Six Months: The Architecture of Change

Six months is not a motivational slogan. It is a practical season of repair.

The human system needs time to replace old inputs with new materials, to retrain appetite, to shift microbial ecology, to stabilize sleep timing, to restore bowel cadence, to strengthen muscle signaling, and to teach the brain that predictability is not deprivation.

Blood cells turn over across months. The intestinal lining renews rapidly, but microbial communities and immune tolerance require repetition. Sleep architecture does not obey one perfect night; it learns from repeated evenings. Muscles do not become metabolically intelligent from one walk; they respond to daily use. Neural pathways are not remade by inspiration; they are engraved by practice.

This is why the plan is gradual. A system that has lived for years under stimulation, irregular meals, fragmented sleep, overwork, and chemical overload often resists sudden purity. It needs structure firm enough to hold, but gentle enough to be trusted. Six months gives the system a new baseline.

The Monthly Arc

The six months are not six identical repetitions. Each month has a distinct clinical mood.

Month 1 clears the room. The patient removes the loudest irritants and discovers how much appetite, mood, sleep, and pain were being shaped by stimulation rather than true need.

Month 2 establishes tempo. Digestion begins expecting meals instead of constant input. The nervous system begins expecting morning light, evening darkness, and regular recovery.

Month 3 builds capacity. Movement, strength, breathing, and controlled dietary expansion test the new foundation without overwhelming it.

Month 4 teaches moderation. The patient learns when to push, when to rest, when to eat raw, when to eat warm, when to speak, and when to be still.

Month 5 proves durability. The practice must survive travel, stress, social meals, work pressure, and emotional weather without collapsing into old chaos.

Month 6 gives the practice a purpose. Recovered energy becomes available for work, family, creativity, leadership, worship, study, service, and the deeper obligations of a meaningful life.

This arc prevents the common mistake of treating healing as a single dramatic cleanse. Sim-Bo is not built on shock. It is built on sequence. The patient does not become well by attacking the old pattern once; the patient becomes well by making the new pattern ordinary enough to repeat under pressure.

How to Begin: Four Laws of Execution

Commit to consistency; release perfection. One imperfect meal does not break the work. Abandoning the pattern does. Healing is trained through return.

Keep a Sim-Bo diagnostic journal. Record meals, mood, digestion, sleep, movement, cravings, skin, pain, and mental clarity. Writing turns vague experience into visible pattern.

- Use simplicity as the compass. When uncertain, ask: Does this reduce friction? Does this make the day easier to repeat? Does this help physiology receive a clearer instruction?
- Shape the environment before relying on willpower. Stock the kitchen with whole foods, remove trigger foods, prepare grains in advance, place walking shoes where they are visible, and make sleep the easiest choice at night.

This journey is not a race back to youth. It is the deliberate rebuilding of trust between choice and physiology. Every repeated act of simplicity tells the system: the emergency is ending.

The Daily Anchor System

Every stage of the plan rests on a small number of anchor behaviors. These anchors are deliberately ordinary because ordinary acts survive stress better than elaborate protocols. A complicated plan collapses when travel, family conflict, work pressure, illness, or fatigue enters the day. A simple anchor survives because it can be performed almost anywhere.

- Morning anchor: outdoor light, warm water, one slow breath cycle, and the first clear decision of the day.
- Meal anchor: a 3:2:1 plate, eaten without digital distraction, with chewing slow enough for the nervous system to register safety.
- Movement anchor: a walk, mobility sequence, or strength practice that brings circulation back into the tissues.
- Evening anchor: dim light, reduced input, written reflection, and a protected sleep window.

These anchors are not decorative rituals. They are the load-bearing beams of the transformation. When the day becomes uncertain, the patient returns to the anchors. When motivation drops, the anchors remain. When results seem slow, the anchors quietly continue to write the new pattern.

Stage 1: Detox (Weeks 1-4)

The Objective: Clear the loudest dietary, sensory, and circadian noise.

The Clinical Focus:

- Return to strict 3:2:1 meals: three parts unrefined grain, two parts fibrous vegetables, and one part whole fruit.
- Remove refined sugar, industrial seed oils, ultra-processed packaged foods, artificial sweeteners, and snack grazing.
- Hydrate steadily with warm water or simple herbal teas; avoid forcing excessive fluid beyond comfort and clinical need.

Walk 15-20 minutes daily with nasal breathing or relaxed diaphragmatic breath.
Anchor morning light and protect an earlier evening shutdown to restore the day-night boundary.

The Clinical Purpose: The first stage lowers stimulation. Taste buds recalibrate. Blood sugar becomes less erratic. Bowel movement begins to organize. The liver receives fewer confusing inputs. The nervous system begins to experience simplicity as relief rather than loss. Early fatigue, cravings, emotional release, or temporary resistance are not failure; they are signs that old chemical habits are losing their grip.

Reflection Directive: "What becomes audible when dietary noise fades?"

The first month is often psychologically revealing. Many patients discover that the craving was not only for sugar, salt, or stimulation; it was for interruption. Processed food interrupts boredom. Constant snacking interrupts anxiety. Late-night screens interrupt silence. Stage 1 removes enough noise for the real pattern to appear. That appearance is not failure. It is the first honest diagnostic moment.

Stage 2: Adapt (Weeks 5-8)

The Objective: Reestablish metabolic flexibility, digestive timing, and autonomic order.

The Clinical Focus:

Maintain three structured meals per day with clear spaces between them, allowing digestion to finish before the next meal begins.
Introduce live fermented foods in modest portions when tolerated: traditional kimchi, sauerkraut, miso, or other culturally appropriate ferments.
Begin light bodyweight strength, mobility, or full-body stretching twice weekly.
Continue morning light and 10-minute post-meal walks to support glucose handling and parasympathetic tone.
Create a digital sunset: reduce screens, bright light, stressful work, and emotional stimulation during the final hour of the day.

The Clinical Purpose: Adaptation teaches the organs what to expect. Insulin becomes less reactive. Cortisol finds a steadier arc. The microbiome receives more consistent fiber and fermentation. The stomach, liver, pancreas, and bowels begin to coordinate around time. Predictability becomes internal safety.

Reflection Directive: "How does predictability feel inside my nervous system?"

Adaptation also teaches the patient to respect the space between meals. The fasting interval is not starvation; it is digestive quiet. The liver can complete unfinished work, bile flow becomes less chaotic, and appetite begins to separate from habit. Hunger becomes more readable. Fullness becomes more trustworthy. This is where the patient learns the difference between a true need and a nervous-system request for stimulation.

Stage 3: Strengthen (Weeks 9-12)

The Objective: Build resilience through controlled, intelligent challenge.

The Clinical Focus:

- Alternate lighter meals with slightly more complex Sim-Bo meals to test digestive flexibility without returning to chaos.
- Add one weekly cardiovascular challenge: hill walking, steady cycling, swimming, or a longer nature walk.
- Perform strength training two to three times weekly using bodyweight, bands, simple weights, or daily functional labor.
- Practice three conscious breathing pauses daily: morning, midday, and evening.
- Reintroduce soaked legumes, sprouted seeds, or other previously avoided foods only when digestion is steady enough to interpret the response clearly.

The Clinical Purpose: This stage develops capacity. Mitochondria receive a reason to become more efficient. Skeletal muscle becomes a stronger glucose sink. Myokines begin to speak through movement. Digestion learns to handle measured variety. Strength, in Sim-Bo, is not strain; it is the ability to meet challenge without losing order.

Reflection Directive: "What does strength feel like when it arrives without punishment?"

Strengthening must remain intelligent. A depleted patient should not imitate an athlete. A sedentary patient should not treat soreness as proof of success. The Sim-Bo approach uses challenge as instruction, not punishment. The correct challenge leaves the patient more awake after recovery, not more inflamed.

Stage 4: Balance (Weeks 13-16)

The Objective: Integrate physical output, rest, digestion, emotion, and season into one operating system.

The Clinical Focus:

Alternate active-output days with deliberate recovery days.

Write a short gratitude entry before sleep to settle attention and complete the emotional day.

Adjust raw and cooked foods according to season, digestion, constitution, and internal temperature.

Identify emotional-eating triggers before they become action. Use breath, hydration, walking, or journaling before reaching for stimulation.

Spend at least 30 uninterrupted minutes weekly in raw nature: walking, sitting, gardening, sunlight, soil, wind, or water.

The Clinical Purpose: Balance is the point where the plan stops feeling like restriction and begins to feel like intelligence. Cravings lose some of their authority. Rest becomes easier to choose. Emotional hunger becomes easier to distinguish from physical hunger. Daily order becomes more valuable than novelty.

Reflection Directive: "How has balance changed my definition of pleasure?"

Balance also reveals the hidden relationship between exertion and contentment. Many patients are skilled at output and poor at recovery. Others avoid challenge and call it rest. Stage 4 teaches the difference. The system learns that work and recovery are not enemies; they are partners in one cadence.

Stage 5: Maintain (Weeks 17-20)

The Objective: Let routine become ordinary enough to survive real life.

The Clinical Focus:

Keep meals simple, seasonal, and mostly home-prepared.

Move daily, alternating strength, cardiovascular flow, mobility, and tissue rest.

Protect consistent sleep and wake times as the foundation of appetite, mood, immunity, and repair.

Continue short breathing rituals before meals and before sleep.

Review supplements and supportive products with clinical judgment; reduce what is no longer needed as food, sleep, movement, and rhythm carry more of the load.

The Clinical Purpose: Maintenance is mastery without drama. The patient is no longer performing health. The architecture has become familiar. The kitchen is predictable. The calendar protects sleep.

Movement is embedded. The journal reveals patterns before symptoms become loud.

Reflection Directive: "What practices now feel natural enough to keep for life?"

Maintenance is where the work becomes honest. A plan can be performed under ideal conditions; a life must be lived under pressure. The patient learns how to stay steady during travel, family gatherings, deadlines, grief, celebration, weather changes, and social friction. A method that cannot survive real life is not medicine; it is theater. Stage 5 removes theatrical effort and tests durability.

The Future of Prescribed Routine

The next frontier of medicine will not be another contest of more data. It will be sequencing: the clinical ordering of light, food, movement, breath, sleep, social contact, and recovery with the same seriousness now given to laboratory numbers.

A prescription can be chemical. It can also be temporal. Morning light at the right hour, a simple first meal, a post-meal walk, a protected evening, and a consistent sleep window are not lifestyle decorations. They are instructions. The future clinician will not only ask what the patient consumes, but when, under what nervous-system state, after what sleep, with what movement, and inside what emotional environment.

Stage 6: Thrive (Weeks 21-24)

The Objective: Turn recovered stability into identity, usefulness, and service.

The Clinical Focus:

Add controlled variety through Sim-Bo meals that explore ancestral herbs, antioxidant colors, seasonal textures, and traditional preparations.
Move with joy: dancing, gardening, hiking, swimming, tai chi, walking with others, or functional movement that reconnects skill with pleasure.
Teach one person a principle you have embodied. Teaching turns private discipline into living knowledge.
Deepen your tolerance for stillness: silent walks, device-free meals, prayer, meditation, or extended reflection.
Evaluate the emotional environment. Protect relationships that create steadiness. Reduce exposure to patterns that keep the nervous

system guarded.

The Clinical Purpose: The final stage turns active healing into character. The plan is no longer a set of rules; it becomes the way you organize the day. Food becomes clear. Movement becomes normal. Sleep becomes protected. Breath becomes available. Energy has a direction.

The purpose of six months is not merely to look better or collect improved numbers. The purpose is capacity. Health gives stamina for vocation, family, leadership, study, service, endurance, and presence. A life that no longer spends all its energy managing symptoms can finally spend energy on meaning.

Reflection Directive: "How will I use recovered energy to serve beyond myself?"

The Weekly Review: Turning Practice into Pattern

Daily discipline creates data. Weekly review creates wisdom.

At the end of each week, sit with the journal and study the preceding seven days without shame or self-congratulation. The question is not, Did I behave perfectly? The question is, What did my system reveal?

Which meal gave the clearest energy?
Which food created heaviness, bloating, itching, pain, cravings, reflux, fatigue, or mental fog?
Which day had the deepest sleep, and what happened during the twelve hours before it?
Which conversation, screen pattern, work demand, or emotional loop disturbed breath and digestion?
Which movement restored clarity without leaving exhaustion?
Which simple practice protected the week when motivation dropped?

This weekly review is where Sim-Bo stops being a rule set and becomes individualized clinical intelligence. The principle remains simple: food, movement, sleep, breath, timing, and emotional order. The personal expression becomes precise: this breakfast, this bedtime, this walking route, this breathing ritual, this level of social exposure, this form of rest.

A patient who reviews weekly becomes difficult to mislead. Marketing loses power. Cravings become legible. Relapse becomes visible before it becomes severe. The journal turns the plan into a mirror.

Troubleshooting Setbacks

Healing is not a straight line. Some days bring fatigue, emotional resistance, digestive change, travel disruption, family pressure, cravings, or discouragement. These moments are not proof that the plan has failed. They are feedback from a system learning a new order.

- When motivation drops: return to one anchor. Choose morning light, the first meal, the evening shutdown, or the post-meal walk. One restored anchor often restores the entire day.
- When emotion overwhelms the system: pause before reaction. Breathe slowly, walk, write, or call a steady person. Emotional charge needs movement, language, and oxygen before it becomes appetite, insomnia, inflammation, or pain.
- When progress plateaus: audit sleep, stress, bowel movement, meal timing, and hidden snacking. The system often stalls when it feels unsafe or overstimulated.
- When digestion reacts: simplify again. Use warm grains, cooked vegetables, ripe fruit, gentle teas, and fewer ingredients until the response becomes clear.
- When cravings return: examine the previous night, not only the current meal. Poor sleep, emotional strain, inadequate hydration, and irregular timing often masquerade as hunger.

The work is not to avoid every difficulty. The work is to return faster, with less shame and more intelligence.

The Sim-Bo Diagnostic Journal: The Daily Mirror

The journal is not a diary of self-criticism. It is a mirror. It teaches the patient to see patterns before those patterns become symptoms.

Do not record only what you ate. Record how the day felt chemically: clarity, heaviness, warmth, coldness, bowel movement, sleep depth, cravings, emotional loops, and physical ease. Over time, the page becomes an honest clinician. It reveals the meal that steadies you, the thought that agitates you, the hour that weakens sleep, and the ritual that restores calm.

Track three daily metrics:

- Physical terrain: digestion, joint mobility, breath, skin, bowel movement, and baseline fatigue.
- Mental loop: the repeated thought or emotional charge that occupied the day.
- Chemical gratitude: one specific, tangible thing that brought steadiness, beauty, relief, or appreciation.

Once each week, write one sentence beginning with: "I am learning that..." That sentence turns experience into instruction. It converts the week from random events into clinical intelligence.

Signs of Transformation

By the end of six months, the most important signs are often quiet. They do not always arrive as spectacle. They arrive as steadiness.

Energy becomes more even from morning to evening, with fewer emergency cravings for caffeine or sugar.
Digestion becomes lighter and more predictable after meals.
Sleep becomes deeper, earlier, and easier to protect.
Morning clarity improves without requiring immediate stimulation.
Skin, mood, and joint comfort often reflect a calmer internal terrain.
The patient becomes less reactive to food, stress, and schedule disruption.
Dependence on stimulants, convenience foods, and unnecessary supportive products often decreases as the foundation strengthens.
Medication decisions, when relevant, remain under the appropriate prescribing clinician; the Sim-Bo goal is not reckless withdrawal, but a life that requires less rescue where clinically appropriate.

These changes are not miracles. They are the predictable result of fewer insults, clearer inputs, better timing, and repeated repair.

Conclusion: The Habit of Harmony

Healing is not a single dramatic event. It is a habit learned through repetition.

The Six-Month Sim-Bo Plan restores trust between intention and physiology. Meals become quieter. Movement becomes cleaner. Sleep becomes protected. Emotional weather becomes easier to observe. The person stops chasing health as a project and begins living it as a pattern.

Six months is not the finish line. It is the point at which effort begins to soften into character. What once required discipline becomes ordinary. What once felt restrictive becomes relief. What once demanded willpower becomes a way of moving through the day.

The most important outcome is not the completion of a calendar. It is the transfer of authority from impulse to observation.

At the beginning, the patient often follows the plan because the old pattern has become unbearable. By the middle, the patient follows because the contrast is unmistakable. By the end, following is no longer the correct word. The practice has become preference. The nervous system prefers the quiet meal. The stomach prefers the earlier dinner. The mind prefers the walk. The evening prefers darkness. The morning prefers light.

Routine is not the enemy of freedom. Routine is what gives freedom a nervous system.

Clinical Case Study 19: Rebuilding the Outer Shield

Restoring Skin, Breath, and Elimination Through Sim-Bo Nutrition, Acupuncture, Emperor's Cupping Therapy®, and Botanical Medicine

Patient: Chloe J., 31-year-old female, data architect.

Chief Concerns: Long-standing atopic dermatitis with cracked and weeping eczema across the neck and flexural surfaces, chronic asthma, and constipation with bowel movements every three to four days. She used topical corticosteroids, oral antihistamines, and an albuterol rescue inhaler for symptom control.

Clinical Presentation

Chloe illustrates a classic border pattern: skin, breath, and elimination speaking through the same terrain. Her work was sedentary and cognitively intense. Her diet was heavy in dairy, refined wheat, packaged snacks, and late meals. Her bowels moved slowly, her breathing felt restricted, and her skin carried the visible expression of internal irritation.

Within Traditional Asian Medicine, the Lung and Large Intestine form a paired axis. The Lung governs breath, surface defense, and the exterior skin. The Large Intestine governs elimination. When bowel movement slows and respiratory tissue dries, the outer shield becomes fragile: skin erupts, breath tightens, and the immune boundary loses clarity.

Initial Findings and TAM Assessment

Oxygen saturation: 93 percent at intake, consistent with restricted breathing during the visit.

Tongue: pale and puffy with a dry, cracked front third and a thick, dry yellow root coating.

Primary pattern: Lung Yin depletion, Large Intestine Heat and Dryness, Phlegm accumulation, and weakened Wei Qi.

Treatment principle: restore elimination, moisten the respiratory terrain, reduce food-derived mucus load, calm skin reactivity, and rebuild the outer defensive layer.

Plan and Intervention

Chloe committed to a twelve-week Sim-Bo respiratory and epidermal restoration protocol.

Sim-Bo dietary correction: industrial dairy and refined wheat were removed. Meals were rebuilt around brown rice, Job's tears, daikon, steamed greens, Asian pear, and Tremella preparations, with emphasis on warm hydration and bowel regularity.
Grain anchor: Job's tears and brown rice were used to create gentle bulk, steady energy, and a more regular elimination pattern.
White/Metal foods: daikon, Asian pear, and Tremella were used to moisten dryness, support the Lung terrain, and soften intestinal stagnation.
Targeted acupuncture: LI11 and LI4 were used to clear surface heat and support the exterior; LU9 and ST36 were used to support Lung Qi, digestion, and constitutional strength.
Emperor's Cupping Therapy®: sliding decompression was applied along the upper thoracic region and BL13 area to reduce myofascial restriction, support rib expansion, and improve the mechanical ease of breathing.
Botanical medicine: Fang Feng Tong Sheng San was used during the early phase to support bowel movement and vent heat through appropriate channels. Yu Ping Feng San was later used to support Wei Qi and the surface defense once elimination improved.
Medication context: dermatology and pulmonary medications were not treated as enemies; changes in medication use remained under the appropriate prescribing clinicians.

Observed Outcomes After Twelve Weeks

Atopic dermatitis: weeping and cracking markedly decreased; the skin barrier appeared calmer and more intact by the end of follow-up.
Asthma symptoms: rescue-inhaler use decreased by patient report, with pulmonary management remaining under prescribing-clinician oversight.
Bowel motility: bowel movements improved from every three to four days to a more regular morning pattern.
Oxygen saturation: SpO2 improved from 93 percent at intake to 99 percent during follow-up measurement.
Tongue presentation: dryness, puffiness, and root coating improved as observed through Traditional Asian Medicine assessment.

The most important intervention in Chloe's case was not the novelty of any single technique. It was the removal of competing inputs. Her meals became cleaner. Her bowel cadence became more regular. Her thoracic tissues softened. Her breath deepened. The skin was no longer asked to carry the unfinished work of the gut and lungs alone.

Reflection on the Case

Chloe's case shows the central lesson of this chapter: routine becomes medicine when it reaches the borders of life. Skin, breath, and bowel movement are not isolated compartments. They form a living perimeter. When the diet became quieter, elimination resumed, thoracic restriction softened, and the respiratory-skin axis received steadier support, the outer shield became less reactive.

The point is not that one food or one needle technique solved a lifetime pattern. The point is that repeated, aligned inputs changed the terrain: food, timing, breath, movement, bowel cadence, acupuncture, cupping, botanical support, and clinical supervision all moved in the same direction. That is the architecture of execution.

Transition: From Routine to Reverence

Six months of practice turns checklists into character. The tracking of meals, the daily walk, the mechanics of breath, and the protection of sleep gradually lose their rigidity. They become a way of inhabiting the day.

When health no longer demands constant negotiation, a deeper question appears: What is this restored energy for?

The answer is not another protocol. It is a posture toward life. Simplicity begins as a therapeutic method, then matures into a way of belonging, creating, leading, and serving. The kitchen and the calendar have done their work. The practice now steps into the wider world.

Part VI

Beyond the Body

The mastery of physiology is never the final destination. It is the ground beneath a life capable of service, clarity, and consequence.

Part VI carries the Sim-Bo principle beyond the plate. Food, movement, breath, sleep, and emotional order are not private trophies. They are preparations for a more coherent life: a life less ruled by appetite, less scattered by noise, less dependent on emergency rescue, and more available to family, community, vocation, and spirit.

When the internal terrain becomes quiet, attention returns. When attention returns, purpose becomes audible. The final expression of Sim-Bo is not merely better laboratory markers. It is a human being restored to usefulness, reverence, and presence.

Chapter 20

Beyond the Diet: Simplicity as a Life Architecture

The Medicine of Less

After years of searching through modern wellness, many serious patients arrive at the same conclusion: lasting repair rarely comes from the frantic addition of more. It comes from the disciplined mastery of needing less.

Simplicity is not poverty. It is clarity. It is the removal of excess inputs until the nervous system can hear its own cadence again. Engineered food, digital noise, constant stimulation, and emotional overcommitment scatter attention and drain the reserves required for repair. When unnecessary inputs are removed, vitality no longer has to fight its way through clutter.

The Sim-Bo philosophy began as a dietary structure, but it was never only a diet. It is a way of organizing life so that physiology, attention, emotion, and purpose no longer contradict one another. To live simply is to live with fewer false emergencies. It is to understand enough not as deprivation, but as medicine.

The Daily Architecture of Enough

Enough is not a vague mood. It is an architecture. It appears in the kitchen when the meal is simple enough to repeat without anxiety. It appears in the calendar when the day contains work, rest, movement, silence, and human contact without constant negotiation. It appears in the mind when desire no longer needs novelty every hour to feel alive.

The modern nervous system is trained to mistrust enough. It is taught to upgrade, scroll, compare, purchase, track, optimize, and expand. Sim-Bo reverses that training. It teaches the patient to recognize sufficiency as a felt state: the exhale after a warm meal, the quiet satisfaction after useful work, the calm of a room without unnecessary objects, the dignity of saying no before resentment begins.

This architecture is not passive. It requires boundaries. It requires a kitchen stocked with food that supports the plan, not food that negotiates against it. It requires a bedroom protected from screens, a morning protected from panic, and a table protected from distraction. Simplicity becomes real only when the environment stops arguing with the intention.

The discipline of enough is also the discipline of energy conservation. Every unnecessary choice spends attention. Every unnecessary object requires maintenance. Every unnecessary commitment divides the nervous system. A simple life returns that scattered expenditure to repair, thought, worship, work, and love.

In clinical practice, this is often the moment patients begin to understand why Sim-Bo works. The meal is not doing everything. The reduced noise around the meal is doing something equally important. The entire day becomes easier for physiology to read.

From Health to Wholeness

Physical health is regulation. Wholeness is coherence.

Once food becomes steady, movement becomes natural, and sleep regains its place, a deeper question rises inside the quieted nervous system: what is this vitality for? Health is not the prize at the end of the path. It is the foundation that allows the path to be walked with strength.

You do not restore metabolism merely to exist longer in private comfort. You restore it to carry responsibility without collapse, to serve without resentment, to think clearly under pressure, to love with steadiness, and to endure the difficult work that meaning requires.

Wholeness does not require sterile perfection. It requires alignment. The food you eat, the work you do, the words you speak, the people you protect, and the values you claim must begin moving in the same direction. A life becomes coherent when its daily actions stop contradicting its deepest commitments.

In this way, Sim-Bo becomes spiritual without becoming abstract. It restores relationship: between the person and the earth, between doing and being, between molecular science and the immeasurable depth of human purpose.

Redefining Success: The Metrics of Lightness

Modern culture measures success by accumulation: money, possessions, titles, visibility, validation, influence. Sim-Bo measures success by lightness.

Can you draw a full diaphragmatic breath without effort? Can you move through a day without heaviness? Can you eat without compulsion, sleep without negotiation, work without constant adrenal pressure, and return to joy without requiring stimulation? These are not sentimental measures. They are clinical signs of a life whose internal load has decreased.

The invisible markers of genuine success are often the most valuable: steady energy, restorative sleep, secure relationships, a calm digestive pattern, unforced gratitude, and the ability to remain present in ordinary moments. A simple home, a clear schedule, a few loyal friendships, meaningful work, and a table where food is eaten slowly may be worth more than the visible symbols of achievement that exhaust the person who owns them.

Stress is not created only by hard work. It is created by work that violates nature, timing, values, and recovery. Simplicity realigns success with sanity.

The Home as a Clinic of Order

A healing life requires a healing environment. The home is not background scenery; it is a daily therapeutic instrument. The kitchen teaches appetite. The bedroom teaches sleep. The entryway teaches whether life begins in rush or in pause. The table teaches whether food is received as fuel, entertainment, or reverence.

A Sim-Bo home does not need luxury. It needs order. Visible fruit. Washed greens. Grains stored plainly. Water available. Lighting that softens in the evening. Space for walking shoes by the door. Fewer objects competing for attention. Fewer digital invitations to leave the present moment. The room itself should make the healthy act easier than the unhealthy one.

This is not aesthetic minimalism for appearance. It is metabolic minimalism for regulation. A crowded home creates a crowded mind. A chaotic kitchen creates chaotic eating. A bedroom used as an office teaches the nervous system that rest and productivity occupy the same territory. A table covered with devices teaches digestion to occur under vigilance.

Healing becomes more durable when the environment becomes an ally. The patient no longer relies on heroic willpower. The house begins to practice with them.

Compassion as Coherence

When personal needs become simpler, the capacity to care expands.

A person who is constantly overstimulated, under-rested, inflamed, and emotionally guarded has little reserve left for compassion. Attention is consumed by survival. But when nourishment becomes steady, sleep becomes protected, and desire becomes less chaotic, care begins to move outward. A well-regulated person becomes a stabilizing presence inside a family, a workplace, a clinic, and a community.

Calm is contagious. Human nervous systems read one another through tone, breath, facial expression, posture, and pace. A grounded person changes the room without argument. They slow the conversation. They reduce the pressure to perform. They remind others, silently, that safety is possible.

This is why personal healing is never merely private. It changes the atmosphere around the person who practices it. Sim-Bo begins with a bowl of rice, vegetables, and fruit, but its final expression is relational: less consumption, more steadiness; fewer demands, more service; less self-occupation, more capacity to nourish others.

Service Without Self-Erasure

A restored life is not a life emptied of obligation. It is a life capable of carrying obligation without losing its center. Many patients confuse service with self-erasure. They give from depletion, then wonder why compassion turns into fatigue, irritability, and silent resentment.

Sim-Bo teaches a different order. Nourish first, then serve. Breathe first, then speak. Sleep first, then lead. Eat in stability, then give from stability. This is not selfishness. It is the physiology of sustainable compassion. A depleted person may still perform duty, but the duty often carries the chemistry of sacrifice. A nourished person serves with less hidden violence.

The world does not need martyrs who collapse while helping others. It needs steady people who can remain useful for decades. Simplicity protects that endurance. It removes the unnecessary so the necessary can be held with grace.

The Spiritual Law of Simplicity

Every serious wisdom tradition has understood the same law in different language: excess fractures attention; simplicity returns it.

The discipline of balance appears in meditation halls, monasteries, fasting traditions, healing kitchens, gardens, and ordinary households where life is lived with restraint and gratitude. Modern physiology names the same pattern through homeostasis, autonomic regulation, circadian timing, inflammatory resolution, and metabolic stability. Different vocabularies. One principle.

Nature heals through ordered cycles. Day and night. Eating and fasting. Effort and rest. Speech and silence. Growth and shedding. A life that ignores those cycles becomes noisy inside. A life that honors them becomes available to grace.

When simplicity matures, daily life stops feeling like crisis management. It becomes participation. Breath, work, food, sleep, prayer, conversation, and service begin to share one cadence.

Community and Co-Regulation

Simplicity is not isolation.

The quieter a life becomes, the more clearly relationships can be felt. When consumption no longer consumes attention, the real weight of human presence returns: the person across the table, the child asking a question, the patient trying to be understood, the elder needing time rather than efficiency.

Healing is incomplete when it leaves a person calm but disconnected. The nervous system settles most deeply in environments of trust. Shared meals, slow listening, familiar voices, eye contact, useful work, and repeated kindness communicate safety in ways no supplement can imitate.

A calm community is medicine at scale. It lowers the ambient pressure of living. It replaces competition with belonging, and belonging gives physiology permission to stop defending itself against the world.

Simplicity and Creativity: The Uncluttered Network

When life is crowded with decisions, alerts, possessions, and unfinished obligations, imagination has no room to breathe.

Simplicity creates the inner space where original thought can return. The mind requires periods of unforced attention: walking without headphones, cooking without hurry, sitting in silence, reading deeply, tending soil, repairing something by hand. These quiet intervals allow hidden associations to rise. Insight appears when the nervous system is no longer spending all of its energy processing noise.

Patients often rediscover creativity during the Sim-Bo process. Not because the protocol injects inspiration, but because energy previously spent on cravings, inflammation, poor sleep, digestive distress, and decision fatigue becomes available again. Curiosity returns. Humor returns. The desire to create returns.

Creativity is not reserved for artists. It is how a person solves problems, repairs relationships, prepares food, organizes a home, teaches a child, leads a team, and perceives meaning in ordinary life. When internal order returns, even humble acts regain artistry.

The Future of Healing: The Era of Alignment

The future of healing will not be defined only by sharper technology. It will be defined by alignment.

Medicine will always need emergency rooms, surgery, diagnostics, antibiotics, pharmaceuticals, and skilled clinicians. Civilization depends on those tools. But the next mature era of health must place daily life back at the center: sunlight, clean food, breathable air, meaningful work, shared meals, sleep protected by darkness, and communities designed for movement and belonging.

Hospitals may become more than places of repair. They may become schools of prevention, teaching patients how to live in a way that reduces the repeated need for rescue. Cities may be judged not only by speed and productivity, but by whether they allow walking, cooking, rest, sunlight, and human connection. Homes may become clinics of rhythm. Kitchens may become the first pharmacy. Tables may become places where nervous systems learn safety.

Sim-Bo is a bridge to that future. It teaches that the pattern of living is often more powerful than any isolated intervention because the pattern repeats every day. What repeats becomes terrain. Terrain becomes destiny.

The Economy of Attention

The final currency of health is attention. What receives attention receives energy. What receives energy grows. A distracted life therefore becomes a malnourished life, even when the plate is full.

Modern life fragments attention into pieces too small to become wisdom. Sim-Bo gathers those pieces back. It asks for enough quiet to chew, enough darkness to sleep, enough stillness to pray, enough movement to feel the limbs, enough honesty to release resentment, and enough humility to eat ordinary food without demanding entertainment from it.

When attention returns, the ordinary becomes luminous. Brown rice is no longer plain starch. It is warmth, texture, patience, mineral, ground.

Vegetables are no longer obligation. They are flow, color, bitterness, fiber, and inner cleansing. Fruit is no longer dessert. It is light, water, sweetness, and refreshment held in structure. A walk is no longer exercise. It is circulation, orientation, and contact with earth.

This is the quiet miracle of simplicity: it does not make life smaller. It restores the ability to perceive how much was already present.

Living as the Medicine

The question at the center of this book is not a slogan of rebellion against medicine. It is a question of design: can a person live with such coherence that the need for constant rescue decreases?

The answer is found in practice. Food becomes instruction when it is simple, whole, and repeated with attention. Movement becomes therapy when it circulates blood, lymph, breath, and emotion without punishment. Sleep becomes treatment when it is protected by darkness and timed with the sun. Emotion becomes chemistry when resentment is released, gratitude is practiced, and the nervous system is allowed to feel safe. Simplicity becomes spirituality when it turns outward as compassion.

To live this way is not to reject medical science. It is to cooperate so deeply with nature that physiology has fewer reasons to cry for rescue. Prevention is not passive. It is daily architecture. It is the disciplined shaping of food, light, movement, rest, breath, relationship, and thought until life itself becomes less inflammatory.

The human organism carries an old intelligence. The frantic mind does not need to command it into repair. It needs to stop interrupting the conditions under which repair becomes possible.

Clinical Case Study 20: Protecting the Sovereign Mind

Restoring Cognitive Clarity Through Metabolic Simplicity, Circadian Repair, Acupuncture, Cupping, and Botanical Medicine

Patient: Eleanor C., 67-year-old female, former chief librarian.

Chief Concerns: accelerating short-term memory difficulty, word-finding problems, spatial confusion, agitation, poor sleep continuity, and digestive intolerance to a prescribed cognitive medication.

Clinical Presentation

Eleanor arrived with the quiet grief of a highly intelligent woman losing trust in her own mind. She had spent her life surrounded by language, order, books, cataloging systems, and memory. Her decline felt to her like a betrayal of identity. She would pause mid-sentence, search for common words, misplace familiar objects, and become suddenly irritable when she could not complete a thought.

Her medical evaluation had identified mild cognitive impairment. A cholinesterase inhibitor had been prescribed, but she reported severe gastrointestinal distress and a dull, apathetic feeling. Medication decisions remained under the care of her prescribing clinician. The Sim-Bo intervention was used to address the terrain around cognition: glucose stability, inflammation, sleep architecture, vascular flow, digestive tolerance, and nervous-system steadiness.

The clinical question was not whether the brain could be forced into clarity by chemical pressure. The question was whether the environment feeding the brain could become more coherent.

Initial Findings and TAM Assessment

Homocysteine: 18.4 micromol/L at intake, indicating elevated vascular and methylation-related strain.

Cognitive pattern: short-term recall difficulty, word-finding pauses, spatial disorientation in unfamiliar settings, and agitation during mental fatigue.

Digestive pattern: medication-related gastrointestinal distress,

irregular appetite, and poor tolerance for heavy meals.
Tongue and pulse: withered, stiff, slightly deviated presentation with red, peeled quality; pulse empty, floating, and wiry. Within Traditional Asian Medicine observation, this pattern suggested Kidney Jing depletion complicated by Liver Wind and Phlegm-Blood Stasis clouding the orifices.

Treatment Principles

The clinical strategy was to reduce neuro-metabolic friction, stabilize daily fuel, support methylation and vascular clarity, improve sleep timing, soften cervical and suboccipital restriction, and nourish the traditional Kidney-Jing axis associated with the Sea of Marrow.

Plan and Intervention

Sim-Bo brain matrix: refined flour, liquid sugar, late-night eating, and unstable oils were removed. Meals were simplified around warm grains, dark vegetables, whole fruit, hydration, and predictable timing.
Black-water anchor: black rice, black sesame, walnuts, sea vegetables, and mineral-rich dark plant foods were used to support the Kidney axis within TAM reasoning while providing fiber, minerals, and polyphenol density.
Vegetable antioxidant layer: dark leafy greens, cruciferous vegetables, purple vegetables, and herbs were emphasized to support vascular integrity, redox reserve, and digestive regularity.
Lipid support: carefully sourced marine lipids and modest unrefined fats were used to support membrane health and steady energy without returning to processed-fat patterns.
Sleep and glymphatic cadence: evening screens were removed, dinner was shifted earlier, and morning outdoor light was used to anchor circadian timing.
Acupuncture: DU20, Sishencong, GB39, KI3, ST36, and SP6 were used to support clarity, marrow/Jing patterns, digestive resilience, and calmer autonomic tone.
Emperor's Cupping Therapy®: gentle decompression was applied along the suboccipital and cervical region to reduce myofascial restriction, support local circulation, and encourage relaxation before sleep.
Botanical medicine: Di Huang Yin Zi was used within the TAM framework to nourish Kidney Jing, support sensory clarity, and assist the pattern of Phlegm obstructing the orifices.

Twelve-Week Observations

Cognitive language: word-finding pauses decreased, and Eleanor became more fluent and confident in conversation by patient and family report.
Short-term memory: daily task independence improved; she required fewer reminders for routine activities.
Spatial orientation: disorientation episodes decreased during the follow-up period.
Mood and agitation: irritability softened, and emotional steadiness improved as sleep and digestion became more predictable.
Homocysteine: improved from 18.4 micromol/L to 8.2 micromol/L during follow-up.
Sleep: sleep onset and continuity improved with earlier meals, reduced evening stimulation, and consistent darkness.
Digestive tolerance: gastrointestinal distress decreased after medication status was reviewed by the prescribing clinician and meals were simplified.
Tongue and pulse: dryness, deviation, peeled quality, and wiry tension softened within TAM observation.

Clinical Logic

Eleanor did not need a more complicated life. She needed a clearer metabolic field for the mind to inhabit. The plan therefore avoided novelty. Meals repeated. Evenings dimmed. Sleep was treated as cognitive medicine. Movement was gentle and rhythmic, chosen for circulation rather than athletic output. The therapeutic emphasis was not stimulation; it was steadiness.

The treatment also respected the grief of cognitive change. Fear can worsen confusion by tightening breath, fragmenting attention, and increasing autonomic pressure. Eleanor was asked to slow her world down: one task at a time, one meal pattern, one evening ritual, one daily walk, one notebook for orientation. The mind was not scolded for faltering. It was given fewer demands and better fuel.

Clinical Insight

Eleanor's case illustrates the final lesson of this book: the mind is not separate from terrain. Memory depends on more than neurotransmitters. It depends on sleep, vascular clarity, glucose stability, inflammation, methylation, digestion, breath, light, and emotional safety.

Her improvement did not come from one heroic intervention. It came from coordinated simplicity. The plate became quieter. The evening became darker. The cervical tension softened. The gut tolerated food more gracefully. The nervous system received fewer conflicting instructions. The sovereign mind did not need to be conquered; it needed a clearer kingdom in which to function.

Conclusion: The Return Home

Radical simplicity brings the journey back to the beginning: to food that can be recognized, breath that can be felt, sleep that can be trusted, movement that can be enjoyed, emotion that can be released, and relationships that can be inhabited without performance.

This is not the end of Sim-Bo. It is the beginning of a life no longer organized around rescue. Health stops being an exhausting metric to chase and becomes a quiet state of participation. A meal becomes prayer. A walk becomes circulation. A boundary becomes medicine. A slow breath becomes an instruction to the immune system. A simple day becomes a sanctuary.

The world does not need more people trapped inside private optimization. It needs people steady enough to serve, clear enough to discern, rested enough to love, and simple enough to remain free.

When you have the courage to live simply, you stop outsourcing healing to complexity. You return to the old intelligence beneath the noise. You learn to eat as medicine, move as medicine, breathe as medicine, sleep as medicine, forgive as medicine, and serve as medicine.

You do not merely take medicine. You become medicine.

Appendices

Appendix A. Nutrient Reference Architecture 306

Appendix B. The Sim-Bo Materia Medica 313

Appendix C. The Sim-Bo Clinical Formularies: Recipes and Procurement 320

Appendix D. Scientific and Philosophical Foundation 324

Appendix E. The Biological Lexicon 328

Appendix A - Nutrient Reference Architecture

The Vocabulary of Nourishment

Nutrients are not inert fragments. They are the working vocabulary of metabolism: fuel, structure, electric charge, enzyme support, microbial instruction, membrane integrity, antioxidant reserve, and hormonal cadence. The Sim-Bo approach studies nutrients without reducing food to isolated pills. The central question is never simply what a compound does in a laboratory. The deeper question is how that compound behaves inside a meal, inside digestion, inside timing, and inside the living terrain of a patient.

This reference architecture organizes the major nutrient families used throughout the book. It is not a pharmaceutical prescription and not an invitation to chase isolated molecules. It is a map of how whole-food patterns create recognizable instruction for metabolism.

I. Macronutrients: Fuel and Framework

Carbohydrates

Role: Primary energy substrate for the brain, skeletal muscle, thyroid-adrenal coordination, and daily ATP production.
Sources: Brown rice, millet, quinoa, barley, oats, root vegetables, legumes, and whole seasonal fruit.
Sim-Bo directive: Choose intact, fiber-bound forms. Refined flour, liquid sugar, and isolated sweeteners deliver speed without structure.

Protein

Role: Structural material for enzymes, immune proteins, connective tissue, peptide hormones, muscle repair, and recovery.
Sources: Lentils, mung beans, adzuki beans, fermented tofu, tempeh, chia, hemp, flax, seeds, nuts, and carefully selected clinical animal sources when appropriate.
Sim-Bo directive: Aim for sufficiency, not worship. Vary sources, protect digestion, and keep protein proportional to metabolic need.

Fats and Lipids

Role: Membrane architecture, myelin support, steroid hormone substrate, bile signaling, satiety, and lipid mediator pathways.

Sources: Olive oil, avocado, walnuts, flax, hemp, chia, sesame, whole nuts, seeds, and clean algae-based omega-3 support when clinically indicated.
Sim-Bo directive: Favor minimally processed fats. Avoid repeatedly heated, oxidized, hydrogenated, or industrially refined oils.

Water

Role: Solvent, transport medium, thermoregulatory support, lymphatic flow, mucosal hydration, and electrolyte balance.
Sources: Filtered water, herbal infusions, mineral broths, cucumber, melon, citrus, pear, and other water-rich produce.
Sim-Bo directive: Sip steadily between meals. Avoid overwhelming digestion with large volumes during meals. Warm or room-temperature fluids are generally gentler for gastric function.

Dietary Fiber

Role: Mechanical bulk, bowel cadence, bile binding, microbial fermentation, short-chain fatty acid production, and satiety.
Sources: Rice bran, oats, legumes, cruciferous vegetables, greens, fruit skins, ground flax, chia, and root vegetables.
Sim-Bo directive: Increase gradually and pair with steady hydration. Fiber is instruction only when motility can move it.

II. Vitamins: Co-Enzymatic Keys

Vitamins are small in volume and large in consequence. They act as coenzymes, redox partners, immune regulators, tissue-repair allies, and timing assistants. The Sim-Bo preference is whole-food delivery first, with targeted supplementation reserved for a defined clinical reason.

Vitamin A Precursors and Carotenoids

Role: Support epithelial surfaces, vision, mucosal barriers, skin resilience, and immune tolerance.
Sources: Carrots, pumpkin, sweet potato, kale, spinach, parsley, winter squash.
Sim-Bo directive: Pair with a small amount of dietary fat to improve absorption.

B-Complex Family

Role: Supports mitochondrial energy, carbohydrate metabolism, methylation, nervous-system steadiness, and stress adaptation.
Sources: Whole grains, legumes, seeds, nuts, greens, mushrooms,

fermented foods, and nutritional yeast when appropriate.
Sim-Bo directive: Stress, alcohol, refined sugar, and poor intake increase demand. Food-first replenishment creates steadier response than isolated megadosing.

Vitamin C

Role: Electron donor for antioxidant recycling, collagen support, immune cell function, wound repair, and tissue integrity.
Sources: Citrus, kiwi, berries, peppers, broccoli, cabbage, parsley.
Sim-Bo directive: Freshness matters. Heat and prolonged storage reduce potency. Use raw or lightly prepared sources daily.

Vitamin D

Role: Secosteroid hormone involved in calcium regulation, immune tone, bone metabolism, mood-related pathways, and circadian-light biology.
Sources: Morning sunlight exposure, UV-exposed mushrooms, and targeted D3 support when clinically indicated.
Sim-Bo directive: Assess context. Pair fat-soluble nutrients with dietary fat. Vitamin K2 and magnesium status matter when calcium metabolism is the therapeutic focus.

Vitamin E

Role: Lipid-phase antioxidant that helps protect cell membranes and supports circulation.
Sources: Almonds, sunflower seeds, avocado, spinach, wheat germ, olive oil.
Sim-Bo directive: Works best as part of the antioxidant network, not as an isolated heroic dose.

Vitamin K1 and K2

Role: Supports clotting physiology, bone-mineral handling, calcium routing, and vascular-mineral balance.
Sources: Kale, broccoli, cabbage, parsley, natto, fermented soy foods.
Sim-Bo directive: Fat-soluble. Requires bile flow and dietary lipids for better absorption. Patients on anticoagulant medication require clinician guidance.

Folate

Role: Supports methylation, DNA synthesis, red-cell formation, fetal development, and homocysteine metabolism.

Sources: Lentils, asparagus, greens, beets, avocado, legumes.
Sim-Bo directive: Prefer food folate and clinically appropriate forms when supplementation is needed. Genetic context and medication status matter.

III. Minerals: Electrical Conductors

Minerals carry charge, create structure, stabilize enzymes, regulate vascular tone, and help the nervous system speak with precision. Deficiency and excess both matter. The Sim-Bo principle is sufficiency within a whole-food matrix.

Calcium

Role: Supports skeletal matrix, neuromuscular contraction, cardiac conduction, and cellular signaling.
Sources: Sesame tahini, bok choy, broccoli, kale, almonds, fortified foods when appropriate.
Sim-Bo directive: Requires vitamin D, magnesium, vitamin K, movement, and acid-base balance. Isolated calcium is not a complete strategy.

Magnesium

Role: ATP stability, smooth-muscle relaxation, bowel motility, insulin signaling, sleep quality, and stress physiology.
Sources: Pumpkin seeds, greens, oats, cacao, legumes, nuts.
Sim-Bo directive: Frequently depleted by stress and poor intake. Supplemental form matters when used clinically.

Potassium

Role: Cellular voltage gradient, vascular tone, muscle contraction, fluid balance, and blood-pressure regulation.
Sources: Potatoes, bananas, avocado, spinach, beans, lentils, squash.
Sim-Bo directive: Balances sodium patterns. Patients with kidney disease or potassium-altering medications require supervision.

Sodium

Role: Blood volume, nerve transmission, adrenal support, muscle contraction, and osmotic balance.
Sources: Mineral salt, sea vegetables, vegetables, broths.
Sim-Bo directive: Use deliberately, not excessively. Highly processed sodium intake behaves differently from mineral-balanced food salt.

Zinc

Role: Immune defense, epithelial repair, taste, skin integrity, stomach-acid support, and enzyme function.
Sources: Pumpkin seeds, lentils, nuts, oats, legumes.
Sim-Bo directive: Balance with copper. Long-term isolated zinc supplementation can disturb mineral relationships.

Iron

Role: Hemoglobin formation, oxygen transport, mitochondrial enzymes, and energy production.
Sources: Lentils, tofu, spinach, blackstrap molasses, beans, seeds; clinical animal sources when appropriate.
Sim-Bo directive: Non-heme iron absorption improves with vitamin C. Iron status requires testing when deficiency or overload is suspected.

Selenium

Role: Glutathione peroxidase activity, thyroid conversion, antioxidant defense, and immune balance.
Sources: Brazil nuts, whole grains, mushrooms, legumes.
Sim-Bo directive: Small amounts are sufficient. Excess intake can be harmful.

Iodine

Role: Raw material for thyroid hormones and baseline metabolic rate.
Sources: Seaweed, iodized salt, seafood where appropriate.
Sim-Bo directive: Use carefully in autoimmune thyroid patterns. More iodine is not always better.

IV. Phytochemicals: Plant Intelligence

Phytochemicals are plant defense compounds that become human regulatory allies. They shape redox balance, immune tone, microbial ecology, detoxification pathways, vascular function, and cellular resilience. Color is not decoration; it is chemistry made visible.

Flavonoids

Role: Support vascular integrity, mast-cell balance, immune modulation, and antioxidant defense.
Sources: Berries, citrus, onion, tea, parsley, herbs.
Sim-Bo directive: Use daily color diversity rather than heroic dosing.

Carotenoids

Role: Support visual tissue, skin, mucosal barriers, and antioxidant protection.
Sources: Carrots, pumpkin, squash, sweet potato, greens.
Sim-Bo directive: Pair with a little fat. Light cooking may improve accessibility in some foods.

Glucosinolates and Sulforaphane

Role: Support phase-II detoxification, Nrf2-related antioxidant defense, and cellular stress response.
Sources: Broccoli sprouts, broccoli, cabbage, kale, cauliflower, mustard greens.
Sim-Bo directive: Chew thoroughly. Light steaming preserves more benefit than boiling into exhaustion.

Polyphenols

Role: Support redox reserve, endothelial function, microbiome diversity, and cognitive resilience.
Sources: Berries, grapes, green tea, cocoa, herbs, purple vegetables.
Sim-Bo directive: Consistency matters. Small daily exposure works better than occasional excess.

Lignans

Role: Support estrogen metabolism, fiber ecology, bowel cadence, and microbial fermentation.
Sources: Freshly ground flaxseed, sesame seed, whole grains.
Sim-Bo directive: Grind flax fresh to improve access to the inner matrix.

V. The Five Laws of Sim-Bo Nutritional Harmony

Whole over isolated: the food matrix delivers cofactors, fiber, water, texture, minerals, and pacing together.
Color is code: every pigment family carries a different protective instruction.
Gentle transformation: steaming, simmering, soaking, sprouting, and fermenting improve digestibility without destroying structure.
Sufficiency before excess: the goal is enough, not maximal intake.
Timing shapes efficacy: food behaves differently when eaten with light, hunger, calm, and digestive readiness.

Summary

Appendix A is a compass, not a rulebook. Exact micrograms belong to clinical assessment. Daily wisdom belongs to the plate: whole structure, steady timing, mineral sufficiency, color diversity, digestive calm, and enough repetition for metabolism to trust the message.

Appendix B - The Sim-Bo Materia Medica

Approved Food Lists and Volumetric Architecture

The Sim-Bo materia medica organizes food by recognition, repeatability, digestive ease, and regulatory order. The goal is not culinary novelty. The goal is to make the meal legible: three parts grain, two parts vegetables, one part fruit, supported by modest protein, clean fat, water, warmth, and timing.

1. The Sim-Bo Paradigm of Selection

3 parts grains: the dense foundation for steady ATP production and cognitive grounding.
2 parts vegetables: the cleansing current of fiber, minerals, color, and elimination support.
1 part fruit: the light element of hydration, natural sweetness, and antioxidant refreshment.

Food is selected for repeatable clarity. A meal that can be recognized, digested, and repeated without inflammatory provocation becomes therapeutic through cadence.

2. Whole Grains - The Anchor

Brown Rice

Role: The core Sim-Bo grain: grounding, fiber-rich, steady, and structurally intact.
Sources: Short-grain or medium-grain brown rice, rinsed and soaked.
Sim-Bo directive: Soak overnight when possible. Cook slowly until the bran softens and the grain becomes tender.

Millet

Role: Light, mild, and useful when digestion needs warmth without heaviness.
Sources: Whole millet, lightly toasted before simmering.
Sim-Bo directive: Good for breakfast bowls, summer transitions, and sensitive stomach patterns.

Quinoa

Role: A mineral-rich seed-grain with a broader amino acid pattern.

Sources: Rinsed quinoa with saponins removed.
Sim-Bo directive: Use as a rotation grain, especially when the patient needs variety without complexity.

Steel-Cut Oats

Role: Beta-glucan fiber, morning satiety, bowel cadence, and lipid-pattern support.
Sources: Steel-cut oats simmered slowly.
Sim-Bo directive: Use with cinnamon, apple, berries, or ground flax.

Buckwheat

Role: A warming, mineral-rich grain-like seed with rutin and earthy density.
Sources: Buckwheat groats.
Sim-Bo directive: Useful in cooler seasons, broths, porridges, and grounding bowls.

Pearl Barley

Role: Soothing mucilage, bowel support, and slow-release structure.
Sources: Soaked barley simmered until fully tender.
Sim-Bo directive: Use in soups and autumn/winter meals.

Avoid white flour, instant grains, and highly processed grain products. Speed of absorption is the issue; intact structure is the medicine.

3. Vegetables - The Green Pharmacy

Leafy Greens

Role: Magnesium, folate, chlorophyll, vitamin K, and lightness.
Sources: Kale, spinach, bok choy, chard, collards.
Sim-Bo directive: Steam lightly or add to soups at the end.

Dense Roots

Role: Grounding energy, minerals, slow starch, and emotional steadiness.
Sources: Carrot, beet, daikon, sweet potato, burdock, turnip.
Sim-Bo directive: Cook until tender. Roots prevent cleansing from becoming depletion.

Crucifers

Role: Glucosinolates, sulforaphane potential, fiber, and phase-II

support.
Sources: Broccoli, cabbage, cauliflower, Brussels sprouts, mustard greens.
Sim-Bo directive: Chew well. Light steam; avoid boiling into exhaustion.

Aromatics

Role: Circulation, warmth, antimicrobial support, and digestive stimulation.
Sources: Garlic, onion, leeks, scallion, ginger.
Sim-Bo directive: Use as accents, not domination.

Sea Vegetables

Role: Iodine, trace minerals, and oceanic mineral depth.
Sources: Nori, wakame, kombu, dulse.
Sim-Bo directive: Use small amounts. Thyroid context matters.

4. Fruit - The Light Element

Apples

Role: Pectin, respiratory support, bowel rhythm, and autumn steadiness.
Sources: Whole apples, preferably with skin when tolerated.
Sim-Bo directive: Use as morning or midday fruit; avoid turning into juice.

Pears

Role: Moistening, cooling, soothing for dry throat and respiratory dryness.
Sources: Asian pear, Bosc pear, ripe seasonal pear.
Sim-Bo directive: Especially useful in autumn dryness.

Dark Berries

Role: Anthocyanins, vascular support, polyphenol density, and cognitive resilience.
Sources: Blueberries, blackberries, raspberries, cherries.
Sim-Bo directive: Use fresh or frozen without added sugar.

Citrus

Role: Vitamin C, brightness, bile flow, and morning refreshment.
Sources: Lemon, orange, grapefruit, tangerine.

Sim-Bo directive: Use whole or freshly squeezed into water; avoid sweetened juices.

Bananas

Role: Potassium, softness, and gastric settling when used in moderation.
Sources: Ripe bananas.
Sim-Bo directive: Use strategically, not as a constant snack.

Papaya and Pineapple

Role: Proteolytic enzymes and tropical digestive assistance.
Sources: Fresh papaya, pineapple.
Sim-Bo directive: Use in small portions; avoid late-night use.

Use whole fruit. Avoid commercial fruit juice, syrups, and heavily sweetened dried fruit.

5. Plant Proteins

Lentils, Mung Beans, and Adzuki Beans

Role: Amino acids, fiber, mineral depth, and bowel support.
Sources: Soaked or sprouted beans cooked until fully tender.
Sim-Bo directive: Combine with grain for completeness and digestibility.

Tofu, Tempeh, Edamame, and Natto

Role: Gentle plant protein with fermented options for microbial support.
Sources: Organic non-GMO soy foods, especially fermented forms.
Sim-Bo directive: Use modest portions. Fermentation improves tolerance for many patients.

Seeds: Chia, Hemp, Flax

Role: ALA omega-3, lignans, soluble fiber, and mineral support.
Sources: Freshly ground flax, hemp hearts, soaked chia.
Sim-Bo directive: Grind flax fresh; protect oils from heat.

Raw Nuts

Role: Dense minerals, healthy fats, and satiety.
Sources: Walnuts, almonds, pumpkin seeds, sesame, Brazil nuts in moderation.
Sim-Bo directive: Use small portions. Avoid oil-fried or heavily salted

mixtures.

Avoid highly processed plant-meat imitations built from isolates, stabilizers, flavor systems, and refined oils. They may be plant-derived but not necessarily whole food.

6. Healthy Fats

Cold-Pressed Olive Oil

Role: Monounsaturated fat, polyphenols, and endothelial support.
Sources: Extra-virgin olive oil.
Sim-Bo directive: Use cold or low heat. Do not repeatedly heat.

Avocado

Role: Whole-food fat matrix with potassium and fiber.
Sources: Ripe avocado.
Sim-Bo directive: Use as a small accent to stabilize meals.

Flax and Hemp Oil

Role: Fragile omega-3-rich oils.
Sources: Cold-pressed oils stored cold.
Sim-Bo directive: Never heat. Use as a post-cooking drizzle.

Sesame Oil

Role: Warming aroma and culinary grounding.
Sources: Unrefined sesame oil, toasted sesame oil as accent.
Sim-Bo directive: Use sparingly for flavor and warmth.

Avoid hydrogenated fats and repeatedly heated industrial oils. Fat quality changes with processing, storage, and heat.

7. Beverages

Warm filtered water: baseline hydration and digestive gentleness.
Herbal infusions: ginger, chamomile, roasted barley, mint, or other gentle teas matched to constitution.
Green tea: antioxidant-rich and mildly stimulating; best used before mid-afternoon.
Vegetable broth: mineral replenishment and a calm medium for sensitive digestion.

Avoid soda, routine alcohol, sweetened beverages, and large iced drinks with meals when digestion is weak.

8. Condiments and Flavor

Core seasonings: mineral salt, fermented tamari, miso, lemon, ginger, garlic, scallion, fresh herbs.
Sweet accents: if needed, use very small amounts of raw honey or maple syrup; train the palate back toward fruit and grain sweetness.
Fermented accents: kimchi, sauerkraut, natto, miso; use small amounts regularly rather than large sporadic servings.
Avoid artificial sweeteners, flavor enhancers, and additive-heavy sauces that override satiety and microbial clarity.

9. Volumetric Geometry and Circadian Timing

Grains: roughly two closed fists together.
Vegetables: the most visible part of the plate; about half the visual field.
Fruit: one palm-sized portion, used as light and refreshment.
Clean protein: approximately a deck-of-cards portion when used as a separate emphasis.
Healthy fat: a thumb-tip portion or small drizzle.
Breakfast: warm primer or hydrating fruit pattern, depending on constitution and season.
Lunch: the largest and most complex meal of the day.
Dinner: lighter, earlier, simpler, and easier to digest before sleep.

10. Exclusions: Removing Metabolic Noise

Refined carbohydrates: rapid absorption, weak satiety, and unstable glucose response.
Processed meats and heavily processed dairy patterns: dense salt, additives, oxidized fats, and high inflammatory potential in many modern diets.
Deep-fried foods: oxidized oils and heat-damaged lipid residues.
Routine alcohol and heavy caffeine dependence: disrupted sleep, stress chemistry, and appetite distortion.
Mindless overeating: even whole food becomes difficult when quantity exceeds digestive capacity.

11. The Calm Kitchen

Cook slowly enough for the nervous system to arrive before the meal does.
Keep visible ingredients simple: grains, roots, greens, fruit, beans, seeds, oils, broths, herbs.
Prepare extra grain and roots in advance so hunger does not drive

convenience choices.

Begin meals with one breath of gratitude. Vagal tone is part of digestion.

Summary

The Sim-Bo materia medica is a living pantry, not a rigid list. Its power comes from repetition, digestibility, intact structure, and calm preparation. When the kitchen becomes quiet, food becomes easier to interpret.

Appendix C - The Sim-Bo Clinical Formularies

Recipes and Procurement

The Sim-Bo kitchen is the home pharmacy of rhythm. Recipes are not entertainment vehicles; they are repeatable clinical forms. Each one reduces decision fatigue, protects digestion, and gives the patient a stable way to practice nourishment.

1. Core Principles of the Sim-Bo Kitchen

Radical minimalism: fewer ingredients, higher quality, clearer digestion.
Thermal harmony: simmer, steam, soak, sprout, ferment, and soften. Avoid burning and repeated high-heat oil damage.
No haste: cooking pace is part of autonomic regulation.
Predictable surplus: cook extra grains and roots to remove the temptation of emergency eating.
Quiet execution: food prepared in agitation often becomes food eaten in agitation.

2. Everyday Sim-Bo Meals

Formulary 1: The Anchoring Brown-Rice Bowl

Yield: 2 servings
Inputs: 1 cup soaked short-grain brown rice; 2 cups filtered water; 1 cup lightly steamed dark greens; 1/2 cup grated carrot; 1 tsp sesame oil; 1 tsp fermented tamari; toasted sesame seeds
Execution: Simmer rice slowly until tender. Layer greens and carrot over the grain. Add oil and tamari after cooking. Chew deliberately.
Clinical role: A complete 3:2:1 anchor: steady grain, green minerals, root sweetness, and a small lipid cue for satiety.

Formulary 2: Morning Millet and Fruit Primer

Yield: 1-2 servings
Inputs: 1/2 cup millet; 1 1/2 cups water or unsweetened oat milk; 1/2 diced apple; Ceylon cinnamon; 1 tsp freshly ground flaxseed
Execution: Toast millet briefly, simmer until soft, fold in apple and cinnamon near the end, then add flax off heat.
Clinical role: A warm morning primer that supports satiety, bowel cadence, and steady energy without heavy digestion.

Formulary 3: Probiotic Miso Infusion

Yield: 2-3 servings
Inputs: 4 cups water or vegetable broth; bok choy or spinach; daikon or carrot; fresh ginger; 1-2 tbsp unpasteurized miso; scallion or seaweed
Execution: Simmer vegetables and ginger. Turn off heat. Dissolve miso separately in warm broth, then return it to the pot without boiling.
Clinical role: A mineral-rich broth with fermented depth, useful after travel, antibiotics, stress, or heavy eating patterns.

Formulary 4: Lentil and Root Grounding Stew

Yield: 3-4 servings
Inputs: 1 cup sprouted lentils; carrot; sweet potato; turmeric; garlic; olive oil; 4 cups water or broth; mineral salt
Execution: Warm oil gently, add garlic and turmeric briefly, then add lentils, roots, and liquid. Simmer until creamy.
Clinical role: Combines plant protein, soluble fiber, root stability, and warming spice in a simple repair meal.

Formulary 5: Stir-Steamed Greens with Fermented Soy

Yield: 2 servings
Inputs: organic tofu or tempeh; 3 cups dark greens; sesame oil; tamari; fresh ginger
Execution: Warm tofu gently, add ginger and greens, cover briefly to steam, then finish with tamari.
Clinical role: A light protein-green pattern that supports minerals, amino acids, and low-friction digestion.

Formulary 6: Golden Mineral Broth

Yield: 4-6 servings
Inputs: yellow onion with skin; carrots; celery; kombu; fresh ginger; 8 cups water
Execution: Simmer for 40 minutes. Strain. Store refrigerated for up to four days.
Clinical role: A mineral broth for hydration, recovery, light evenings, and sensitive digestion.

Formulary 7: Cellular Hydration Tonic

Yield: 1 serving
Inputs: 1/2 cucumber; 1 green apple; handful spinach; juice of 1/2

lemon; 1 cup water

Execution: Blend and sip slowly. Strain only when the digestive system needs a lighter texture.

Clinical role: A morning or post-heat hydration option built from water, potassium, vitamin C, and green minerals.

3. Seasonal Cooking Architecture

Spring: barley or quinoa; asparagus and tender greens; strawberries and citrus; light steaming and brief sauteing.

Summer: millet or brown rice; zucchini and cucumber; melons and berries; raw integration, blanching, and cooling broths.

Autumn: brown rice and oats; pumpkin and carrot; apples and pears; slow simmering, soups, and grounding bowls.

Winter: buckwheat and barley; roots and cabbage; citrus and persimmon; stews, broths, ginger, and warming preparations.

Seasonal cooking aligns texture, temperature, and digestive demand with the environment.

4. Seven-Day Sim-Bo Clinical Protocol

Monday: millet porridge with pear; brown-rice bowl with steamed greens; lentil-root stew with mineral broth.

Tuesday: steel-cut oats with berries; tofu stir-steam with brown rice; miso soup with roots.

Wednesday: rice porridge with banana; quinoa salad with miso broth; brown rice with bitter greens.

Thursday: green hydration tonic with nuts; collard-leaf lentil wrap with fruit; millet bowl with golden broth.

Friday: warm oats with apple; brown-rice bowl with tempeh; vegetable stew.

Saturday: slow congee with papaya; quinoa salad with avocado; barley soup with greens.

Sunday: ginger tea with almonds; simple brown-rice bowl; early light dinner and rest.

The seven-day structure is intentionally repetitive. Repetition is not culinary failure. It is metabolic training.

5. Master Procurement List

Foundational Pantry

Brown rice, millet, quinoa, barley, oats.

Lentils, mung beans, adzuki beans.

Tamari, miso, seaweed, ginger, garlic, mineral salt.
Olive oil, sesame oil, flax, chia, hemp, walnuts, pumpkin seeds.

Living Produce

Dark leafy greens, bok choy, kale, spinach, chard, cabbage.
Roots: carrot, beet, daikon, sweet potato, burdock, turnip.
Seasonal fruit: apple, pear, berries, citrus, melon, papaya when appropriate.
Avocado, lemon, fresh herbs, cucumber.

Refrigerated Matrix

Organic tofu, tempeh, natto where tolerated.
Kimchi, sauerkraut, miso.
Unsweetened single-ingredient plant milk without emulsifier-heavy additives.

Targeted Supports

Ginger, roasted barley, chamomile, mint, nettle, dandelion, and other constitution-appropriate teas.
Algae-based omega-3 support when clinically indicated.
Nutritional yeast when B-vitamin support is useful and tolerated.

6. The Kitchen as Somatic Therapy

The movements of the Sim-Bo kitchen are deliberately ordinary: rinse, soak, slice, simmer, steam, breathe, serve, chew, repeat. These gestures re-teach the nervous system that nourishment does not have to be urgent. A calm kitchen is not aesthetic decoration. It is the first phase of digestion.

Cook with simplicity. Eat with slowness. Repeat with discipline. This is how food becomes practice.

Appendix D - Scientific and Philosophical Foundation

The Architecture of Evidence

The Sim-Bo method is built from clinical observation, traditional medical reasoning, and modern research on inflammation, metabolism, circadian biology, the microbiome, movement, stress physiology, and lifestyle medicine. The works below are provided as a research foundation for readers who want to study the scaffolding beneath the method.

I. Systemic Inflammation and Chronic Disease

Calder, P. C. (2020). Omega-3 fatty acids and inflammatory processes: From molecules to man. Biochemical Society Transactions, 48(1), 51-59.

Furman, D., et al. (2019). Chronic inflammation in the etiology of disease across the life span. Nature Medicine, 25(12), 1822-1832.

Hotamisligil, G. S. (2017). Inflammation, metaflammation and immunometabolic disorders. Nature, 542(7640), 177-185.

Libby, P. (2021). The changing landscape of atherosclerosis. Nature, 592(7855), 524-533.

II. Nutrition and Mitochondrial Metabolism

Hu, F. B., & Willett, W. C. (2019). Dietary patterns and long-term survival. New England Journal of Medicine, 381(9), 856-865.

Levine, B., & Kroemer, G. (2019). Biological functions of autophagy genes: A disease perspective. Cell, 176(1-2), 11-42.

Li, Y., et al. (2020). Timing of eating and metabolic risk. Current Nutrition Reports, 9, 1-11.

Longo, V. D., & Mattson, M. P. (2014). Fasting: Molecular mechanisms and clinical applications. Cell Metabolism, 19(2), 181-192.

Mozaffarian, D., & Liu, J. (2018). Plant-based foods and cardiometabolic health. Progress in Cardiovascular Diseases, 61(1), 1-10.

Satija, A., et al. (2016). Healthful and unhealthful plant-based diets and the risk of coronary heart disease. Journal of the American College of Cardiology, 70(4), 411-422.

III. Gut Health and the Microbiome

Clemente, J. C., et al. (2012). The impact of the gut microbiota on

human health: An integrative view. Cell, 148(6), 1258-1270.
Lynch, S. V., & Pedersen, O. (2016). The human intestinal microbiome in health and disease. New England Journal of Medicine, 375(24), 2369-2379.
Sommer, F., & Backhed, F. (2013). The gut microbiota - masters of host development and physiology. Nature Reviews Microbiology, 11(4), 227-238.
Wang, Z., et al. (2011). Gut flora metabolism of phosphatidylcholine promotes cardiovascular disease. Nature, 472(7341), 57-63.
Zhao, L., et al. (2018). Gut bacteria selectively promoted by dietary fibers alleviate type 2 diabetes. Science, 555(7695), 62-67.

IV. Plant-Dominant and Anti-Inflammatory Eating

Barnard, N. D., et al. (2019). A Mediterranean diet and low-fat vegan diet to improve body weight and cardiometabolic risk factors: A randomized, cross-over trial. Journal of the American College of Nutrition, 149(3), 573-582.
Esselstyn, C. B. (2014). A plant-based diet and coronary artery disease: A mandate for effective therapy. Journal of Geriatric Cardiology, 12(3), 171-177.
McDougall, J. (2012). The Starch Solution. Rodale Books.
Ornish, D., et al. (2013). Effect of comprehensive lifestyle changes on telomerase activity and telomere length in men with biopsy-proven prostate cancer. The Lancet Oncology, 14(11), 1112-1120.

V. Mind, Emotion, and Psychoneuroimmunology

Black, D. S., & Slavich, G. M. (2016). Mindfulness meditation and the immune system: A systematic review of randomized controlled trials. Annals of the New York Academy of Sciences, 1373(1), 13-24.
Davidson, R. J., & McEwen, B. S. (2012). Social influences on neuroplasticity: Stress and interventions to promote well-being. Nature Neuroscience, 15(5), 689-695.
Kabat-Zinn, J. (2013). Full Catastrophe Living. Bantam.
Sapolsky, R. M. (2004). Why Zebras Don't Get Ulcers. Holt Paperbacks.
Tracey, K. J. (2002). The inflammatory reflex. Nature, 420(6917), 853-859.

VI. Movement and Cellular Exercise

Booth, F. W., et al. (2012). Lack of exercise is a major cause of chronic diseases. Comprehensive Physiology, 2(2), 1143-1211.
Langevin, H. M., et al. (2001). Mechanical signaling through connective tissue: A mechanism for the therapeutic effect of

acupuncture. The FASEB Journal, 15(12), 2275-2282.
Nieman, D. C., & Wentz, L. M. (2019). The compelling link between physical activity and the body's defense system. Journal of Sport and Health Science, 8(3), 201-217.
Pedersen, B. K., & Saltin, B. (2015). Exercise as medicine - evidence for prescribing exercise as therapy in 26 different chronic diseases. Scandinavian Journal of Medicine & Science in Sports, 25(S3), 1-72.

VII. Sleep Architecture and Circadian Health

Chaput, J. P., et al. (2018). Sleep timing, sleep consistency, and health in adults: A systematic review. Applied Physiology, Nutrition, and Metabolism, 19(S1), 27-38.
Czeisler, C. A., et al. (2019). Circadian biology and human health. Science, 365(6453), 1006-1007.
Panda, S. (2020). The Circadian Code. Rodale Books.
Walker, M. P. (2017). Why We Sleep. Scribner.
Xie, L., et al. (2013). Sleep drives metabolite clearance from the adult brain. Science, 342(6156), 373-377.

VIII. Integrative and Lifestyle Medicine

Bland, J. (2014). The Disease Delusion. Harper Wave.
Hyman, M. (2020). Food Fix. Little, Brown Spark.
Li, Q. (2018). Forest Bathing. Viking.
Weil, A. (2017). Mind Over Meds. Little, Brown and Company.

IX. Eastern Philosophy and Ancestral Perspectives

Kaptchuk, T. J. (2000). The Web That Has No Weaver. McGraw-Hill.
Lao Tzu. Tao Te Ching. Various annotated translations.
Ni, M. (1995). The Yellow Emperor's Classic of Medicine. Shambhala.
Pitchford, P. (2002). Healing with Whole Foods. North Atlantic Books.

X. Environment and Behavioral Epigenetics

Frumkin, H., et al. (2017). Nature contact and human health: A research agenda. Environmental Health Perspectives, 125(7), 075001.
Glanz, K., et al. (2015). Built environment and obesity: An assessment of the evidence. Annual Review of Public Health, 36, 243-271.
Harvard T.H. Chan School of Public Health. (2023). The Nutrition Source: The Healthy Eating Plate. https://www.hsph.harvard.edu/nutritionsource

XI. Pharmacology of Traditional Botanical Medicine

Chen, J. K., & Chen, T. T. (2004). Chinese Medical Herbology and Pharmacology. Art of Medicine Press.

Wang, X., et al. (2018). Systems pharmacology unravels the active mechanisms of traditional Chinese medicine. Nature Communications, 9(1), 1-9.

Appendix E - The Biological Lexicon

The Language of the Living System

This lexicon defines the core medical, nutritional, and physiological terms used throughout the book. The purpose is not to make life feel clinical. It is to remove fear from language. Once a patient can name a process, that process becomes easier to observe, discuss, and change.

A

Amino Acids: The small units that build protein. They form enzymes, antibodies, connective tissue, muscle, neurotransmitter precursors, and repair proteins.

Antioxidants: Compounds and enzyme systems that neutralize reactive oxygen species and support redox balance. They work as a network rather than as isolated heroes.

Autoimmunity: A state in which immune tolerance becomes impaired and the immune system begins reacting against self-tissue. It may involve genetics, infection history, gut barrier integrity, stress chemistry, and inflammatory load.

B

Beta-Carotene: A carotenoid pigment found in orange roots and dark greens. It can serve as a precursor to vitamin A activity and supports epithelial and visual tissues.

Blood Sugar: Circulating glucose used for energy. When repeated spikes exceed regulatory capacity, glycation, insulin resistance, vascular strain, and fatigue become more likely.

C

C-Reactive Protein (hs-CRP): A liver-derived inflammatory marker used clinically to estimate low-grade inflammatory activity, especially in cardiovascular and metabolic contexts.

Circadian Rhythm: The roughly 24-hour timing system coordinated by light, darkness, sleep, eating, movement, temperature, and hormonal cycles.

Cortisol: A survival hormone that mobilizes energy and coordinates stress adaptation. It is useful acutely and costly when chronically elevated.

D

Detoxification: The liver-centered process of transforming, binding, and eliminating metabolic waste, hormones, medications, and environmental compounds. It requires bile, protein, micronutrients, fiber, hydration, and bowel movement.

Dysbiosis: An imbalanced microbial ecology in which resilience, diversity, and barrier support decline while irritation, gas, reactivity, or inflammation may increase.

E

Endorphins: Neuropeptides that modulate pain, reward, movement-related well-being, laughter, and stress adaptation.

Enzymes: Biological catalysts that allow metabolic reactions to occur efficiently, including digestion, energy production, detoxification, and repair.

F

Fiber: Plant carbohydrate that resists digestion in the small intestine and supports bowel bulk, bile binding, satiety, microbial fermentation, and short-chain fatty acid production.

Free Radical / Reactive Oxygen Species: Reactive molecules generated during normal metabolism, immune defense, pollution exposure, stress, and mitochondrial activity. Problems arise when production exceeds antioxidant capacity.

G

Gastrointestinal Tract: The boundary where external food is broken down, interpreted, absorbed, rejected, or transformed into tissue, energy, immunity, and microbial chemistry.

Gut-Brain Axis: The two-way communication network between gut, microbiome, vagus nerve, immune system, endocrine signals, and mood circuits.

H

Homeostasis: Dynamic internal regulation: temperature, pH, blood pressure, glucose, immune tone, and fluid balance held within functional ranges.

Hormesis: Adaptive strengthening that can occur after manageable stress, such as movement, heat, cold, fasting windows, or effort, when followed by adequate recovery.

I

Inflammation: A protective immune response used for injury, infection, and repair. It becomes harmful when the alarm remains active without resolution.

Insulin Resistance: A metabolic state in which tissues respond less efficiently to insulin, often associated with energy excess, ectopic fat, inflammation, inactivity, and mitochondrial strain.

Intestinal Permeability: A change in gut-barrier regulation that may allow increased passage of microbial fragments or incompletely digested proteins into immune surveillance.

L

Lymphatic System: The low-pressure fluid network that transports immune cells, tissue fluid, and metabolic byproducts. It depends heavily on movement and diaphragmatic breathing.

M

Macronutrients: Carbohydrates, proteins, and fats: the major fuel and structural inputs required in larger amounts.

Magnesium: A mineral involved in ATP stability, muscle relaxation, nerve conduction, bowel motility, sleep quality, and hundreds of enzyme reactions.

Microbiome: The microbial ecosystem of bacteria, fungi, archaea, and viruses living largely in the gut. It shapes fermentation, immune education, barrier integrity, and metabolic signaling.

Mindfulness: Disciplined attention to the present moment. Clinically, it supports nervous-system regulation, breath awareness, emotional digestion, and behavior change.

N

Nitric Oxide: A signaling molecule produced by endothelial cells that supports vascular relaxation, circulation, and blood-flow regulation.

O

Omega-3 Fatty Acids: Essential fats involved in membrane function and pro-resolving lipid mediator pathways. Sources include flax, chia, hemp, walnuts, and algae-derived EPA/DHA support.

Oxidative Stress: A state in which reactive species outpace antioxidant defense, contributing to membrane damage, mitochondrial strain, inflammation, and aging patterns.

P

Phytochemicals: Plant compounds such as polyphenols, flavonoids, carotenoids, and glucosinolates that help regulate redox balance, detoxification, microbes, and immune tone.

Probiotics: Beneficial microbial strains used temporarily to support microbial diversity and gut ecology. They work best when paired with prebiotic fiber and a hospitable diet.

Polyphenols: Pigmented plant compounds found in berries, tea, herbs, cocoa, grapes, and colorful vegetables. They support antioxidant defense and microbial signaling.

R

Resilience: The capacity to meet stress and return to regulation without prolonged collapse.

S

Serotonin: A neurotransmitter and peripheral signaling molecule involved in mood, motility, satiety, and gut-brain communication. Much serotonin is produced in the gut, while brain serotonin is regulated separately.

Sim-Bo Diet™: Simple and Boring: a disciplined 3:2:1 pattern of grains, vegetables, and fruit designed to reduce dietary noise and restore regulatory order.

Subclinical Inflammation: Low-grade inflammatory activity that may persist before overt disease is diagnosed. It often appears as fatigue, stiffness, bloating, sleep disturbance, or poor recovery.

T

Thermogenesis: Heat production through metabolism, food digestion, muscle activity, and adaptive processes.

Thyroid Hormone: A major regulator of metabolic rate, temperature, energy, and tissue turnover. It depends on iodine, selenium, iron, protein, stress status, and circadian rhythm.

V

Vagus Nerve: Cranial nerve X, a major parasympathetic pathway connecting brain, heart, lungs, gut, immune tone, and emotional regulation.

Vitamin D: A secosteroid hormone made through sunlight exposure and available through supplementation when indicated. It supports bone, immune, mood, and mineral pathways.

W

Whole Food: Food consumed close to its intact structure, retaining fiber, water, minerals, phytochemicals, texture, and natural pacing.

Z

Zinc: A trace mineral important for immunity, taste, skin repair, stomach acid, reproductive health, and enzyme function.

Closing Note

These definitions are a working language for daily practice. They turn vague fear into observable process. The more clearly a patient understands metabolism, inflammation, digestion, sleep, movement, and emotional chemistry, the easier it becomes to live with discipline instead of confusion.

Practical Use Notes for the Appendices

The appendices are meant to be used at the counter, in the kitchen, in the clinic, and in the weekly review. They are not decorative back matter. They convert the philosophy of Sim-Bo into a practical operating language. A reader should be able to open these pages and decide what to buy, how to cook, how to simplify, how to rotate, how to observe, and when to stop adding complexity.

How to Use Appendix A

Appendix A should be read as a nutrient map, not a supplement catalog. Its purpose is to help the reader understand why whole foods repeatedly produce broader clinical effects than isolated compounds. A carrot is not beta-carotene alone. It is fiber, water, potassium, carotenoids, texture, sweetness, chewing time, microbial substrate, and digestive pace. Brown rice is not carbohydrate alone. It is starch inside bran, germ, B-vitamins, minerals, resistant starch, aroma, warmth, and slow release. This is the difference between a molecule and a meal.

Use the macronutrient section to build the plate: grain for ground, vegetables for flow, fruit for light, and modest protein and fat for structure and satiety.
Use the vitamin and mineral sections to recognize patterns of insufficiency, not to self-diagnose from symptoms alone.
Use the phytochemical section to remember that color diversity is not visual luxury. It is a practical way of widening antioxidant and microbial instruction.
Use the Five Laws when confused. Whole structure, color, gentle preparation, sufficiency, and timing settle most nutritional debates before they become complicated.

The most common misuse of a nutrient reference is to turn it into another source of anxiety. Sim-Bo does the opposite. It removes obsessive arithmetic and brings the reader back to pattern recognition. If the plate is structurally whole, colorful, warm enough for digestion, timed with the day, and repeated with steadiness, the nutrient architecture is already speaking clearly.

How to Use Appendix B

Appendix B is the practical materia medica of the Sim-Bo kitchen. It identifies the foods most compatible with the method and organizes them by function. A materia medica is not a shopping trend. It is a disciplined relationship with ingredients. The patient learns which foods anchor, which foods move, which foods hydrate, which foods warm, which foods cool, and which foods create unnecessary noise.

Begin with the anchor grain. For most readers, brown rice or millet provides the easiest baseline.
Choose two vegetable directions at each main meal: one leaf or crucifer for lift and flow, one root for ground and stability.
Choose one fruit in whole form. Keep fruit simple rather than turning it into a chaotic bowl of competing sugars and fibers.
Add plant protein when the meal needs structure. Use fermented soy, lentils, or seeds with attention to tolerance.
Add fat as an accent. Fat should carry, soften, and stabilize the meal; it should not dominate the plate.
Use fermented foods like punctuation, not the entire sentence. Small daily exposure is often better tolerated than large sporadic servings.

The exclusion section should be understood as noise reduction. It is not a moral list. It is a clinical list of inputs that commonly distort appetite, sleep, bowel rhythm, glucose regulation, microbial balance, and inflammatory tone. Removing them creates the silence required to hear what the remaining food is doing.

How to Use Appendix C

Appendix C turns principle into repetition. The recipes are intentionally plain. Their power is not novelty. Their power is that they can be cooked again tomorrow with the same calm result. A patient who is exhausted, inflamed, anxious, or metabolically unstable does not need culinary entertainment. The patient needs a formula that can be trusted.

Choose one breakfast formula and repeat it for seven days before changing it.
Choose one lunch bowl and one evening soup or stew for the week.
Batch-cook grain twice weekly, not daily. This prevents hunger from becoming an emergency.
Wash greens immediately after purchase and store them ready to cook. Preparedness protects discipline.
Keep broth available. A simple mineral broth can prevent late-night snacking and support lighter dinners.
Repeat the same menu long enough to observe cause and effect. Constant variety hides patterns.

The recipes may be modified for season and constitution, but the architecture should remain intact. The grain should remain whole. The vegetables should remain dominant. The fruit should remain whole. The cooking should remain gentle. The eating should remain slow. When the architecture is preserved, the formula survives variation.

Clinical Adjustment Notes

Sim-Bo simplicity does not mean every patient receives the same plate forever. It means the clinician adjusts from a stable baseline rather than from chaos. Once the baseline is clear, refinements become accurate.

Cold, depleted digestion may need warmer grains, soups, ginger, stews, and fewer raw vegetables for a period of rebuilding.
Heat, irritability, constipation, bitter taste, or red skin patterns may need more greens, pears, cucumber, bitter vegetables, and earlier dinners.
Gas and bloating may require smaller legume portions, longer soaking, more thorough cooking, and a temporary reduction in raw fiber.
Blood-sugar instability may require stricter meal timing, post-meal walking, lower fruit quantity at night, and more vegetable volume.
High stress patterns require breath before meals as seriously as they require food selection.
Sleep disruption requires the evening meal to become earlier, lighter, warmer, and simpler.

The advanced clinician does not add complexity first. The clinician first asks what the current plate is asking the digestive system to manage. Most patients improve when the demand becomes smaller, the timing steadier, and the food easier to interpret.

Procurement Discipline

Shopping is part of treatment. A chaotic grocery trip becomes a chaotic kitchen, and a chaotic kitchen becomes a chaotic plate. Procurement should be done with the same seriousness as prescribing. The goal is not abundance. The goal is readiness.

Buy fewer categories and better quality.
Prioritize the foods that can be repeated without fatigue: rice, millet, greens, roots, apples, pears, berries, lentils, tofu, miso, ginger, broth ingredients.
Keep emergency foods simple: cooked rice, steamed roots, broth, apples, roasted barley tea, miso soup.
Do not stock foods that require willpower to resist. Environment is stronger than intention.
Use glass jars and visible storage. Seeing the raw ingredients lowers the friction of cooking.
Rotate grains and vegetables by season, not by online trends.

The pantry should feel quiet. When the pantry becomes quiet, the patient stops negotiating with hunger. The meal becomes almost inevitable, and inevitability is one of the hidden strengths of the Sim-Bo method.

Recipe Substitution Rules

Substitution is useful when it preserves function. It becomes disruptive when it chases novelty. The following rules keep substitutions inside the Sim-Bo architecture.

Substitute grain for grain: brown rice, millet, oats, barley, quinoa, buckwheat.
Substitute leaf for leaf: kale, spinach, bok choy, chard, cabbage, collards.
Substitute root for root: carrot, beet, daikon, sweet potato, turnip, burdock.
Substitute fruit by function: apples for pectin and steadiness, pears for moistening, berries for polyphenols, citrus for brightness, melon for summer hydration.
Substitute protein by digestibility: lentils, tofu, tempeh, mung beans, adzuki, seeds, or clinically appropriate animal sources when

required.

Substitute fat by stability: olive oil, sesame oil, avocado, nuts, seeds, or algae-based omega-3 when indicated.

Every substitution should answer one question: does this preserve the meal's instruction? If it does, it belongs. If it adds stimulation, confusion, or heaviness without purpose, it does not.

How to Use Appendix D

Appendix D is not meant to interrupt the reading experience. It is the foundation beneath the floor. The main manuscript speaks in clinical and literary form; the references provide the research terrain behind that voice. Readers who want the direct path can practice Sim-Bo without reading every study. Readers who want the deeper scaffolding can return to Appendix D and trace the scientific threads.

Use the inflammation references to understand why low-grade immune activation connects chronic disease patterns.

Use the nutrition and metabolism references to study timing, fasting physiology, plant-dominant diets, and mitochondrial strain.

Use the microbiome references to deepen the gut chapters and the food-matrix argument.

Use the movement references to understand skeletal muscle as a metabolic and immune organ.

Use the sleep references to support the circadian sections and the master-clock framework.

Use the traditional medicine references as philosophical and clinical context, not as a substitute for practitioner training.

The manuscript does not ask the reader to worship authority. It asks the reader to observe pattern. Appendix D is included because good clinical philosophy should stand on a floor that can be inspected.

Additional Lexicon Terms

Allostatic Load: The cumulative strain created when the stress response is repeatedly activated without adequate recovery. It explains why small daily stressors can become physiologically significant over time.

Autophagy: A cellular recycling process that helps clear damaged components and maintain internal quality control. It is influenced by fasting windows, energy status, exercise, sleep, and nutrient signaling.

Bile: A digestive fluid made by the liver and stored in the gallbladder. It emulsifies fats, carries waste products, and supports bowel movement when flow is adequate.

Butyrate: A short-chain fatty acid produced by fiber-fermenting gut microbes. It supports colon cells, barrier integrity, immune regulation, and microbial resilience.

Coenzyme Q10: A mitochondrial electron carrier involved in energy production and antioxidant defense. It is especially relevant in cardiovascular and mitochondrial discussions.

Glycation: A nonenzymatic reaction in which sugar binds to proteins or lipids, forming advanced glycation end-products that can stiffen tissues and increase oxidative stress.

Glutathione: A major intracellular antioxidant and detoxification molecule. It depends on amino acids, sulfur metabolism, minerals, and cellular redox demand.

Glymphatic System: A brain-cleaning fluid-exchange system that becomes more active during sleep and supports clearance of metabolic waste from neural tissue.

mTOR: A nutrient-sensing pathway involved in growth, protein synthesis, repair, and autophagy regulation. It is useful in growth and recovery, but excessive growth signaling can become poorly matched to adult repair needs.

Myokines: Signaling molecules released by contracting muscle. They help explain why movement affects inflammation, metabolism, mood, and immune regulation.

Nrf2: A transcriptional regulator involved in antioxidant and detoxification response. Colorful plants, hormetic stressors, and redox signals can influence this pathway.

PRAL: Potential Renal Acid Load, a way of estimating the acid or alkaline load of foods after metabolism. Vegetables and fruits generally help buffer acid-producing patterns.

Randle Cycle: A fuel-competition model describing how glucose and fatty acid metabolism interact. It helps explain why constant mixed excess can impair metabolic flexibility.

Short-Chain Fatty Acids: Microbial metabolites such as acetate, propionate, and butyrate produced through fermentation of fiber. They influence gut barrier function, immunity, and energy metabolism.

TMAO: Trimethylamine N-oxide, a liver-derived compound produced from microbial metabolism of certain nutrients such as choline and carnitine. It is discussed in cardiovascular and microbiome research.

Zonulin: A regulator of tight-junction dynamics in the intestinal barrier. It is often discussed in relation to intestinal permeability, though barrier regulation involves many pathways.

Final Use Principle

The appendices should make the reader less dependent on confusion, not more dependent on rules. They are here to reduce friction. When deciding what to eat, return to the simplest architecture: grain for ground, vegetables for current, fruit for light, water for flow, breath for digestion, and timing for trust. When deciding what to remove, remove what creates noise. When deciding what to add, add only what supports the foundation. This is the practical discipline of Sim-Bo.

Weekly Review Architecture

The appendices become most useful when they are paired with a simple weekly review. The review should not feel like surveillance. It should feel like returning to the map. The patient observes whether the food architecture is still clear, whether the kitchen is still quiet, whether the bowels are moving with consistency, whether sleep is arriving on time, and whether cravings are decreasing or increasing. This is how the method remains alive rather than becoming another rigid diet.

Food structure: Did most meals preserve the 3:2:1 pattern? If not, which meals lost proportion first?

Digestive response: Was there bloating, reflux, constipation, urgency, heaviness, or clearer post-meal comfort?

Energy response: Did the morning feel steadier? Did the afternoon crash soften? Did caffeine become less necessary?

Sleep response: Did dinner timing support rest, or did late eating keep the nervous system active?

Emotional response: Did simple meals reduce decision fatigue, irritability, guilt, or compulsive snacking?

Kitchen response: Was the refrigerator prepared, or did convenience food enter because the kitchen lacked structure?

A weekly review turns observation into correction. If digestion is heavy, simplify dinner. If cravings return, strengthen breakfast and lunch. If sleep becomes restless, move dinner earlier and protect darkness. If bowel rhythm slows, increase warm fluids, cooked greens, roots, and walking. The review is not punishment. It is the practice of staying in relationship with physiology.

Clinician Use Notes

Clinicians using these appendices should avoid turning Sim-Bo into another complicated protocol. The value of the system is that it creates a clear baseline. Once the baseline is established, the practitioner can see what is truly needed: more warmth, more fiber, less raw food, more protein, less evening density, more sleep protection, more breath before meals, or more movement after eating. A complex patient does not always require complex food. Often the patient requires food simple enough for the clinical picture to become visible.

Start with one stable breakfast, one stable lunch, and one stable dinner pattern before adding refinements.
If symptoms flare after adding a food, remove the food and return to baseline rather than adding another intervention.
When using herbs, supplements, acupuncture, or cupping, maintain the food structure so outcomes can be interpreted.
When medications are involved, keep prescribing clinicians informed and avoid positioning food as a unilateral substitute for necessary care.
When patients become obsessive, reduce tracking and increase embodied practices: cooking, walking, chewing, sleeping, and journaling.

The strongest clinical use of the appendices is not memorization. It is disciplined simplification. The practitioner teaches the patient to recognize the few variables that matter most, then to repeat them long enough for regulatory order to return.

The Final Appendix Principle

A reference section can become another form of clutter if the reader uses it to chase perfection. Sim-Bo asks for the opposite. Learn the categories, then return to the bowl. Understand vitamins, then eat the greens. Understand minerals, then cook the broth. Understand microbiome science, then feed it with fiber. Understand research, then sleep earlier. Understand the glossary, then breathe before the meal. Knowledge earns its place only when it simplifies action.

The entire appendix can be reduced to one disciplined sequence: procure clean ingredients, prepare them calmly, eat them slowly, repeat them predictably, observe the response, and remove whatever creates noise. This is not less sophisticated than advanced nutrition. It is the architecture beneath it.

Use these appendices with patience. Their purpose is not to create another system of perfection, but to make daily choices repeatable. The reader should not attempt to master every nutrient, recipe, and definition at once. Begin with the plate, then the pantry, then the kitchen rhythm, then the weekly review. As the daily pattern becomes steadier, the technical language becomes easier to understand because it is no longer abstract; it is being lived. This is the practical end of the Sim-Bo method: knowledge returning to the bowl, the breath, the walk, the sleep, and the ordinary meal prepared again with care.

The final measure of these appendices is not how much information they contain, but how much unnecessary thinking they remove. A patient should be able to stand before a simple bowl and know why it works: grain for steady energy, vegetables for mineral current, fruit for light and hydration, water for flow, breath for digestion, movement for circulation, and sleep for repair. That knowledge does not need to be shouted. It becomes powerful when it is repeated quietly.

The Sim-Bo way is deliberately plain because physiology does not need entertainment in order to heal. It needs recognizable inputs, a prepared kitchen, a calmer nervous system, and the dignity of ordinary repetition. These pages exist to support that dignity. Return to them when confusion returns. Then close the book, cook the meal, and practice the medicine of enough.

About the Author and Cover Designer

Dr. Choi is a Doctor of Acupuncture and Oriental Medicine, Functional Nutritionist, Certified Emperor's Cupping Therapist®, and founder of Precision Acupuncture, Inc. in Long Beach, California.

His clinical work focuses on chronic inflammation, metabolic dysfunction, digestive imbalance, pain patterns, stress physiology, and lifestyle-related disease. Through decades of patient care, Dr. Choi has developed a practical system that integrates Eastern medical philosophy, functional nutrition, circadian rhythm, food simplicity, acupuncture, Emperor's Cupping Therapy®, breath regulation, and behavioral consistency.

As the developer of the Sim-Bo Diet™, Dr. Choi teaches that many chronic health patterns are not isolated failures of individual organs, but signs of a living system operating under excessive physiological load. His method emphasizes clean nutritional inputs, predictable timing, digestive rest, nervous-system regulation, emotional steadiness, and the reduction of unnecessary inflammatory friction.

In clinical practice, the patient is not treated as a broken machine requiring endless correction, but as an intelligent biological system requiring the right internal and external conditions for repair.

The Medicine of Less represents the culmination of Dr. Choi's clinical observations and educational mission: to help readers understand how food, simplicity, movement, sleep, emotional regulation, and daily cadence can support the body's natural capacity for resilience.

광야 : the wilderness [Gwang-ya]
의학 : the medicine [Ui-hak]

Cover design by Sharon Choi

www.ingramcontent.com/pod-product-compliance
Lightning Source LLC
LaVergne TN
LVHW052034200926
848481LV00005B/1674